Orbit and Neuro-ophthalmic Imaging

Editors

JUAN E. GUTIERREZ
BUNDHIT TANTIWONGKOSI

NEUROIMAGING CLINICS OF NORTH AMERICA

www.neuroimaging.theclinics.com

Consulting Editor
SURESH K. MUKHERJI

August 2015 • Volume 25 • Number 3

ELSEVIER

1600 John F. Kennedy Boulevard • Suite 1800 • Philadelphia, Pennsylvania, 19103-2899

http://www.neuroimaging.theclinics.com

NEUROIMAGING CLINICS OF NORTH AMERICA Volume 25, Number 3
August 2015 ISSN 1052-5149, ISBN 13: 978-0-323-39344-7

Editor: John Vassallo (j.vassallo@elsevier.com)
Developmental Editor: Casey Jackson

Neuroimaging Clinics of North America (ISSN 1052-5149) is published quarterly by Elsevier Inc., 360 Park Avenue South, New York, NY 10010-1710. Months of issue are February, May, August, and November. Business and editorial offices: 1600 John F. Kennedy Blvd., Suite 1800, Philadelphia, PA 19103-2899. Business and editorial offices: 6277 Sea Harbor Drive, Orlando, FL 32887-4800. Periodicals postage paid at New York, NY, and additional mailing offices. Subscription prices are USD 360 per year for US individuals, USD 514 per year for US institutions, USD 180 per year for US students and residents, USD 415 per year for Canadian individuals, USD 655 per year for Canadian institutions, USD 525 per year for international individuals, USD 655 per year for international institutions and USD 260 per year for Canadian and foreign students and residents. To receive student/resident rate, orders must be accompanied by name of affiliated institution, date of term, and the *signature* of program/residency coordinator on institution letterhead. Orders will be billed at individual rate until proof of status is received. Foreign air speed delivery is included in all *Clinics* subscription prices. All prices are subject to change without notice. POSTMASTER: Send address changes to *Neuroimaging Clinics of North America*, Elsevier Health Sciences Division, Subscription **Customer Service, 3251 Riverport Lane, Maryland Heights, MO 63043. Telephone: 1-800-654-2452 (U.S. and Canada); 314-447-8871 (outside U.S. and Canada). Fax: 314-447-8029. E-mail: journalscustomer service-usa@elsevier.com (for print support); journalsonlinesupport-usa@elsevier.com (for online support).**

Reprints. For copies of 100 or more of articles in this publication, please contact the Commercial Reprints Department, Elsevier Inc., 360 Park Avenue South, New York, NY 10010-1710. Tel.: 212-633-3874; Fax: 212-633-3820; E-mail: reprints@elsevier.com.

Neuroimaging Clinics of North America is covered by *Excerpta Medical/EMBASE,* the RSNA Index of Imaging Literature, *MEDLINE/PubMed (Index Medicus),* MEDLINE/MEDLARS, SciSearch, Research Alert, and Neuroscience Citation Index.

PROGRAM OBJECTIVE

The goal of *Neuroimaging Clinics of North America* is to keep practicing radiologists and radiology residents up to date with current clinical practice in radiology by providing timely articles reviewing the state of the art in patient care.

TARGET AUDIENCE

Practicing radiologists, radiology residents, and other healthcare professionals who utilize neuroimaging findings to provide patient care.

LEARNING OBJECTIVES

Upon completion of this activity, participants will be able to:

1. Review the applications of diagnostic ophthalmic ultrasound and optical coherence tomography for radiologists.
2. Discuss the role of Neuro-Ophthalmic Imaging in conditions such as visual cortex disorders, optic neuropathy, and chiasmal syndromes.
3. Recognize the use for neuroimaging in orbital traumas and pediatric orbital diseases.

ACCREDITATION

The Elsevier Office of Continuing Medical Education (EOCME) is accredited by the Accreditation Council for Continuing Medical Education (ACCME) to provide continuing medical education for physicians.

The EOCME designates this enduring material for a maximum of 15 *AMA PRA Category 1 Credit*(s)™. Physicians should claim only the credit commensurate with the extent of their participation in the activity.

All other health care professionals requesting continuing education credit for this enduring material will be issued a certificate of participation.

DISCLOSURE OF CONFLICTS OF INTEREST

The EOCME assesses conflict of interest with its instructors, faculty, planners, and other individuals who are in a position to control the content of CME activities. All relevant conflicts of interest that are identified are thoroughly vetted by EOCME for fair balance, scientific objectivity, and patient care recommendations. EOCME is committed to providing its learners with CME activities that promote improvements or quality in healthcare and not a specific proprietary business or a commercial interest.

The planning committee, staff, authors and editors listed below have identified no financial relationships or relationships to products or devices they or their spouse/life partner have with commercial interest related to the content of this CME activity:

Han Cheng, OD, PhD; Roberto Alejandro Cruz, MD; Timothy Duong, PhD; Anjali Fortna; Dan Gombos, MD; Juan E. Gutierrez, MD; John R. Hesselink, MD, FACR; Kim O. Learned, MD; Mahmood M. Mafee, MD, FACR; Suyash Mohan, MD; Suresh K. Mukherji, MD, MBA, FACR; Farbod Nasseri, MD; Nimesh B. Patel, OD, PhD; Noriko Salamon, MD, PhD; Jade S. Schiffman, MD, FAAO, FAAN; Karthikeyan Subramaniam; Megan Suermann; Rosa A. Tang, MD, MPH, MBA; Bundhit Tantiwongkosi, MD; Behroze A. Vachha, MD, PhD; John Vassallo; Blair A. Winegar, MD; Fang Yu, MD.

The planning committee, staff, authors and editors listed below have identified financial relationships or relationships to products or devices they or their spouse/life partner have with commercial interest related to the content of this CME activity:

Cynthia J. Kendall, **BMET, ROUB, CDOS** is a consultant/advisor for Quantel Medical USA.

Thomas C. Prager, PhD, MPH is a consultant/advisor for, and receives roylaties/patents from, ClearScan, manufactured by ESI, Inc.

Caroline D. Robson, **MBChb** receives royalties/patents from Amirsys, Inc.

UNAPPROVED/OFF-LABEL USE DISCLOSURE

The EOCME requires CME faculty to disclose to the participants:

1. When products or procedures being discussed are off-label, unlabelled, experimental, and/or investigational (not US Food and Drug Administration [FDA] approved); and
2. Any limitations on the information presented, such as data that are preliminary or that represent ongoing research, interim analyses, and/or unsupported opinions. Faculty may discuss information about pharmaceutical agents that is outside of FDA-approved labelling. This information is intended solely for CME and is not intended to promote off-label use of these medications. If you have any questions, contact the medical affairs department of the manufacturer for the most recent prescribing information.

TO ENROLL

To enroll in the *Neuroimaging Clinics of North America* Continuing Medical Education program, call customer service at 1-800-654-2452 or sign up online at http://www.theclinics.com/home/cme. The CME program is available to subscribers for an additional annual fee of USD 235.

METHOD OF PARTICIPATION

In order to claim credit, participants must complete the following:
1. Complete enrolment as indicated above.
2. Read the activity.
3. Complete the CME Test and Evaluation. Participants must achieve a score of 70% on the test. All CME Tests and Evaluations must be completed online.

CME INQUIRIES/SPECIAL NEEDS

For all CME inquiries or special needs, please contact elsevierCME@elsevier.com.

NEUROIMAGING CLINICS OF NORTH AMERICA

RELATED INTEREST

Radiologic Clinics of North America, January 2015 (Vol. 53, No. 1)
Head and Neck Imaging
Richard H. Wiggins III and Ashok Srinivasan, *Editors*
Available at: http://www.radiologic.theclinics.com/

THE CLINICS ARE AVAILABLE ONLINE!
Access your subscription at:
www.theclinics.com

NEUROIMAGING CLINICS OF NORTH AMERICA

Contributors

CONSULTING EDITOR

SURESH K. MUKHERJI, MD, MBA, FACR
Professor and Chairman, Walter F. Patenge
Endowed Chair, Department of Radiology,
Michigan State University; Chief Medical
Officer and Director of Health Care Delivery,
Michigan State University Health Team, East
Lansing, Michigan

EDITORS

JUAN E. GUTIERREZ, MD
Director of Neuroradiology Division, Centro
Avanzado de Diagnostico Medico CEDIMED,
Medellin, Colombia, South America

BUNDHIT TANTIWONGKOSI, MD
Assistant Professor of Radiology and
Otolaryngology, Neuroradiology Division,
University of Texas Health Science Center at
San Antonio; Imaging Service, South Texas
Veterans Health Care System,
San Antonio, Texas

AUTHORS

HAN CHENG, OD, PhD
MS Eye CARE, University Eye Institute, College
of Optometry, University of Houston, Houston,
Texas

ROBERTO ALEJANDRO CRUZ, MD
MS Eye CARE, University Eye Institute,
University of Houston School of Optometry,
University of Houston, Houston, Texas

TIMOTHY DUONG, PhD
Research Imaging Institute, San Antonio,
Texas

DAN GOMBOS, MD
Section of Ophthalmology, Department of
Head and Neck Surgery, MD Anderson Cancer
Center, Houston, Texas

JUAN E. GUTIERREZ, MD
Director of Neuroradiology Division, Centro
Avanzado de Diagnostico Medico CEDIMED,
Medellin, Colombia, South America

JOHN R. HESSELINK, MD, FACR
Division of Neuroradiology, Department of
Radiology, UCSD Medical Center, San Diego,
California

**CYNTHIA J. KENDALL, BMET,
ROUB, CDOS**
Ophthalmic Ultrasound Consultant,
Sacramento, California

KIM O. LEARNED, MD
Neuroradiology Division, Department of
Radiology, Hospital of the University of
Pennsylvania, Perelman School of Medicine
at University of Pennsylvania, Philadelphia,
Pennsylvania

MAHMOOD F. MAFEE, MD, FACR
Division of Neuroradiology, Department of
Radiology, University of California, San Diego,
San Diego, California

SUYASH MOHAN, MD
Neuroradiology Division, Department of
Radiology, Hospital of the University of
Pennsylvania, Perelman School of Medicine
at University of Pennsylvania, Philadelphia,
Pennsylvania

FARBOD NASSERI, MD
Neuroradiology Division, Department of
Radiology, Hospital of the University of
Pennsylvania, Perelman School of Medicine at
University of Pennsylvania, Philadelphia,
Pennsylvania

NIMESH B. PATEL, OD, PhD
Research Assistant Professor, University of
Houston School of Optometry, University of
Houston, Houston, Texas

THOMAS C. PRAGER, PhD, MPH
The Methodist Hospital Research Institute,
Weill Cornell Medical College, Houston,
Texas

CAROLINE D. ROBSON, MBChB
Division Chief of Neuroradiology,
Department of Radiology, Boston Children's
Hospital; Associate Professor of Radiology,
Harvard Medical School, Boston,
Massachusetts

NORIKO SALAMON, MD, PhD
Division of Neuroradiology, Department of
Radiology, University of California Los Angeles,
Los Angeles, California

JADE S. SCHIFFMAN, MD, FAAN, FAAO
Co-Director of MS Eye CARE, University Eye
Institute, University of Houston School of
Optometry, University of Houston; Co-Director
of The Optic Nerve Center, Houston, Texas

ROSA A. TANG, MD, MPH, MBA
Co-Director of MS Eye CARE, University Eye
Institute, University of Houston School of
Optometry, University of Houston; Co-Director
of The Optic Nerve Center; Research
Professor, University of Houston School of
Optometry, University of Houston, Houston,
Texas

BUNDHIT TANTIWONGKOSI, MD
Assistant Professor of Radiology and
Otolaryngology, Neuroradiology Division,
University of Texas Health Science Center at
San Antonio; Imaging Service, South Texas
Veterans Health Care System, San Antonio,
Texas

BEHROZE A. VACHHA, MD, PhD
Department of Radiology, Massachusetts
General Hospital, Harvard Medical School,
Boston, Massachusetts

BLAIR A. WINEGAR, MD
Neuroradiology Fellow, Department of
Radiology, University of Utah, Salt Lake City,
Utah

FANG YU, MD
Department of Radiology, University of Texas
Health Science Center, San Antonio, Texas

Contents

> Ophthalmic ultrasound is an invaluable tool that provides quick and noninvasive evaluation of the eye and the orbit. It not only allows the clinicians to view structures that may not be visible with routine ophthalmic equipment or neuroimaging techniques but also provides unique diagnostic information in various ophthalmic conditions. In this article, the basic principles of ophthalmic ultrasound and examination techniques are discussed. Its clinical application is illustrated through a variety of ocular pathologic abnormalities (eg, narrow angles, ciliary body tumor, detached retina, choroidal melanoma, and papilledema).

> Optical coherence tomography is an imaging technique using low coherence light sources to produce high-resolution cross-sectional images. This article reviews pertinent anatomy and various pathologies causing optic atrophy (eg, compressive, infiltrating, demyelinating) versus optic nerve swelling (from increased intracranial pressure known as *papilledema* or other optic nerve intrinsic pathologies). On optical coherence tomography, optic atrophy is often associated with reduced average retinal nerve fiber layer thickness, whereas optic nerve swelling is usually associated with increased average retinal nerve fiber layer thickness.

> Vision is one of our most vital senses, deriving from the eyes as well as structures deep within the intracranial compartment. MR imaging, through its wide selection of sequences, offers an array of structural and functional imaging tools to interrogate this intricate system. This review describes several advanced MR imaging sequences and explores their potential clinical applications as well as areas for further development.

> Optic neuropathy involves loss of visual acuity, color vision, and visual field defect with a swollen, pale, anomalous, or normal optic disc seen on fundoscopy. Chiasmal

disorders classically present with gradual onset of vision loss, bitemporal hemianopsia, and occasionally, endocrinopathy if the pituitary gland and/or hypothalamus are the causes or are involved. Advance in neuroimaging, especially magnetic resonance MR imaging, can reveal pathologic conditions previously detected only clinically. Some entities have imaging characteristics, leading to appropriate treatment without requiring tissue biopsies. Imaging also provides disease surveillance and posttreatment assessment, with computed tomography and MR imaging being complementary to each other.

Retrochiasmal visual pathways include optic tracts, lateral geniculate nuclei, optic radiations, and striate cortex (V1). Homonymous hemianopsia and field defect variants with relatively normal visual acuity suggest that the lesions involve retrochiasmal pathways. From V1, visual input is projected to higher visual association areas that are responsible for perception of objects, faces, colors, and orientation. Visual association areas are classified into ventral and dorsal pathways. Damage to the ventral stream results in visual object agnosia, prosopagnosia, and achromatopsia. Balint syndrome, visual inattention, and pure alexia are examples of dorsal stream disorders. Posterior cortical atrophy can involve ventral and dorsal streams, often preceding dementia.

Eye movement is controlled by ocular motor pathways that encompass supranuclear, nuclear, and infranuclear levels. Lesions affecting certain locations may produce localizing signs that help radiologists focus on specific anatomic regions. Some pathologic conditions, such as aneurysms and meningiomas, have unique imaging characteristics that may preclude unnecessary tissue biopsies. Some conditions are life-threatening and require urgent or emergent imaging. MR imaging is the imaging of choice in evaluation of ocular motor palsy, with magnetic resonance angiography or computed tomography angiography indicated in cases of suspected aneurysms or neurovascular conflicts.

Diagnostic imaging has become critical in the care of patients suffering from traumatic or nontraumatic emergent orbital conditions. Multidetector computed tomography (MDCT) has become the standard imaging modality for assessing orbital trauma because of its accurate assessment of orbital skeletal and soft tissues injuries. Contrast-enhanced MR imaging is the first-line examination in the assessment of nontraumatic orbital conditions given its excellent evaluation of the orbital soft tissues. Conventional angiography is necessary in some vascular orbital complications and allows for endovascular treatment. This article discusses the spectrum of orbital pathology encountered in the imaging of orbital trauma and nontraumatic orbital emergencies.

Imaging evaluation of the postoperative orbit remains challenging even for the expert neuroradiologist. This article provides a simplified framework for understanding the complex postoperative appearances of the orbit, in an attempt to enhance the diagnostic accuracy of postoperative computed tomography and MR imaging of the orbit. Readers are familiarized with the normal appearances of common eye procedures and orbit reconstructions to help avoid interpretative pitfalls. Also reviewed are imaging features of common surgical complications, and evaluation of residual/recurrent neoplasm in the setting of oncologic imaging surveillance.

This article reviews a variety of congenital and developmental disorders of the pediatric orbit with particular emphasis on ocular lesions, followed by a description of developmental and neoplastic orbital and ocular masses. The relationship of these diseases to various syndromes and/or known genetic mutations is also highlighted.

Foreword
Orbit and Neuro-ophthalmic Imaging

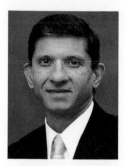

Suresh K. Mukherji, MD, MBA, FACR
Consulting Editor

Mankind has been fascinated with the eye and how it functions since before the birth of Christ. Our greatest thinkers, including Plato, Euclid, and Galen, felt that visual power emanated from the eye outward and allowed objects to be perceived. It was not until DaVinci did we finally understand that the visual stimulus reaches the eye and causes transduction of a nerve pulse along the optic nerve, eventually reaching the primary visual cortex.

Dr Juan E. Gutierrez has provided a practical and clinical approach to interpreting various diseases affecting globe, orbit, and visual pathways. He has assembled an excellent group of contributing authors who have contributed articles on a variety of disorders and imaging techniques, including CT, MR, ultrasound, and optical coherent tomography. I am sure this excellent issue will be very helpful for both radiologists and ophthalmologists.

Juan is not only an excellent colleague but also a very close friend whom I have known for over 20 years. He is a superb neuroradiologist and an even better person. I always can find Juan at RSNA because he is usually in his office. I probably should not reveal the location of his RSNA office, but I am sure he will be there next year. For those who want to make an appointment to hang out with Juan and me at RSNA next year, you will need to ask Juan the location on your own. See you next year, my friend!

Suresh K. Mukherji, MD, MBA, FACR
Department of Radiology
Michigan State University
Michigan State University Health Team
846 Service Road
East Lansing, MI 48824, USA

E-mail address:
mukherji@rad.msu.edu

http://dx.doi.org/10.1016/j.nic.2015.06.002
1052-5149/15/$ – see front matter © 2015 Published by Elsevier Inc.

neuroimaging.theclinics.com

Preface
Orbit and Neuro-ophthalmic Imaging

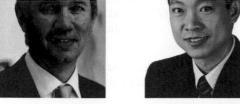

Juan E. Gutierrez, MD   Bundhit Tantiwongkosi, MD

Editors

Being able to perceive images in meaningful ways is a fundamental element to the survival of all of us. Light enters the globe through its delicate optics and is transmitted to the primary visual cortex via the retinotopic visual pathways. Higher visual association areas interpret visual information from the primary visual cortex, yielding precise perception of objects, faces, colors, and orientation. Visual stimuli subsequently activate the ocular motor pathways that control eye movement.

Multiple diseases may affect these pathways, resulting in variable patterns of visual impairment and eye movement disorders. Useful tools that clinicians utilize to evaluate the patients range from simple visual acuity charts to sophisticated optical coherence tomography. Radiologists are more familiar with CT and MR imaging, which are highly valuable in lesion characterization and in providing a differential diagnosis. Advances in neuroimaging, especially MR imaging, can reveal pathologic abnormalities previously assessed only clinically. Some entities have characteristic imaging features leading to appropriate treatment without the need for tissue biopsies.

The main goal of this *Neuroimaging Clinics* issue is to provide a practical approach to image interpretation of diseases affecting both afferent and efferent visual pathways. We were able to recruit an excellent group of contributing authors who developed a practical approach to the different subjects we felt were relevant for this particular issue; this includes articles on optical coherent tomography and orbital ultrasound, dedicated to radiologists, followed by an article focused on techniques and emerging clinical applications of advanced MR sequences, including retinal MR imaging, diffusion weighted imaging, magnetization transfer, high-resolution imaging of lateral geniculate nucleus, diffusion tensor imaging of optic radiation, and retinotopic mapping of the visual cortex. The remaining articles focus on the anatomy and imaging characteristic of diseases/postoperative changes in both adults and children, with clinical correlation.

It was an honor and a real pleasure to build and coordinate this issue. We would like to thank Dr Suresh Mukherjee and Elsevier Inc for the opportunity to guest edit this issue and contribute some articles. We appreciate our expert authors for their time and contributions. We hope our

Neuroimag Clin N Am 25 (2015) xv–xvi
http://dx.doi.org/10.1016/j.nic.2015.06.001
1052-5149/15/$ – see front matter © 2015 Published by Elsevier Inc.

audience, both radiologists and clinicians, will find this issue helpful in day-to-day practice and beneficial for patient care.

DEDICATION

I dedicate this issue to my parents and the rest of my family for their unconditional love, endless support, and thoughtful advice throughout the years. Without them, I will never have today. — B.T.

I dedicate this issue to my mother and father, who have been my support and teachers over the years. Also, to my beloved wife Catalina, and our amazing children, Emilio, Federico, and Gabriel, for their patience and continued encouragement during all the big and great changes in our lives. — J.E.G.

Juan E. Gutierrez, MD
Neuroradiology Section
Centro Avanzado de Diagnostico
Medico CEDIMED
Calle 18 AA sur # 29 C 340
Medellín, Colombia, South America

Bundhit Tantiwongkosi, MD
Neuroradiology Division
University of Texas Health
Science Center San Antonio
7703 Floyd Curl Drive, MC 7800
San Antonio, TX 78230, USA

E-mail addresses:
gutierrezje@cedimed.com (J.E. Gutierrez)
tantiwongkos@uthscsa.edu (B. Tantiwongkosi)

Diagnostic Ophthalmic Ultrasound for Radiologists

Cynthia J. Kendall, BMET, ROUB, CDOS[a], Thomas C. Prager, PhD, MPH[b],
Han Cheng, OD, PhD[c], Dan Gombos, MD[d], Rosa A. Tang, MD, MPH, MBA[c,e,*],
Jade S. Schiffman, MD[c,e]

KEYWORDS

- Ultrasonography • Standardized A-scan of the eye • B-scan of the eye • UBM
- Ultrasound biomicroscopy • Ocular ultrasound • Orbital ultrasound

KEY POINTS

- Ultrasound biomicroscopy provides high-resolution images of the anterior segment of the eye, allowing examination of iris, angles, ciliary body, and intraocular lens.
- Ophthalmic B-scan is commonly used to evaluate the posterior segment of the eye in the presence of opaque optical media. It helps in detecting optic nerve head drusen, retinal detachments, and tumors and is useful for examining the eye and the orbit.
- Ophthalmic A-scan is commonly used for measuring axial eye length in order to calculate intraocular lens power for implantation during cataract surgery.
- Standardized A, a special type of A-scan, is primarily used for differentiating ocular tumors and measuring optic nerve sheath diameters and extraocular muscle sizes.

BASIC PRINCIPLES

Ophthalmic ultrasound (A-scan and B-scan) is performed primarily for the 3 following reasons:

1. When opaque media prevent direct view of the ocular fundus and periphery, ultrasound determines the presence or absence of ocular tumors, retinal detachment, foreign bodies, or other pathologic abnormality.
2. When media are clear, ultrasound allows imaging of intraocular and extraocular structures, such as optic nerve head drusen, orbital structures and lesions, and internal structure of intraocular lesions.
3. Ultrasound allows the measurement of axial length before cataract surgery in order to determine intraocular lens power.

B-mode, or brightness mode, is a 2-dimensional sector image used to characterize ocular structures and determine the status of the globe and orbit.[1–3] These gray-scale images are generated by changes in tissue medium that reflect sound. In ophthalmology, sector images of the globe are displayed 90° from traditional medical ultrasound. Body ultrasound images are oriented with the probe surface at the top of the display, whereas ophthalmic images display the probe surface on

Disclosures: None.
[a] Ophthalmic Ultrasound Consultant, PO BOX 19536, Sacramento, CA 95819-0536, USA; [b] The Methodist Hospital Research Institute, Weill Cornell Medical College, Houston, TX, USA; [c] MS Eye CARE, University Eye Institute, College of Optometry, University of Houston, 4901 Calhoun, 505 JDA Bldg, Houston, TX 77204-2020, USA; [d] Section of Ophthalmology, Department of Head and Neck Surgery, MD Anderson Cancer Center, Houston, TX 77025, USA; [e] The Optic Nerve Center, Houston, TX 77025, USA
* Corresponding author. Optic Nerve Center, Eye Wellness Center, 2617 C West Holcombe Boulevard #575, Houston, TX 77025.
E-mail address: rtang@neuroeye.com

Neuroimag Clin N Am 25 (2015) 327–365
http://dx.doi.org/10.1016/j.nic.2015.05.001
1052-5149/15/$ – see front matter © 2015 Elsevier Inc. All rights reserved.

the left. **Fig. 1** shows the orientation difference between abdominal and ophthalmic ultrasound image presentations. A probe orientation marker indicates the top of the display, so a B-scan with the marker line facing the nose would have the nasal retina at the top of the screen and temporal retina displayed in the lower aspect of the screen (see **Fig. 1**). Traditional ophthalmic ultrasound frequencies for globe and orbit imaging are 10 to 12 MHz. High-frequency posterior probes are 17 to 20 MHz and are focused to provide highest resolution at the optic nerve/retina surface, but have minimal orbital penetration.

B-scans are systematically performed to examine all clock hours with both transverse (across several clock hours) and longitudinal (along a single meridian) scans. In **Fig. 1**, placing the probe on the cornea with the marker line facing the nose performs an axial transverse scan. It shows nasal structures at the top of the screen and temporal structures below, a curved bright

line from posterior lens capsule, and a V-shaped acoustic shadow from the optic nerve. Sound is systematically swept through all ocular quadrants obtaining transverse scans of several clock hours at once. Longitudinal scans image along just one clock hour, or meridian, from the optic nerve to the anterior periphery. They are used to document anterior/posterior extent of anatomy and pathologic abnormality. Examples are found later in the Basic Examination and Clinical Cases sections in this article.

High-frequency ophthalmic ultrasound, for anterior segment imaging, is referred to as UBM, ultrasound biomicroscopy,[4–6] and uses 35 to 70 MHz with 50 MHz being the most common. The higher frequency provides higher resolution but less tissue penetration. Its shallow depth of penetration would not be useful for evaluation of the optic nerve, but rather to show, in detail, structures, such as the cornea, anterior chamber, angles, iris, and ciliary body (**Figs. 2** and **3**). The UBM is

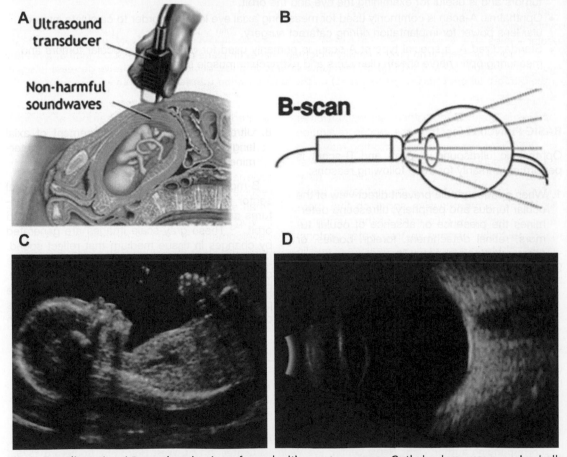

Fig. 1. Two-dimensional B-scan imaging is performed with a sector scanner. Opthalmology uses a mechanically driven transducer (*B, D*). Many abdominal ultrasound units (*A, C*) use a series of fixed transducers, sequentially fired, to generate the sector appearance. (*From* Kendall CJ. Ophthalmic Echography. Thorofare, NJ: Slack Incorporated; 1990; with permission.)

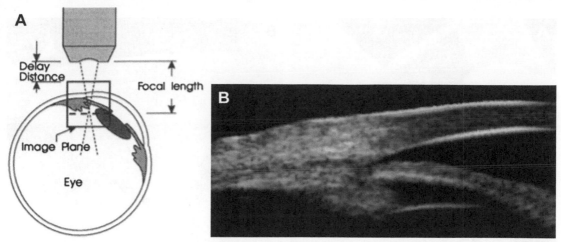

Fig. 2. UBM produces high-resolution images from a 50-MHz transducer, but depth of penetration is very shallow (A). In eyes with clear or minimally cataractous lenses, the posterior lens capsule may often be seen. Useful imaging depth is approximately 6 to 8 mm depending on tissue type. Focal zone also is very small, 2 to 3 mm in the center of the image from top to bottom where image quality is optimal. Probe distance to ocular structure is modified in order to place the tissue of interest within the focal zone as seen the image of the iridociliary angle (B). (From Kendall CJ. Ophthalmic Echography. Thorofare, NJ: Slack Incorporated; 1990; with permission.)

ideal for examining the eye for narrow or closed angles and structures behind the iris, such as cysts, tumors, and dislocated crystalline and intraocular lenses.[7] UBM is performed with a sterile, fluid-filled ClearScan bag[8] or a saline-filled plastic or silicon shell resting on the sclera (Fig. 4). Axial and other transverse scans are routinely performed to document normal tissue or the extent

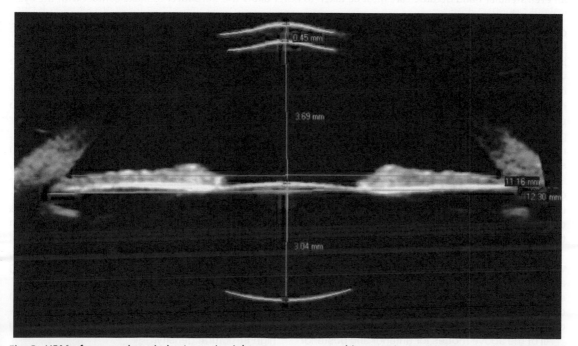

Fig. 3. UBM of a normal eye in horizontal axial transverse scan. In this example, 35 MHz was used to image and measure ocular structures in the anterior segment. This axial scan displays anterior-posterior cornea thickness on top (0.45 mm) as 2 white curved lines, the iris and pupillary space, the anterior chamber depth (3.69 mm), a bright curved anterior lens capsule surface in the pupillary space, and a weaker posterior lens capsule at the bottom (3.04 mm). Additional measurements are made of the anterior chamber diameter (11.16 mm) and the sulcus-to-sulcus measurement (12.30 mm). Detailed measurements are used to evaluate patients for various refractive procedures such as introducing an additional lens into the normal phakic eye to correct for high refractive error. These are called an intraocular contact lens (ICL). (Courtesy of W.A. Kohn, COT, CRA, CDOS, ROUB, Austin, TX.)

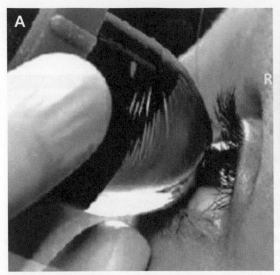
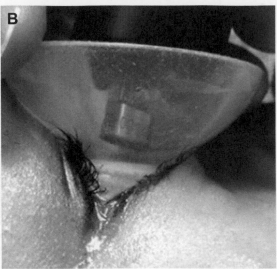

Fig. 4. (A) UBM is performed with a sterile fluid-filled "bag," ClearScan Cover. Insertion of the probe into the cover produces pressurized fluid. It also positions the moving transducer several millimeters away from the ocular surface. Releasing fluid to produce wrinkles also reduces pressure applied to the eye and is important for examination of patients with low intraocular pressure (IOP). Low pressure in the bag is also helpful to allow the membrane to drape over more of the cornea for a wider axial view. Anterior segment structures such as the angle, iris, ciliary body, and lens are imaged in high resolution. (B) Another examination technique uses a saline-filled plastic or silicon shell resting on the sclera. The transducer is placed into bubble-free fluid, because bubbles would interfere with sound transmission. This technique is useful for patients who cannot control their blink reflex but requires an even steadier hand because care must be taken to never allow the transducer to make contact with the eye.

of pathologic abnormality (see Fig. 2, left). Scans for examining the angle between cornea and iris in glaucoma patients are performed primarily with longitudinal scans (see Fig. 2, right). Most ophthalmic UBM probes use sector scanning, but some use linear transducer movement. Sector probes pivot a single transducer so that sound is generated in a fan-shaped display. Sector scans make sense for the eye because it allows the sound waves to be more perpendicular to a wider area of the fundus, thereby producing more clinically useful data. Linear probes are sometimes used in UBM scans. They also have a single transducer, but it is moved back and forth linearly, thereby producing a rectangular image (Figs. 5–8).

A-mode, or Amplitude, scans are also displayed with the ocular surface at the left of the screen and are one-dimensional, up-and-down spikes. Axial eye lengths measured by A-scan are used to calculate intraocular lens power for implantation during cataract surgery.[9,10]

All of the above modes for anterior and posterior B-scans and eye length A-scans use fixed-focus transducers. The only exception is a second, very specific A-mode, referred to as Standardized A-scan, that uses a transducer emitting parallel sound beam and a unique amplifier (Fig. 9).[11,12] This mode is used to characterize a lesion's internal structure and to perform measurements of intraocular and extraocular structures. The operator determines tissue or tumor structure by interpreting the relative amplitude of each.[13] Tissue reflection and absorption produce an A-scan pattern of varying heights or amplitudes. For example, choroidal melanoma produces a low to medium height of echoes from within the tumor due to the homogeneity of the cells. In contrast, a choroidal hemangioma will show an echo pattern from within the lesion of high-amplitude echoes, because of the irregular cellular pattern. Solid tumors such as melanomas have a steeper and uniform falloff of echoes from within the lesion than a vascular lesion. Vascular lesions present with an irregular pattern of both high and low echoes. Although extremely useful in experienced hands, the examination technique has a steep learning curve and is not universally used.

The relationship between A-scan and B-scan echoes is that a tall echo on A-scan will correspond to a bright echo on B-scan, both indicating high structural density.

Diagnostic ultrasound is significantly different from low-frequency, high-power therapeutic ultrasound in the following 2 ways:

1. It does not generate heat in ocular tissues with the US Food and Drug Administration (FDA) required low energy limits.

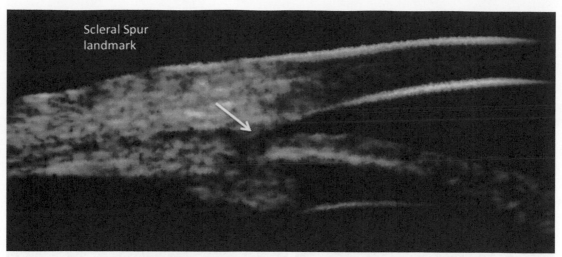

Fig. 5. Narrow anterior chamber angle is confirmed by visualization of iris insertion in relationship to the scleral spur landmark. (*Courtesy of* W.A. Kohn, COT, CRA, CDOS, ROUB, Austin, TX.)

2. The frequency is in the megahertz range of millions of cycles per second, whereas therapeutic ultrasound is in the kilohertz range of thousands of cycles per second.

Ophthalmic ultrasound uses a fixed energy system, whereas other forms of body scanning may use equipment that allows the operator to adjust the amount of sound energy that is being directed into tissue. The FDA limits power levels for sound energy used in ocular examinations. However, confirmation should be made with the Regulatory Department if there are any limits in effect for using superficial scanning probes on the eye. Some small probes on general ultrasound systems may be labeled "For Ophthalmic Use" and would be the optimal choice if available.

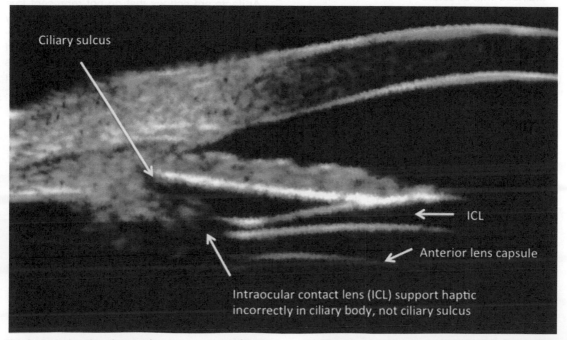

Fig. 6. Anterior chamber angle imaged to visualize the ciliary body. The patient has an ICL placed in front of the crystalline lens. Haptics are the suspension plates surrounding the artificial lens and are represented by the first 2 lines below the iris. This malposition could result in damage to the ciliary body. (*Courtesy of* W.A. Kohn, COT, CRA, CDOS, ROUB, Austin, TX.)

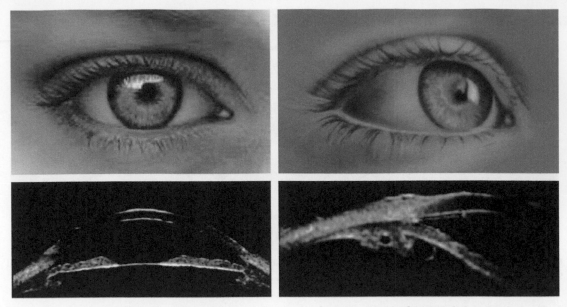

Axial scan, probe marker nasal   Angle view of iridociliary cysts

Fig. 7. (*left*) Axial scan of the anterior segment with the eye in the primary gaze. Probe orientation marker is directed nasally. (*right*) Longitudinal scan of iridociliary cysts with the eye looking to the side. Probe orientation marker is directed toward the cornea at any clock hour.

A clinically useful echo display depends on the 3 following factors (see **Fig. 3**):

1. Angle of incidence between sound beam and interface with structure
2. Difference between structural mediums at the interface
3. Surface condition of the interface

Very dissimilar mediums produce larger echoes (**Fig. 10A**), whereas mediums that are closer in consistency produce smaller echoes (see **Fig. 10B**). Note that if the probe is not perpendicular, then there will be marked weakening of the reflected sound (see **Fig. 10C, D**).

Artifacts are echoes that do not represent true structures. The eye's crystalline lens is a primary culprit for producing an abnormally curved peripheral retina due to attenuation and scattering of sound waves as they travel through the lens. This particular artifact is found in axial B-scans that

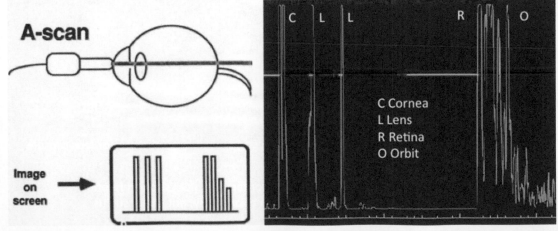

Fig. 8. One-dimensional A-scan imaging is performed with a small pencil-sized 10- to 12-MHz probe. Displayed image shows vertical deflections representing echoes from each interface with a new tissue. The most common use for A-scan is axial eye length biometry for calculating artificial lens power before cataract surgery. (*From* Kendall CJ. Ophthalmic Echography. Thorofare, NJ: Slack Incorporated; 1990; with permission.)

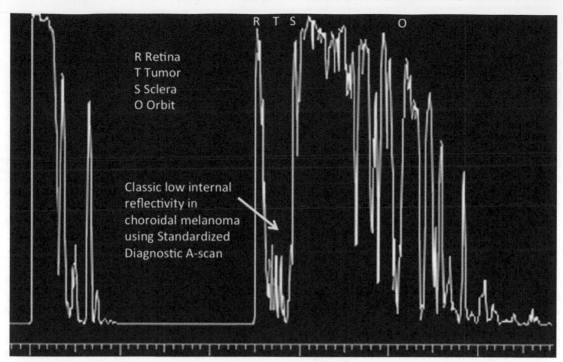

R Retina
T Tumor
S Sclera
O Orbit

Classic low internal
reflectivity in
choroidal melanoma
using Standardized
Diagnostic A-scan

Fig. 9. Standardized diagnostic A-scan is a rarely used, but a powerfully useful A-mode in experienced hands. It uses a parallel beam 8-MHz probe with a very specific set of amplifier characteristics. Low reflectivity of echoes from within a small, pigmented lesion is seen between the arrows, making it suspicious for melanoma. The primary use of standardized A-scan is to differentiate intraocular and extraocular lesions and perform measurements of optic nerve diameter and muscles. A focused probe used for precataract measurements cannot be used to characterize tissue and lesions.

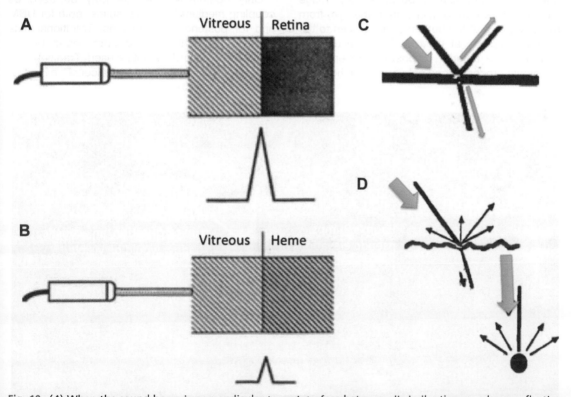

Fig. 10. (*A*) When the sound beam is perpendicular to an interface between dissimilar tissues, a large reflection will be produced. (*B*) A small difference between the tissues at an interface produces smaller echoes. (*C*) Lack of perpendicularity causes reduced reflections. (*D*) Irregular tissue surface or spherical foreign body impacts echo amplitude due to scattering and weakening of reflected sound even when perpendicular. Large arrows represent incident beam, smaller echoes represent reflected echoes of lower amplitude. (*From* Kendall CJ. Ophthalmic Echography. Thorofare, NJ: Slack Incorporated; 1990; with permission.)

direct sound through the lens and is called Baum bumps (**Fig. 11**) for Gilbert Baum, MD, a pioneer in medical ultrasound imaging from the 1960s forward.[14]

Another example of artifact is shown in **Fig. 12**. In the case of calcified optic nerve head drusen, it is common to see a weaker duplicate drusen echo in the orbit. The reverberation artifact is displayed at the same distance to the right of the actual drusen echo as the real drusen is from the probe surface. A low gain setting is important to differentiate drusen from the surrounding highly reflective orbital tissue.

BASIC EXAMINATION TECHNIQUE

Examinations performed in a consistent manner ensure a thorough and accurate observation of all parts of the globe and orbit[15]; this is accomplished by using 2 essential scan planes that in ophthalmology are named transverse and longitudinal, as previously described. Transverse scans will image a plane across about 4 clock hours of the globe. Depending on how the probe is orientated, they are called horizontal, vertical, oblique, and axial. Longitudinal scans, sometimes called radial scans, are named because they image only one clock hour or meridian in the eye, from the optic nerve at the bottom of the screen to the anterior periphery at the top. They are used to document the anterior or posterior extent of a pathologic process along only one clock hour.

Transducers in B-probes move back and forth, toward and away from the orientation mark generating and displaying sound waves in a pie-shaped sector format. Each image's interpretation is based on knowing where the probe is placed on the eye, where the patient is looking, and where the orientation marker is directed. A B-scan can be thought of as a 2- to 3-mm "slice" of sound directed into the tissue of interest.

These longitudinal scans are extremely useful for analysis of the disc (see the later section Clinical Cases of the Optic Nerve). They allow the sound beam to scan around the crystalline lens, thereby reducing retinal surface artifacts. Papilledema is additionally imaged from the side with longitudinal scans allowing the sound beam to be perpendicular to the papilledema's outwardly curved surface, and the shape will be clearly shown from another perspective.[16]

In all posterior ocular scans, the probe is placed on an anesthetized sclera opposite the area being imaged. Images are labeled as to where the echoes are located, not where the probe is placed. Conversely, with UBM, the probe is placed directly over the area being scanned and is labeled with that clock hour.

Only ophthalmic tear gel may be used as coupling medium for ocular scans, both for UBM and for posterior examinations. Traditional blue or clear ultrasound gel is not approved for use on the globe or lid and cannot be used. Traditional ultrasound gel may contain alcohol or other

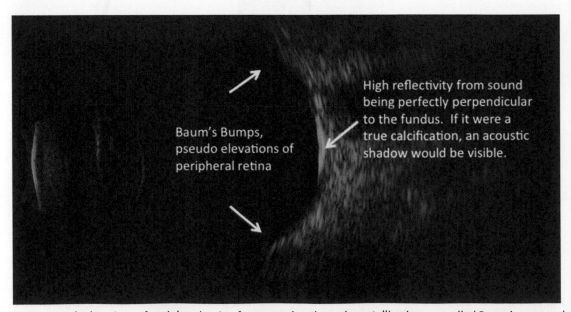

Fig. 11. Pseudoelevations of peripheral retina from scanning through crystalline lens are called Baum bumps and do not represent true ocular fundus curvature. This is a horizontal axial transverse scan with the top of display nasal and the bottom temporal. (See Basic Examination Technique section for details).

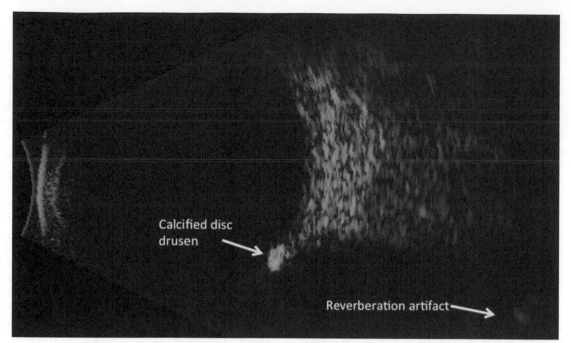

Calcified disc
drusen

Reverberation artifact

Fig. 12. A calcified optic nerve head drusen creates a weaker duplicate drusen echo far into the orbit as seen here. The reverberation artifact is displayed at the same distance to the right of the actual drusen echo because the real drusen is from the probe surface.

chemicals that could damage or irritate ocular tissues (Fig. 13).

For each of the 4 primary positions of transverse scans, direct the patient to look as far away from the probe as possible and hold their gaze. The probe is initially placed at the peripheral edge of cornea at 6:00, 12:00, 9:00, and 3:00. Sound is initially directed posteriorly toward the nerve. Once the nerve shadow is seen, shift the probe away from the cornea in an arc to maintain contact with the sclera. This shift will direct the sound beam away from the disc, toward the equator and then the anterior periphery of the globe and orbit. In this way, all quadrants of the eye and orbit will be screened.

It is routine to document the retinal surface at the macula, where detailed vision occurs, with a longitudinal scan as part of a complete examination. Macula scans do not require extreme gaze and are best with the patient in either primary

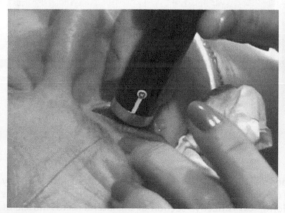
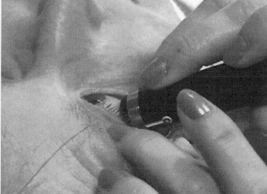

Fig. 13. (left) Vertical transverse scan at the initial position to locate optic nerve shadow. (right) Vertical transverse scan near the end of the nasal quadrant sweep with sound directed toward the eye's equatorial region. Orientation mark is directed superior for vertical transverse and nasal for horizontal transverse scans. Only ophthalmic tear gel may be used as coupling medium.

gaze or only slightly temporal in gaze. This gaze permits better centering of the macula within the image for improved resolution. When imaging the temporal meridian where the macula is found (Fig. 14), display the optic nerve near the bottom of the screen and the dark inserting tendon of lateral rectus muscle near the equator of the globe. The optic nerve and muscles appear hollow because sound waves are not scattered when reflecting from the parallel fibers of the optic nerve or from striated muscle tissue. The top of the screen is the temporal anterior periphery; near the bottom of screen is the optic nerve. The macula appears approximately 5 mm above the center of optic nerve shadow. If pathologic abnormality is detected, additional oblique transverse and longitudinal scans are performed in order to center the pathologic abnormality within the scan for optimal resolution and clinical information.

To image a cross-section of the optic nerve approximately 3 mm behind the globe, direct the patient to look in primary gaze and perform a vertical transverse with probe placed at the edge of the temporal cornea. Locate the nerve and slowly shift the probe to direct the sound beam to cross the nerve just behind the globe. The optic nerve's natural slightly nasal position usually permits an image in this way. A vertical nasal approach may also be performed (see Fig. 13, left).

Quadrant Screening Examination

Probe position 1: Horizontal transverse of superior aspect with probe marker nasal.

Probe position 2: Horizontal transverse of inferior aspect with probe marker nasal.

Probe position 3: Vertical transverse of nasal aspect, with probe marker superior.

Probe position 4: Vertical transverse of temporal aspect, with probe marker superior.

Probe position 5: Longitudinal macula 9 o'clock (L9) for the right eye and 3 o'clock (L3) for the left eye with probe marker directed temporally.

CLINICAL APPLICATION

In general, the most common use of ultrasound is by the general ophthalmologist who, before cataract surgery, performs an A-scan, in order to measure the size of the eye for calculating the power of the intraocular lens implant (IOL). More recently, with the advent of the UBM, the high-frequency ultrasound is helpful in examining the anterior segment of the eye to determine whether the angle of the eye is narrow or closed and requires treatment (laser vs surgery). In addition, this technology helps with lesions of the iris, ciliary body, and lens. When an eye has a cataract that is so dense that there may be no view of the posterior pole, B-scan ultrasound is useful to confirm that there is no retinal detachment, ocular malignancy, or foreign body before the procedure. In cases of ocular trauma where view is impaired, although ocular ultrasound may be an excellent procedure, it is contraindicated when there is an open globe. If there were an ocular tumor, the procedure would be avoided until an ocular oncologist evaluates the patient. Ophthalmologists, in particular those who are retinal experts or ocular oncologists, use ultrasound frequently to determine the consistency of lesions that they see in the eye,

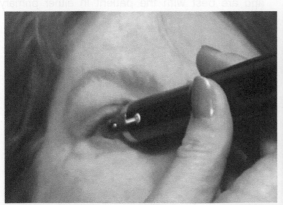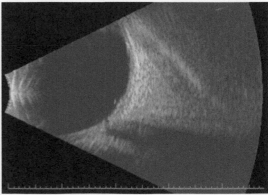

Fig. 14. (Left) Longitudinal macula scan of the 9:00 meridian of the right eye with the patient looking only slightly temporally. Probe marker is directed toward the clock hour to be imaged. (Right) A 10-MHz B-scan shows the insertion of the optic nerve at the bottom, and the long, low reflective section of the lateral rectus muscle at the top. A sector scanner transducer moves toward and away from the probe orientation marker. In this section, when the transducer is by the marker, the anterior periphery is at the top of the screen. When the transducer swings back to the opposite side of the probe, the sound beam crosses the optic nerve. Alignment of the optic disc and the long section of lateral rectus ensure imaging of the macula.

that helps to determine if it is a malignant versus benign entity. For example, choroidal pigmentation is a frequent finding in patients. Most cases of choroidal pigmented lesions are benign nevi. Some of these nevi undergo malignant degeneration and become uveal melanomas. Nevi that are flat are most likely benign, and pigmented choroidal lesions that are elevated may also be benign; however, there is more of a concern that it may be, or evolve into, a malignant melanoma. Serial ultrasound is very helpful in determining elevation and, if there is growth over time, to assist in differential diagnosis. In general, melanocytic lesions greater than 2.5 to 3.0 mm in thickness are highly suspected for being neoplastic. The resolution of ultrasound makes it the preferred modality for assessment of these ocular lesions over computed tomography (CT) or MR imaging. Using a scanning technique, one determines if the lesion is confined to the globe or extended into the orbit. Extraocular extension can occur in a focal area on ultrasound and may be missed by CT or MR imaging. The cuts used in these latter 2 techniques may miss the largest dimension of the tumor. Adjacent shallow retinal detachments (often serous) can be best visualized with ultrasound. Most uveal melanomas are dome-shaped but some may have a collar button or mushroom configuration. Collar button or mushroom configuration occurs when the tumor breaks through Bruch membrane and is highly correlative with a diagnosis of melanoma.

Retinoblastoma is one particular intraocular neoplasm best assessed with ultrasound. These tumors are often associated with calcification, although in one-third of the cases calcification may not be present. Calcification is easily identified with ocular echography due to both bright echoes and attenuation of sound waves posterior to the lesion (see **Figs. 44** and **45**).[17] The examination can be performed on a cooperative infant without anesthesia. Historically, CT scans were used to confirm intraocular calcification in any child thought to harbor retinoblastoma. However, a significant percentage of these patients harbor the RB1 gene defect that is thought to increase the risk of radiation-induced secondary malignancies as well as tumors in the pineal region. As a result, most clinicians avoid CT scans and use ultrasound, followed by MR imaging of the brain and orbit to confirm the diagnosis, assess the midbrain, and avoid radiation exposure.

When considering the optic nerve and orbit, ultrasound has certain advantages over CT and MR imaging in particular, when assessing the optic nerve for calcification (as seen with optic nerve drusen). Ultrasound is more sensitive than other imaging modalities in detecting buried optic nerve drusen. Although CT scans may demonstrate drusen, they can be missed between cuts of the scan. Irrespective, patients who have optic nerve drusen and elevated optic nerves may also have superimposed papilledema that may be difficult to ascertain, so in cases where an underlying neurologic problem may be a cause of raised intracranial pressure (ICP), the presence of drusen does not negate the need for neuroimaging and neurologic workup.

In terms of imaging the orbital component of the optic nerve, the 30° test using standardized A-scan[18,19] is a technically challenging procedure requiring a very well-trained individual. This test allows one to determine if the optic nerve is thickened due to fluid (which often is due to raised ICP) or if it is thickened due to infiltrative process (see the section Clinical Cases of the Optic Nerve).

Regarding imaging of the orbit, CT and MR imaging in general tend to be superior tests to that of orbital ultrasound, because the sound does not penetrate deeply enough into the orbit. CT and MR imaging are better choices when one is assessing for an orbital mass or extension to adjacent structures such as the sinuses. Posterior scleritis is one situation where ultrasound is helpful and can be diagnostic. Although the anterior globe may appear normal, inflammation and fluid posteriorly create a T sign, which in association with severe ocular pain and redness correlates with the diagnosis (see **Fig. 53**).

The following are typical cases of ocular pathologic abnormality seen using ultrasonography. Cases are presented beginning distally at the cornea and proceeding back through the globe and into the orbit.

CLINICAL CASES OF THE ANTERIOR SEGMENT

Figs. 15–29.

CLINICAL CASES OF THE POSTERIOR SEGMENT

Figs. 30–45.

CLINICAL CASES OF THE OPTIC NERVE

Figs. 46–58.

CLINICAL CASES OF THE ORBIT

Figs. 59–69.

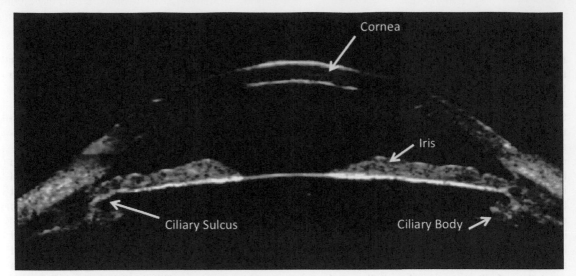

Fig. 15. Axial scan of normal anterior segment.

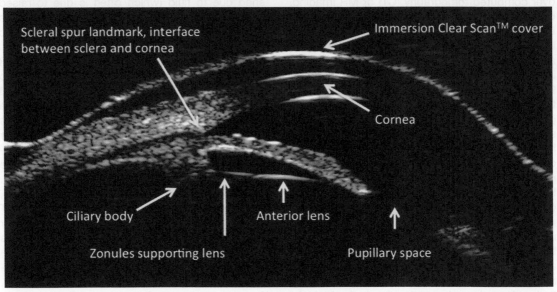

Fig. 16. Longitudinal scan of normal anterior segment with clearly seen scleral spur. Extra tear gel is applied to separate the bag echo from the cornea, thereby providing a clearer image of the anterior corneal surface. Tear gel also protects the cornea and encourages gentle contact with the ocular surface.

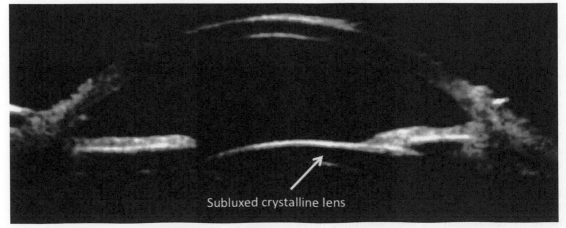

Fig. 17. Axial scan of subluxed crystalline lens.

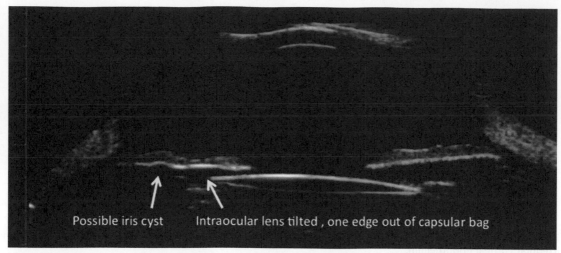

Possible iris cyst   Intraocular lens tilted , one edge out of capsular bag

Fig. 18. Axial scan of the patient with tilted IOL. The edge of the lens has slipped out of the capsular bag on the left and is at risk for rubbing on the posterior iris sloughing off pigment cells that can clog the trabecular meshwork drainage system.

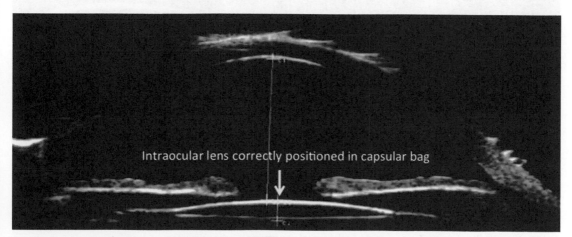

Intraocular lens correctly positioned in capsular bag

Fig. 19. Axial scan of patient with normal IOL position.

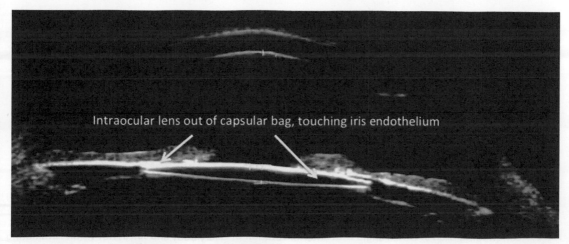

Intraocular lens out of capsular bag, touching iris endothelium

Fig. 20. Axial scan of poorly positioned IOL in contact with iris.

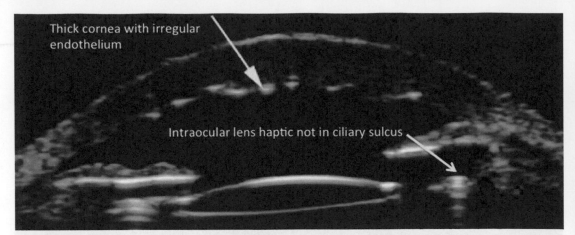

Fig. 21. Axial scan of poorly positioned IOL with haptic in contact with ciliary body and thickened cornea with irregular corneal endothelium.

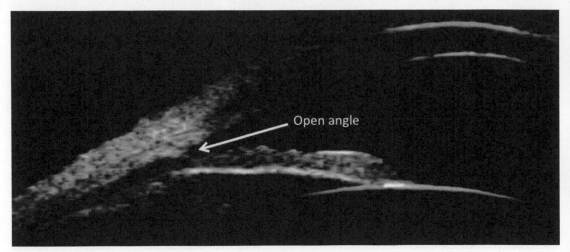

Fig. 22. Longitudinal scan of open angle and normal structures.

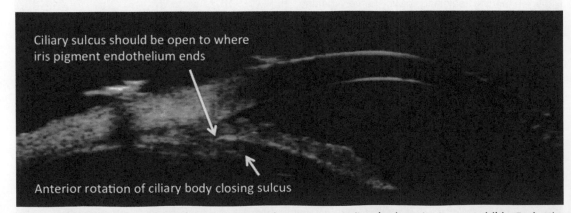

Fig. 23. Longitudinal scan of closed angle with anterior rotation of ciliary body and sulcus not visible. Evaluating ciliary body as rotated or not can direct appropriate laser procedure as needed.

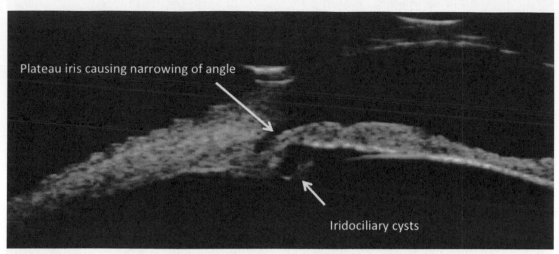

Fig. 24. Longitudinal scan of plateau iris and small iridociliary cysts causing narrow angle.

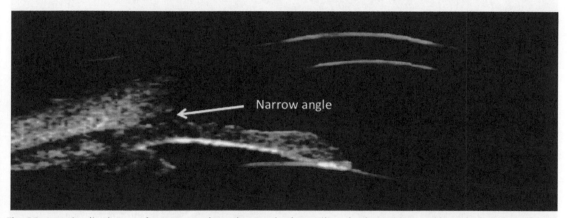

Fig. 25. Longitudinal scan of narrow angle and normal sulcus. Ciliary body position and lens thickness evaluation contribute to selecting an appropriate intervention.

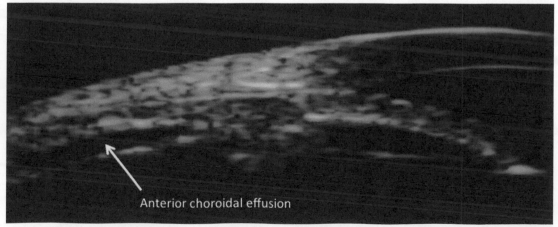

Fig. 26. Longitudinal scan of choroidal effusion shows a separation of the ciliary body from the sclera, a possible cause of reduced intraocular pressure.

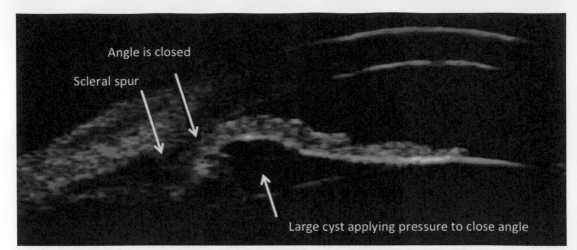

Scleral spur

Angle is closed

Large cyst applying pressure to close angle

Fig. 27. Longitudinal scan of large iridociliary cyst causing closure of angle.

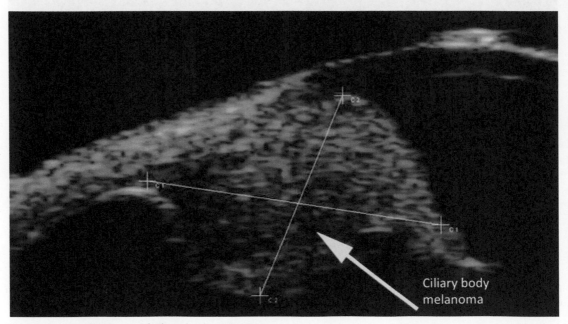

Ciliary body melanoma

Fig. 28. Longitudinal scan of ciliary body melanoma.

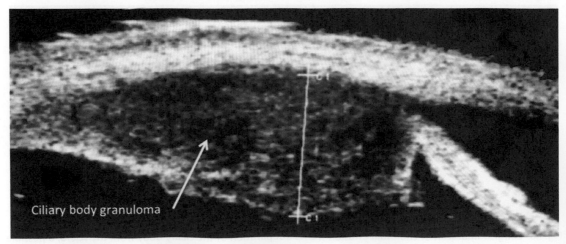

Ciliary body granuloma

Fig. 29. Longitudinal scan of ciliary body granuloma.

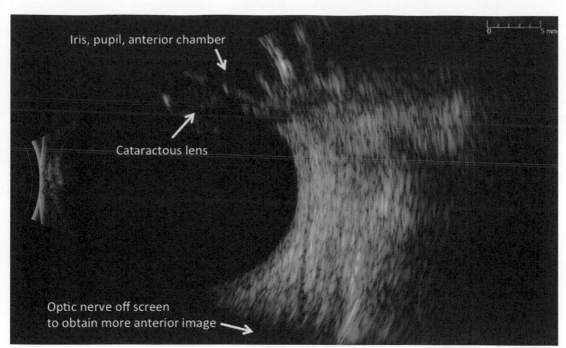

Fig. 30. A longitudinal scan of the nasal meridian provides the best opportunity to image the anterior segment with a posterior segment probe. With no nose or brow bone to limit probe angle, combined with eye position, the sound beam can be directed very anteriorly so that anterior structures appear in the center of the display and therefore in focus. The optic nerve shadow is now off the screen. A dense cataract is seen at the top of the image with the iris and pupillary space above. This scan plane can be useful to detect rupture of the posterior lens capsule.

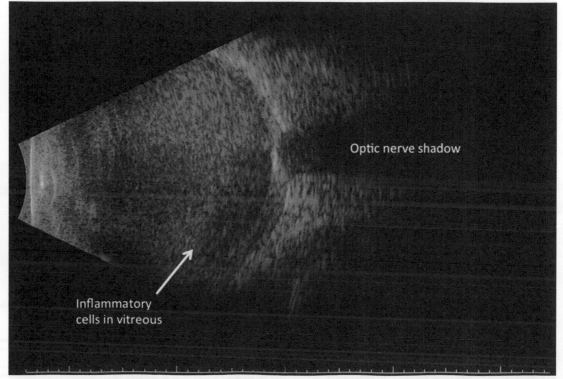

Fig. 31. Transverse scan of inflammatory cells filling the vitreous cavity. It can be difficult to differentiate blood cells from inflammatory cells only with B-scan. Other clinical findings will be needed to support a diagnosis.

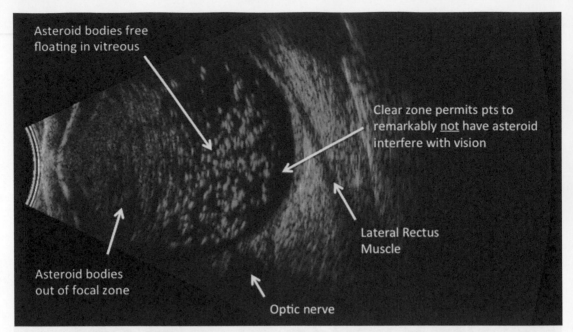

Asteroid bodies free floating in vitreous

Clear zone permits pts to remarkably <u>not</u> have asteroid interfere with vision

Lateral Rectus Muscle

Asteroid bodies out of focal zone

Optic nerve

Fig. 32. Longitudinal macula scan of asteroid hyalosis, with calcium soaps deposited in vitreous. Optic cup at the bottom of the screen with low reflective long section of lateral rectus muscle. The white line on right is the temporal orbital bone. Asteroid bodies in the first one-third of scan appear blurry because they are in the near field of the sound beam and therefore out of the focal zone. The center one-third of a B-scan is the focal zone of the ocular probes. Pts, patients.

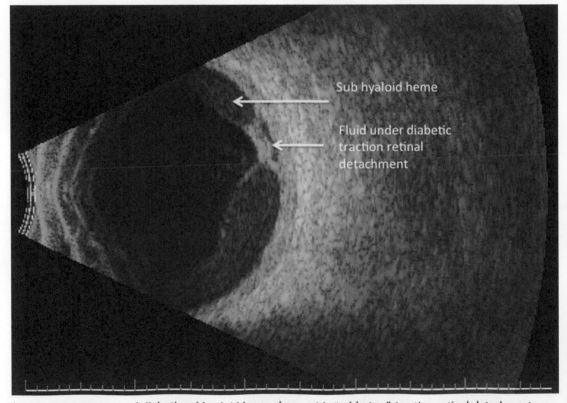

Sub hyaloid heme

Fluid under diabetic traction retinal detachment

Fig. 33. Transverse scan of diabetic subhyaloid hemorrhage with "table top" traction retinal detachment.

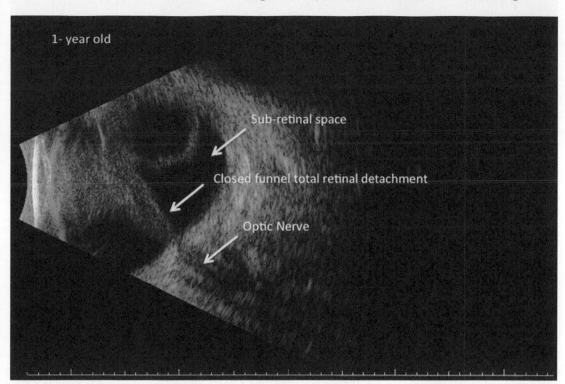

Fig. 34. Longitudinal scan of a 1-year-old child with totally detached, closed funnel retinal detachment (RD). RD is seen inserting into the optic nerve with bullous area of retina anteriorly that is seen in pediatric RDs and is often called a morning glory configuration.

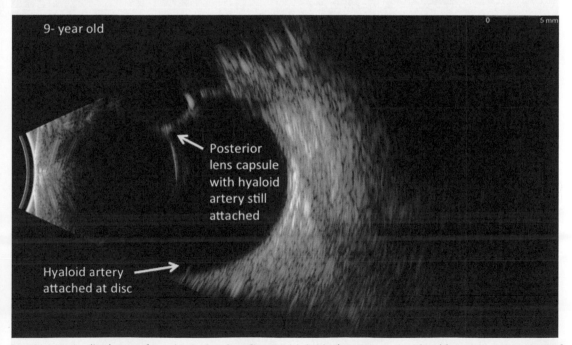

Fig. 35. Longitudinal scan of nasal meridian in a 9-year-old child who presented with subluxed crystalline lens of unknown origin. Longitudinal scan of nasal meridian shows an intact posterior hyaloid artery still attached at the apex of the posterior lens capsule and a small part also seen at the optic nerve. Traction caused by attachment of artery to the lens caused subluxation. Optic nerve shadow is nearly off the screen so that more of the anterior segment tissues would be imaged. In a transverse scan, a small white dot representing cross-section of the artery will be seen moving through the vitreous as sound plane images it during the sweep from posterior to anterior aspect during basic examination.

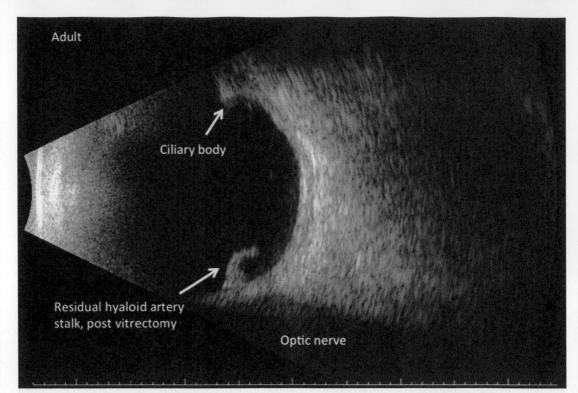

Fig. 36. Adult with primary fetal vasculature. A thick residual vascular stalk is seen attached to the disc, following lensectomy and vitrectomy for cosmesis. The eye was blind, and a dense cataract was removed to provide a more normal eye appearance. The surgeon did not completely remove the stalk due to its vascularity.

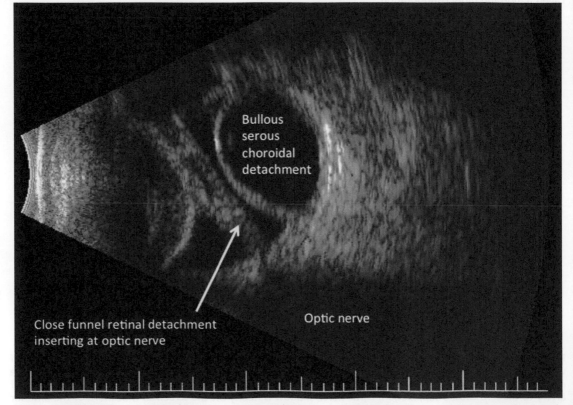

Fig. 37. Longitudinal scan of total retinal and serous choroidal detachments with underlying serous fluid. Tight funnel retinal detachment is seen inserting into the optic nerve, whereas a detached choroid always inserts at the vascular arcades.

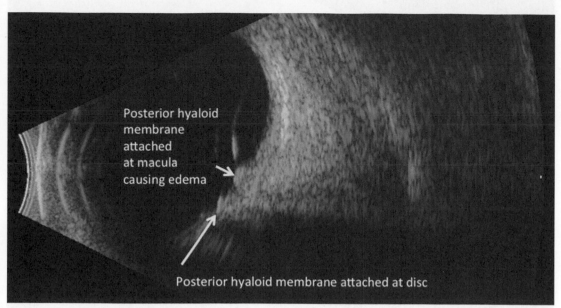

Fig. 38. Longitudinal scan of macula meridian demonstrates vitreomacular traction causing macular edema. Posterior hyaloid membrane is seen inserting at the disc, macula, and equator. Longitudinal scans are required to image delicate vitreous membranes by directing the sound in a perpendicular fashion.

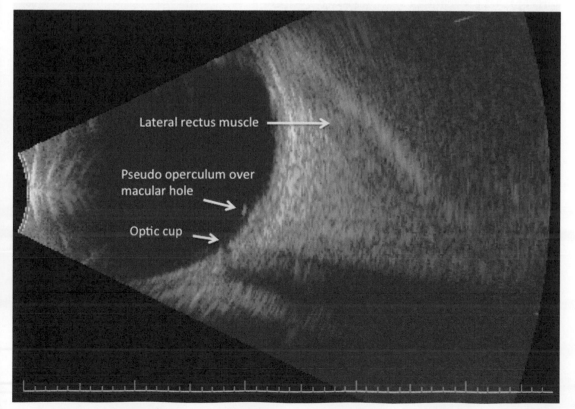

Fig. 39. Longitudinal scan of macula meridian demonstrates an optic cup. In addition, there is a pseudo-operculum over the macula. Pseudo-operculum comprises dense vitreous.

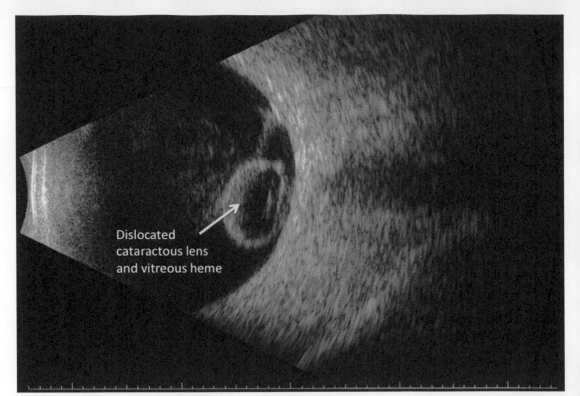

Fig. 40. Traumatic dislocation of cataractous lens into the posterior segment with vitreous hemorrhage and posterior vitreous detachment. With eye movement during a dynamic examination, the lens is seen sliding on the retinal surface.

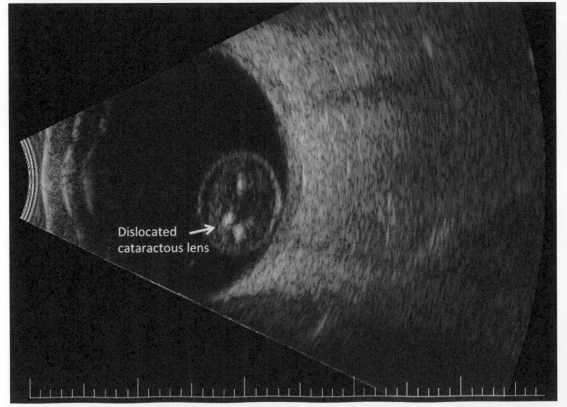

Fig. 41. Another case of traumatic dislocation of cataractous lens into the posterior segment, without hemorrhage. With eye movement during a dynamic examination, the lens is seen sliding on the retinal surface.

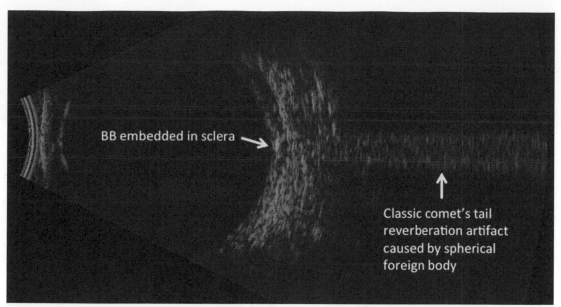

Fig. 42. Transverse scan of a pellet embedded in the sclera. On radiograph, it could not be distinguished if the foreign body was in the eye or the orbit. Once the classic comet's tail reverberation from a spherical object was detected, the patient was directed to follow a target very slowly. The reverberation echo moved at the same rate as the eye, so it was determined that the pellet was embedded within the eye wall.

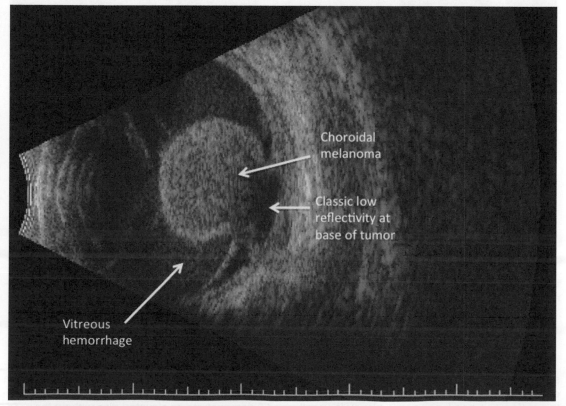

Fig. 43. Transverse scan of a choroidal melanoma's mushroom-shaped configuration. This shape is caused by the tumor breaking through the Bruch membrane in the retina as it stretched during growth. Adjacent retinal detachment and vitreous hemorrhage are also present. There was no ophthalmoscopic view into this eye. The appearance of a mushroom-shaped lesion is highly correlative of a uveal melanoma.

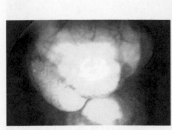 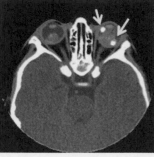 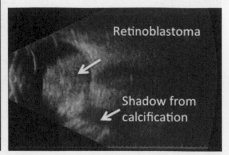

Fig. 44. Large retinoblastoma as seen on fundoscopy, CT, and B-scan. Characteristic calcification is clearly seen on CT and causes multiple shadowing artifacts on B-scan, making tumor dimensions more difficult to determine. *Arrows* on CT in center show bright areas of calcification. Although well imaged on CT, ultrasound and MR imaging are the preferred techniques for this malignancy in order to avoid radiation exposure in these vulnerable patients.

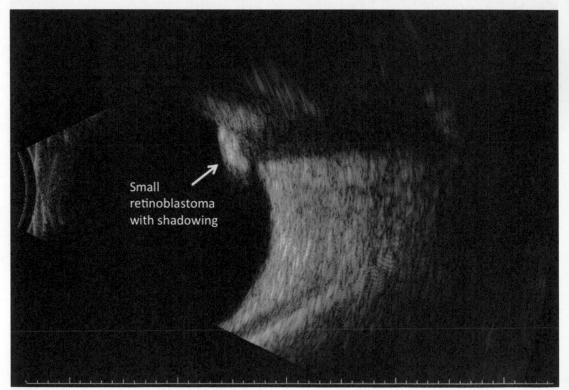

Fig. 45. Small retinoblastoma's characteristic calcification is clearly seen as shadowing artifact posterior to the tumor. A reduplication artifact from the highly reflective calcium can be seen within the shadow.

Differential diagnosis of optic nerve diseases is sometimes challenging because opthalmoscopy examination is limited to the anterior surface of the optic nerve head, and tissue biopsy is usually not available. Ultrasound imaging of the optic nerve head and the retrobulbar optic nerve may provide diagnostic information. On B-scan echography, the optic nerve is a low-reflective homogenous tubular structure surrounded by a distinctly high-reflective dural sheath. **Figs. 56–58** demonstrate an elevated disc without the presence of drusen.

A common use of orbital ultrasound is for detecting buried optic nerve head drusen. Although drusen on the anterior surface of the optic nerve head is easily visible as yellow hyaline bodies on ophthalmoscopy, the appearance of the optic nerve head with buried drusen resembles that of true optic nerve swelling.[20,21] Correctly differentiating optic nerve head drusen from true optic disc edema will avoid unnecessary expensive and sometimes invasive testing and decrease patient anxiety. On B-scan echography, the calcified optic nerve head drusen is identified as a highly reflective echo (see **Fig. 12**; **Figs. 46** and **47**). B-scan is reported to be more reliable in detecting optic nerve head drusen compared with CT or autofluorescence (**Fig. 48**) performed with pre-injection photography for fluorescein angiography.[22] It is important to turn down the B-scan gain in order to observe the characteristically bright reflection and to avoid missing a drusen that is surrounded by highly reflective orbital tissue. The gain setting depends on the instrument design and frequency of the probe (see **Figs. 46** and **47**; **Fig. 49**).

Recently, orbital ultrasound has been considered a noninvasive, low-cost test for detection of increased ICP.[24] The retrobulbar optic nerve sheath diameter (ONSD) measured at 3 mm behind the ocular globe has been shown in early human studies to expand quickly under increased cerebrospinal fluid (CSF) pressure.[25,26] This expansion is not surprising because the optic nerve sheath is contiguous with the intracranial dura, and the retrobulbar part of the dura is surrounded by orbital fat only, which allows the optic nerve sheath to widen with an increase in ICP. A recent prospective blinded observational study in 65 patients requiring invasive ICP monitoring reported that ONSD greater than 4.8 mm showed 96% sensitivity and 94% specificity for detection of ICP greater than 20 mm Hg.[27] Although the criterion for the cutoff ONSD value varied among different studies, a good correlation between ONSD and invasively measured ICP has been consistently reported.[24,27–29]

The 30° test developed by Ossoinig and colleagues is performed with a standardized A-scan technique. This technique is used in order to determine if a larger than normal ONSD measured by ultrasound is due to increased subarachnoid fluid (as occurs most commonly from raised ICP) or from a solid/infiltrated optic nerve as might occur with a meningioma or glioma, among other causes.[30] The ONSD is first measured when the patient looks straight ahead (at primary gaze) and then again at about 30° or more lateral gaze

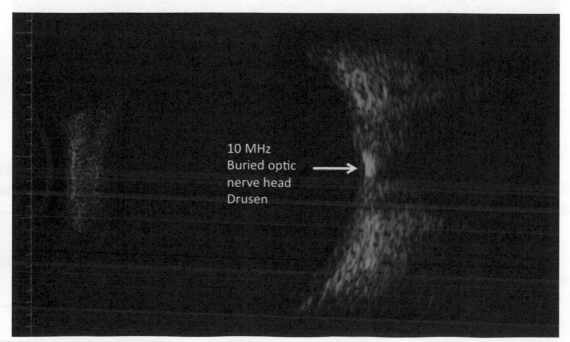

10 MHz
Buried optic
nerve head
Drusen

Fig. 46. Transverse scan of buried calcified drusen at 10 MHz with low gain. With high gain, a drusen can be missed when surrounded by highly reflective orbital tissues. Low gain now shows tissue overlying the calcification. In addition, the artifact of a wide-appearing optic nerve is due to the drusen blocking sound and creating an acoustic shadow. A highly reflective spot at low gain and a wide nerve shadow are a classic presentation of disc drusen.

(Fig. 50). In a normal optic nerve, the ONSD remains the same at different gazes. If the ONSD is widened from increased CSF, there will be a reduction in the widening when the optic nerve and its sheath are stretched at lateral gaze presumably because of a redistribution of the increased amount of CSF over a greater area. In the presence of a large amount of fluid, a 25% to 30% reduction in ONSD may be observed. A greater than 10% reduction in ONSD is considered a positive 30° test,[27] although a higher percentage cutoff has been used by others. Fig. 52 shows an example of a positive 30° test in a patient with papilledema. The ONSD, measured as the distance between the 2 arachnoid sheath spikes (vertical arrows), is 5.74 mm at primary gaze (left side) and decreases to 4.11 mm at lateral gaze (right side). Carter and colleagues[19] and a retrospective study from the authors' own clinic (data to be published) showed that ONSD combined with the 30° test is sensitive in

differentiating papilledema from pseudopapilledema, such as optic nerve drusen, hyperopic disc, or titled optic nerve head (Fig. 51).

Optic nerve tumors (eg, glioma and meningioma) are found in a series of 8% of 1264 patients with orbital tumors.[31] An enlarged normal optic nerve shadow is the most important diagnostic feature on B-scan (Fig. 52).[32–34] The 30° test is usually negative unless there is increased subarachnoid fluid anterior to the tumor. Despite its usefulness, the 30° test is not widely available because it requires a very highly skilled examiner.

B-scan ultrasound is also used for the diagnosis of posterior scleritis, a condition that may present with nonspecific clinical symptoms, such as pain, redness, and photophobia.[35,36] Diffuse thickening of the sclera with fluid in the Tenon space creates a low reflective area between the outer sclera and the orbital fat, called a T sign, in the peripapillary region (Figs. 53–58).

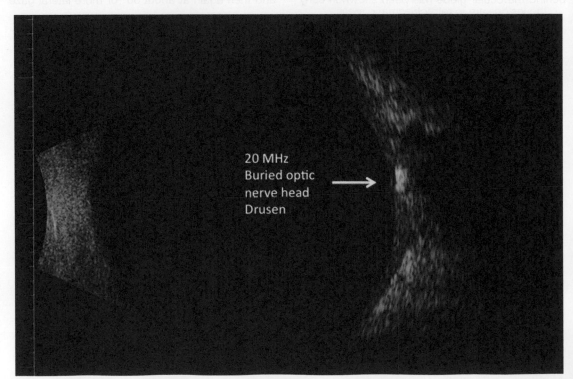

20 MHz
Buried optic
nerve head
Drusen

Fig. 47. Transverse scan of buried calcified drusen at 20 MHz with maximum gain. Full gain is needed in order to obtain maximum penetration into the orbit due to the absorption rate being higher as the frequency increases. Examinations must be performed on the anesthetized sclera with ophthalmic tear gel. When available, a 20-MHz posterior probe provides higher resolution images of retina, choroid, scleral layers and the disc surface, but is less useful for deeper nerve pathologies.

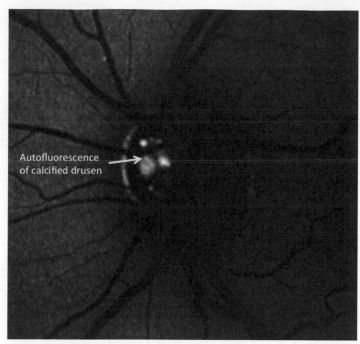

Fig. 48. Surface calcified drusen demonstrates autofluorescence with scanning laser imaging system. (*Courtesy of* E. Redenbo, CRA, CDOS, ROUB, Sacramento, CA.)

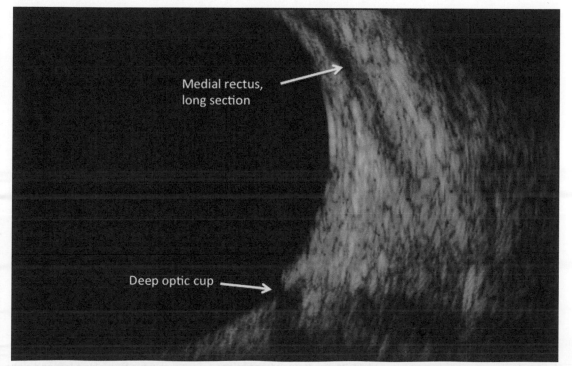

Fig. 49. Longitudinal scan demonstrates deep cup in an eye with dense cataract and no view. It is suggestive of advanced glaucoma.[23] When media are clear, cupping is best observed with slit-lamp examination.

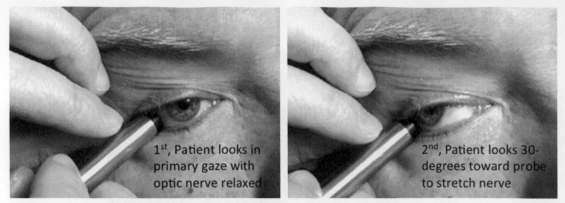

Fig. 50. *(Left)* To determine baseline optic nerve diamter in a relaxed state, patient gaze to primary first. *(Right)* After exercise, patient looks toward the probe. Similar measurements indicate no fluid within the sheath.

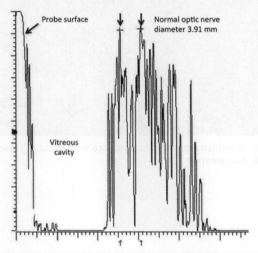

Fig. 51. In either gaze position, a normal nerve will not change in measurement. This normal nerve measured 3.91 mm.

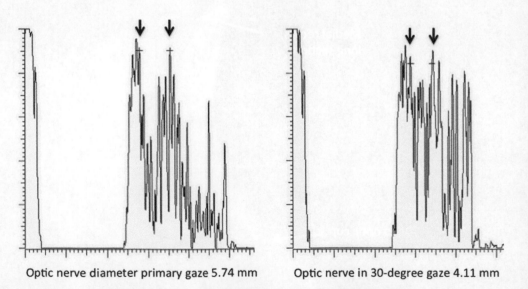

Optic nerve diameter primary gaze 5.74 mm   Optic nerve in 30-degree gaze 4.11 mm

28% reduction in diameter exceeds 20% therefore positive

Fig. 52. In primary gaze, nerve measured 5.74 mm *(left)*. After patient exercises the eye by looking left and right for a period, the nerve is remeasured with the gaze 30° toward the probe as shown in **Fig. 50** *(right)*. Resultant simultaneous measurement of 4.11 mm is a 28% change and therefore positive for fluid within the sheath. *Arrows* indicate optic nerve sheath diameters.

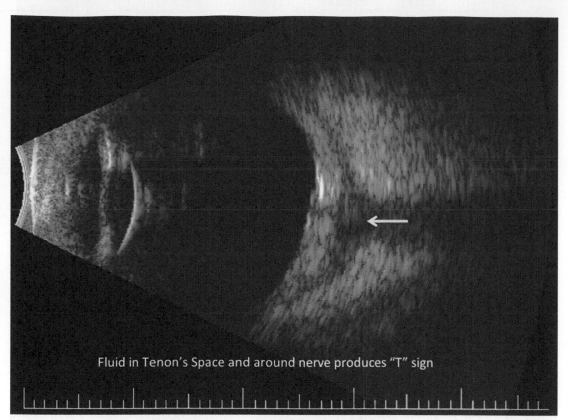

Fluid in Tenon's Space and around nerve produces "T" sign

Fig. 53. Axial scan shows a T sign T sign of low reflectivity (*arrow*) indicating fluid in Tenon's space and around optic nerve. (*Courtesy of* E. Redenbo, CRA, CDOS, ROUB, Sacramento, CA.)

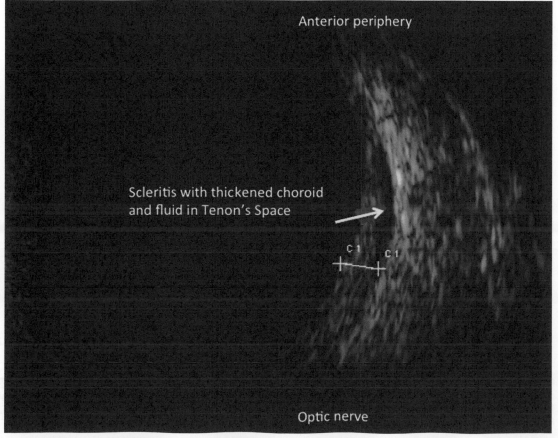

Anterior periphery

Scleritis with thickened choroid and fluid in Tenon's Space

Optic nerve

Fig. 54. Scleritis with thickened choroid and fluid in Tenon space.

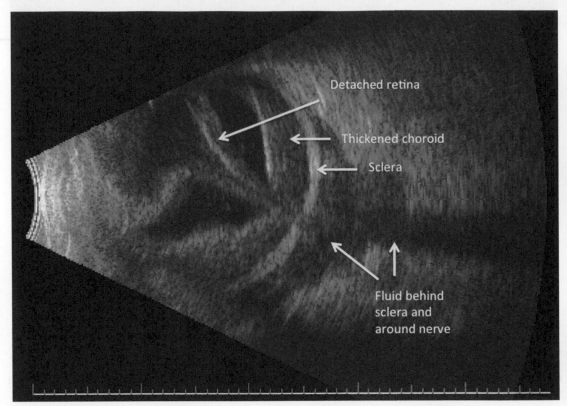

Fig. 55. Choroidal and orbital effusion caused by lymphoma substantially improved after treatment.

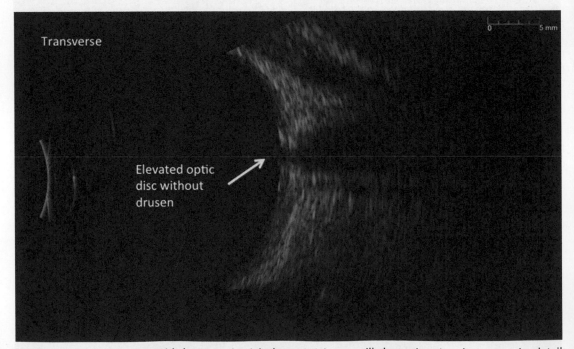

Fig. 56. Elevated optic disc, with horizontal axial plane. Axial scan will show elevation, but may miss details regarding the shape due to ultrasound perpendicularity requirements. It is important to scan the anatomy from 2 scan planes in order to fully appreciate the details needed. (*Courtesy of* E. Redenbo, CRA, CDOS, ROUB, Sacramento, CA.)

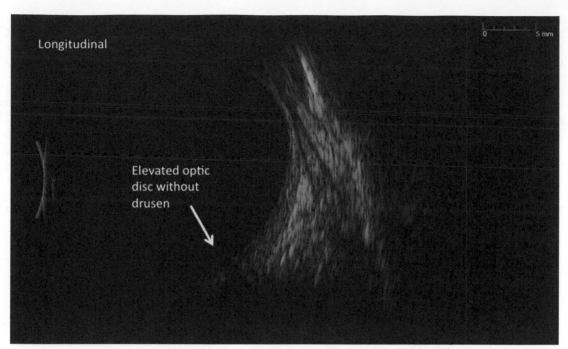

0 5 mm

Longitudinal

Elevated optic
disc without
drusen

Fig. 57. Longitudinal scans for imaging the disc allow sound to image the shape of elevation from the side to improve perpendicularity of sound. The image always has the optic nerve on bottom and the anterior periphery on top. The long section of medial rectus is in the center of the display. (*Courtesy of* E. Redenbo, CRA, CDOS, ROUB, Sacramento, CA.)

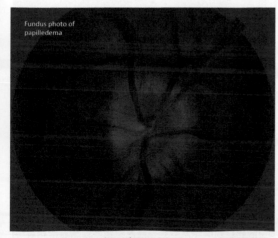

Fundus photo of
papilledema

Fig. 58. Color fundus photo of papilledema seen in the same patient as in **Figs. 56** and **57**. (*Courtesy of* E. Redenbo, CRA, CDOS, ROUB, Sacramento, CA.)

Thyroid orbitopathy is the most common cause of extraocular muscle enlargement. When examining the thyroid patient, who often presents with proptosis or diplopia, B-scan is the initial examination to rule out a space-occupying mass.[37,38] A B-scan of the orbit is performed in all quadrants, transversely and longitudinally. B-scan uses a probe focused at the retina so it is possible to miss a 2- to 4-mm lesion in the muscle apex. Fluid-filled lesions, such as a mucocele, show both the front and the back surfaces in contrast to a solid lesion that can absorb sound waves with no visualization of the posterior margin. B-scans of orbital fat typically show uniformity, except for dilated blood vessels or masses. The inferior rectus is usually the muscle first to be enlarged in thyroid eye disease, followed by the medial, superior, and then lateral rectus muscles.

Typically, more than one muscle is affected and both orbits are involved. B-scan muscle enlargement is most easily seen at the belly and more posteriorly with relative sparing of the insertion. **Fig. 59** shows an enlarged medial rectus muscle in thyroid orbitopathy compared with a normal eye (**Fig. 60**). In contrast, orbital myositis is sometimes unilateral, usually affects a single muscle with thickening in the belly as well as the insertion.[39]

Standardized A-scan can be more precise when measuring muscles, but the display of one-dimensional spikes is more abstract than a 2-dimensional B-scan image.[40] The skill required to obtain accurate A-scan measurements far exceeds what is required for a B-scan. Mistakes can lead to the withholding of treatment. The A-scan must be perpendicular to the belly of the muscle, the widest part. Consequently, multiple measurements must be taken of each muscle to establish reproducibility and a reliable average. In general, patients suspected of thyroid ophthalmopathy will often have a CT or MR imaging to confirm the diagnosis; however, very experienced ultrasonographers may determine enlargements of the extraocular muscles that may be sensitive in the detection of orbitopathy. Experienced examiners' hands may be more sensitive in detecting mild muscle enlargement undetected by other neuroimaging techniques.

Additional orbital diseases detected by B-scan are shown in **Figs. 61–69**.

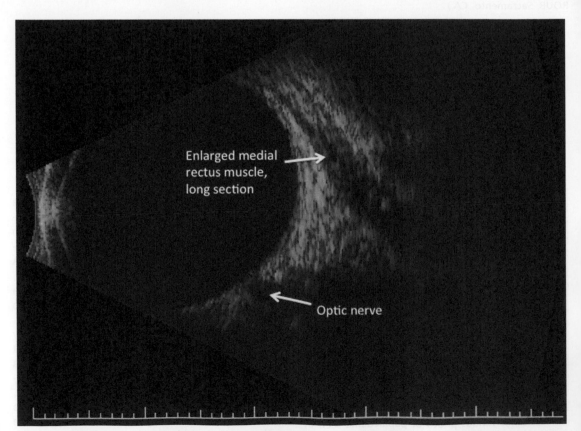

Fig. 59. Longitudinal scan of the nasal meridian with low gain shows optic nerve at the bottom and long section of lower reflective enlarged medial rectus on the top.

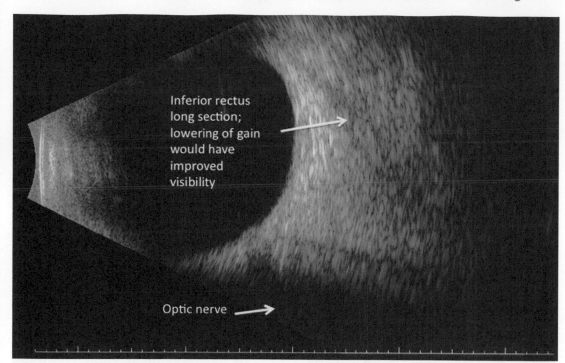

Inferior rectus
long section;
lowering of gain
would have
improved
visibility

Optic nerve

Fig. 60. Longitudinal scan of 6:00 with high gain shows the optic nerve at the bottom and the long section of the lower reflective normal inferior rectus. Part of a posterior vitreous detachment is seen as a thin gray line. Lower gain and higher contrast settings may allow extraocular muscles to be visualized more clearly within orbital fat, but finer echoes such as floaters or the posterior vitreous hyaloid will disappear.

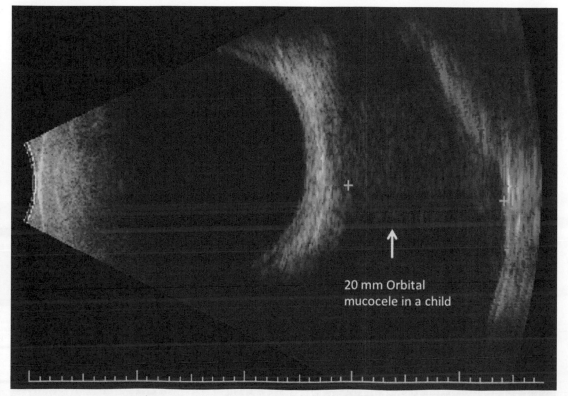

20 mm Orbital
mucocele in a child

Fig. 61. A child with 20-mm low-reflective orbital mucocele in one eye. Fellow eye (**Fig. 62**) shows no lesion, but a dialated orbital vein.

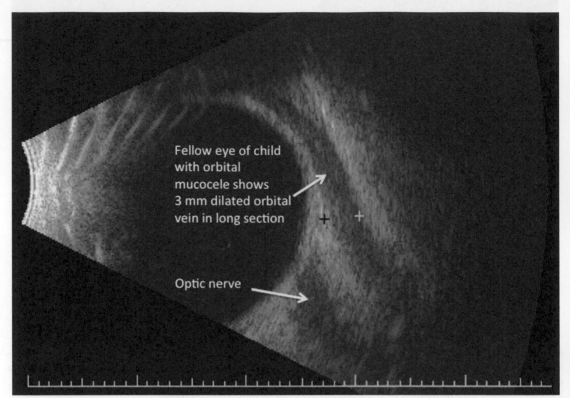

Fig. 62. The fellow eye of the child with mucocele (Fig. 61) shows a 3-mm dilated orbital vein imaged in long section.

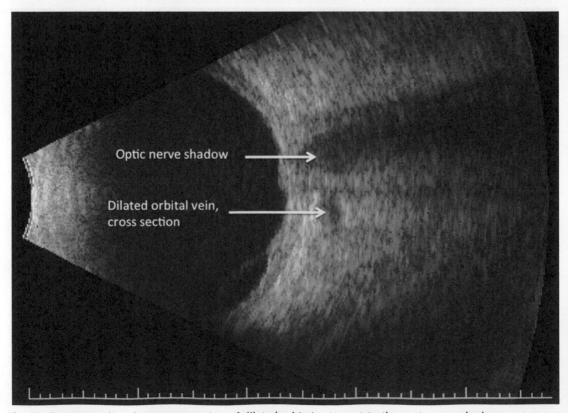

Fig. 63. Transverse view shows cross-section of dilated orbital vein next to the optic nerve shadow.

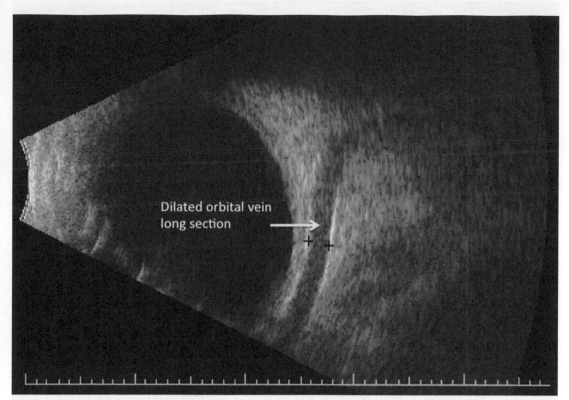

Dilated orbital vein
long section

Fig. 64. Longitudinal scan of the same patient as in **Fig. 63** with dilated orbital vein next to the optic nerve shadow.

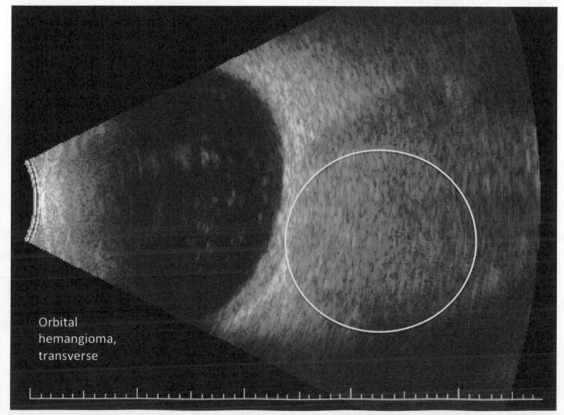

Orbital
hemangioma,
transverse

Fig. 65. Transverse scan of an orbital cavernous hemangioma, one of the most common orbital tumors.[41] Vitreous opacities, often called floaters, are seen at high gain. The tumor is so large that the posterior margin is not visible.

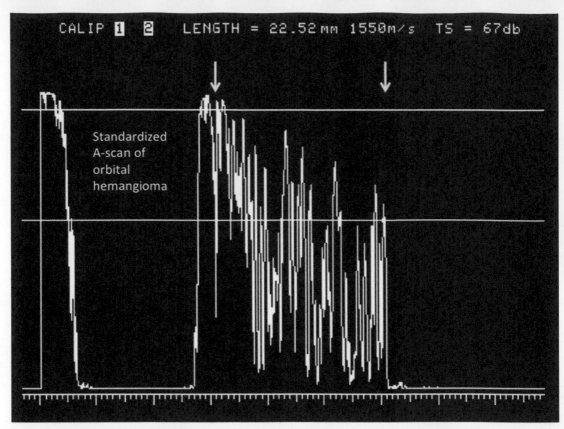

CALIP 1 2   LENGTH = 22.52 mm 1550m/s   TS = 67db

Standardized
A-scan of
orbital
hemangioma

Fig. 66. Standardized diagnostic A-scan of the hemangioma in **Fig. 67** demonstrates classic high internal reflectivity as the A-scan passes through vessel walls and lumen. *Arrows* indicate tumor borders.

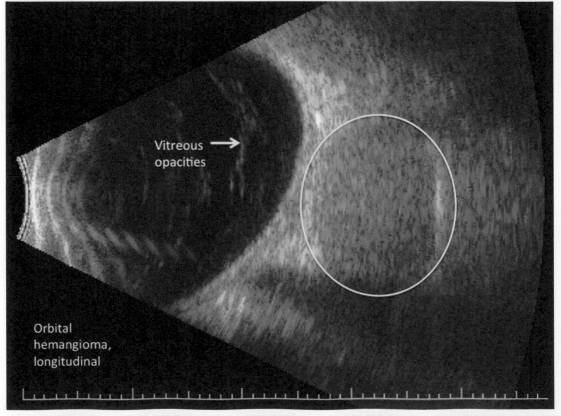

Vitreous →
opacities

Orbital
hemangioma,
longitudinal

Fig. 67. Longitudinal scan of a smaller orbital cavernous hemangioma. Low reflective tumor is indicated by *circle*.

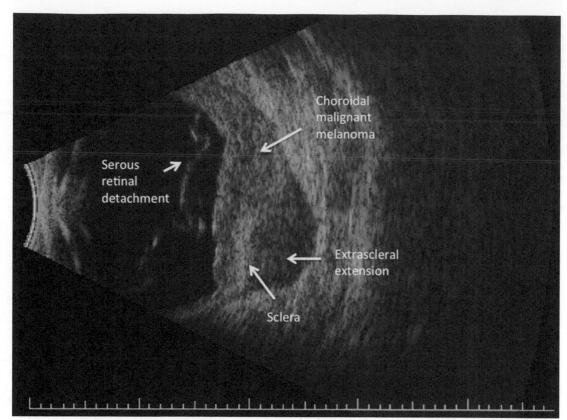

Fig. 68. Extrascleral extension in a metastatic lesion with overlying serous retinal detachment.

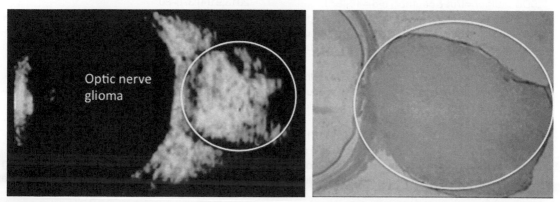

Fig. 69. B-scan image of an optic nerve glioma causing significant enlargement of nerve. On standardized A-scan (not shown), a tall, smooth retinal echo indicates reflection from a smooth surface. Within the lesion, there is a decrease in echo height due to its uniform structure. In contrast, a meningioma's irregular surface displays a jagged surface echo with medium to high internal lesion echoes. On ultrasound, left, and in the pathology section, right, tumor is indicated by circle.

SUMMARY

The basic concepts of ocular and orbital ultrasound were reviewed. This technique is invaluable to measure the eye for placement of intraocular lenses and for cases of an eye with no internal view. Ultrasound has recently gained acceptance for visualizing the anterior segment for narrow angle, iris, ciliary, and lenticular pathologic abnormalities. Ultrasound is excellent for assessing an eye that has no view from a dense cataract and serious retinal and choroidal pathologic abnormalities. Ultrasound is extremely helpful in monitoring pigmented lesions in the eye for growth and malignant conversion. It is helpful in determining if a lesion is benign or malignant. It is the best method to detect optic nerve head drusen. Techniques to image the retrobulbar optic nerve are difficult, but in trained hands, the optic nerve can be evaluated to determine if it is enlarged because of subarachnoid fluid versus infiltration. Scleritis can be detected with the useful T sign. Orbital imaging with ultrasound requires trained hands and can detect pathologic abnormality, including extraocular muscle enlargement as well as anterior orbital lesions; however, in general, CT or MR imaging tends to be a better choice in most of these cases.

REFERENCES

1. Coleman DJ. Reliability of ocular and orbital diagnosis with B-scan ultrasound. 1. Ocular diagnosis. Am J Ophthalmol 1972;73(4):501–16.
2. Ossoinig KC, Bigar F, Kaefring SL. Malignant melanoma of the choroid and ciliary body. A differential diagnosis in clinical echography. Bibl Ophthalmol 1975;83:141–54.
3. Fuller DG, Snyder WB, Hutton WL, et al. Ultrasonographic features of choroidal malignant melanomas. Arch Ophthalmol 1979;97(8):1465–72. Available at: http://www-ncbi-nlm-nih-gov.ezproxyhost.library.tmc.edu/pubmed/?term=Vaiser%20A%5BAuthor%5D&cauthor=true&cauthor_uid=464871.
4. Allemann N, Coleman DJ, Pavlin CJ, et al. Imaging the anterior segment: high-frequency ultrasound and anterior segment OCT. J Ophthalmol 2013; 2013:398715.
5. Velazquez-Martin JP, Krema H, Fulda E, et al. Ultrasound biomicroscopy of the ciliary body in ocular/oculodermal melanocytosis. Am J Ophthalmol 2013;155(4):681–7.
6. Dada T, Mohan S, Bali SJ, et al. Ultrasound biomicroscopic assessment of angle parameters in patients with primary angle closure glaucoma undergoing phacoemulsification. Eur J Ophthalmol 2011;21(5):559–65.
7. Pavlin CJ, Harasiewicz K, Sherar MD, et al. Clinical use of ultrasound biomicroscopy. Ophthalmology 1991;98(3):287–95.
8. Bell NP, Feldman RM, Zou Y, et al. New technology for examining the anterior segment by ultrasonic biomicroscopy. J Cataract Refract Surg 2008;34(1):121–5.
9. Whang WJ, Jung BJ, Oh TH, et al. Comparison of postoperative refractive outcomes: IOLMaster® versus immersion ultrasound. Ophthalmic Surg Lasers Imaging 2012;43(6):496–9.
10. Raymond S, Favilla I, Santamaria L. Comparing ultrasound biometry with partial coherence interferometry for intraocular lens power calculations: a randomized study. Invest Ophthalmol Vis Sci 2009; 50(6):2547–52.
11. Ossoinig KC. Standardized echography: basic principles, clinical applications, and results. Int Ophthalmol Clin 1979;19(4):127–210.
12. Ossoinig KC. Quantitative echography–the basis of tissue differentiation. J Clin Ultrasound 1974;2(1):33–46.
13. Collaborative Ocular Melanoma Study Group, Boldt HC, Byrne SF, Gilson MM, et al. Baseline echographic characteristics of tumors in eyes of patients enrolled in the collaborative ocular melanoma study: COMS report no. 29. Ophthalmology 2008;115(8): 1390–7.
14. Goldberg BB. Gilbert Baum, MD, 1922–2002, a pioneer in ultrasound. J Ultrasound Med 2003;22(6): 660–2.
15. Harrie RP, Kendall CJ. Part II basic principles. In: Clinical ophthalmic echography. 2nd edition. New York: Springer; 2014. p. 47–74.
16. Sadun AA, Green RL, Nobe JR, et al. Papillopathies associated with unusual calcifications in the retrolaminar optic nerve. J Clin Neuroophthalmol 1991; 11(3):175–80 [discussion: 181–2].
17. Sterns GK, Coleman DJ, Ellsworth RM. The ultrasonographic characteristics of retinoblastoma. Am J Ophthalmol 1974;78(4):606–11.
18. Neudorfer M, Ben-Haim MS, Leibovitch I, et al. The efficacy of optic nerve ultrasonography for differentiating papilloedema from pseudopapilloedema in eyes with swollen optic discs. Acta Ophthalmol 2013;91(4):376–80.
19. Carter SB, Pistilli M, Livingston KG, et al. The role of orbital ultrasonography in distinguishing papilledema from pseudopapilledema. Eye 2014;28(12): 1425–30.
20. Flores-Rodríguez P, Gili P, Martín-Ríos MD. Ophthalmic features of optic disc drusen. Ophthalmologica 2012;228(1):59–66.
21. Komur M, Sari A, Okuyaz C. Simultaneous papilledema and optic disc drusen in a child. Pediatr Neurol 2012;46(3):187–8.
22. Kurz-Levin MM, Landau K. A comparison of imaging techniques for diagnosing drusen of the optic nerve head. Arch Ophthalmol 1999;117(8):1045–9.
23. Singh AD, Hayden BC. Glaucoma. In: Ophthalmic ultrasonography. New York: Elsevier Saunders; 2012. p. 95.
24. Merceron S, Geeraerts T. Ocular sonography for the detection of raised intracranial pressure. Expert Rev Ophthalmol 2008;3(5):497–500.
25. Hansen HC, Helmke K. Validation of the optic nerve sheath response to changing cerebrospinal fluid pressure: ultrasound findings during intrathecal infusion tests. J Neurosurg 1997;87(1): 34–40.
26. Helmke K, Hansen HC. Fundamentals of transorbital sonographic evaluation of optic nerve sheath

expansion under intracranial hypertension. I. Experimental study. Pediatr Radiol 1996;26(10):701–5.

27. Rajajee V, Vanaman M, Fletcher JJ, et al. Optic nerve ultrasound for the detection of raised intracranial pressure. Neurocrit Care 2011;15(3):506–15.

28. Kimberly HH, Shah S, Marill K, et al. Correlation of optic nerve sheath diameter with direct measurement of intracranial pressure. Acad Emerg Med 2008;15(2):201–4.

29. Geeraerts T, Launey Y, Martin L, et al. Ultrasonography of the optic nerve sheath may be useful for detecting raised intracranial pressure after severe brain injury. Intensive Care Med 2007;33(10): 1704–11.

30. Bryne SF, Green RL. Ultrasound of the eye and orbit. 2nd edition. St Louis (MO): Mosby; 2002. p. 419–23.

31. Shields JA, Shields C, Scartozzi R. Survey of 1264 patients with orbital tumors and simulating lesions. Ophthalmology 2004;111(5):997–1008.

32. Gans MS, Byrne SF, Glaser JS. Standardized A-scan echography in optic nerve disease. Arch Ophthalmol 1987;105(9):1232–6.

33. de Keizer RJ, de Wolff-Rouendaal D, Bots GT, et al. Optic glioma with intraocular tumor and seeding in a child with neurofibromatosis. Am J Ophthalmol 1989;108(6):717–25.

34. Doro D. Optic neuropathies: diagnostic role of standardized echography. Metab Pediatr Syst Ophthalmol 1990;13(2–4):67–71.

35. Cheung CM, Chee SP. Posterior scleritis in children: clinical features and treatment. Ophthalmology 2012;119(1):59–65.

36. Maggioni F, Ruffatti S, Viaro F, et al. A case of posterior scleritis: differential diagnosis of ocular pain. J Headache Pain 2007;8(2):123–6.

37. Cekić S, Stanković-Babić G. Application of ultrasound in diagnosing and follow-up of endocrine orbitopathy. Med Pregl 2010;63(3–4):241–8.

38. Rabinowitz MP, Carrasco JR. Update on advanced imaging options for thyroid-associated orbitopathy. Saudi J Ophthalmol 2012;26(4):385–92.

39. Dick AD, Nangia V, Atta H. Standardised echography in the differential diagnosis of extraocular muscle enlargement. Eye 1992;6(Pt 6):610–7.

40. Byrne SF, Gendron EK, Glaser JS, et al. Diameter of normal extraocular recti muscles with echography. Am J Ophthalmol 1991;112(6):706–13.

41. Coleman DJ, Silverman RH, Lizzi FL, et al. Orbital diagnosis. In: Ultrasonography of the eye and orbit. 2nd edition. Philadelphia: Lippincott Williams & Wilkins; 2006. p. 154.

Optical Coherence Tomography for the Radiologist

Jade S. Schiffman, MD[a,b], Nimesh B. Patel, OD, PhD[c],
Roberto Alejandro Cruz, MD[a], Rosa A. Tang, MD, MPH, MBA[a,b,*]

KEYWORDS

- Optical coherence tomography • Optic nerve imaging • Macular imaging • Macular volume
- Circumpapillary retinal nerve fiber analysis • Retinal nerve fiber bundle defect • Ganglion cell layer
- Optic nerve swelling • Optic atrophy

KEY POINTS

- Optical Coherence Tomography (OCT) has revolutionized imaging of the retina and optic nerve and has enhanced our ability to diagnose and manage patients.
- OCT of the retina simulates to some degree an anatomic replica of a histological section of the retina treatment of macular degeneration, diabetic macular edema amongst other pathologies.
- OCT of the retina quantitates the thickness of the retinal nerve fiber layer (average retinal nerve fiber analysis), which is adjacent to the optic nerve (known as the circumpapillary retinal nerve fiber layer), and this is an indirect quantitative analysis of one's complement of optic nerve fibers.
- The OCT average retinal nerve fiber analysis is very helpful in following optic nerve pathologies, for example glaucoma, MS, compressive optic neuropathies, however this technique does not distinguish between swollen and normal nerves, therefore, one may be given a false sense that the nerve is normal, when it fact it is swollen, thus missing that there is a reduced complement of retinal nerve fibers.
- The OCT average retinal nerve fiber analysis is a helpful technique in monitoring disc edema over time.
- OCT of the optic nerve gives a morphological view of the optic nerve as well as certain measurements that are helpful to follow over time.

INTRODUCTION

The eye is unique in that through its optics and utilization of devices that use these optics (eg, ophthalmoscope, retinal cameras, optical coherence tomography [OCT]), the neural and vascular tissues of the retina and optic nerve can be assessed by using noninvasive methods, making it ideal for detecting early changes associated with neural diseases. Although most information necessary for diagnosis can be obtained using ophthalmoscopy, imaging technologies with improved transverse and axial resolution are available to aid in the quantification of the morphology of the posterior pole (optic nerve and macula of the retina) yielding information that often is not appreciated solely with ophthalmoscopy. OCT offers good transverse and excellent axial resolution that has revolutionized eye care (**Fig. 1**).

Disclosures: None.
[a] MS Eye CARE, University Eye Institute, UHCO, University of Houston, 4901 Calhoun Street, Houston, TX 77204, USA; [b] The Optic Nerve Center, Neuro-ophthalmology of Texas at the Medical Clinic of Houston, 1701 Sunset Blvd, Houston, TX 77005, USA; [c] UHCO, University of Houston, 4901 Calhoun Street, Houston, TX 77204, USA
* Corresponding author. 2617 C West Holcombe Boulevard #575, Houston, TX 77025.
E-mail address: rtang@neuroeye.com

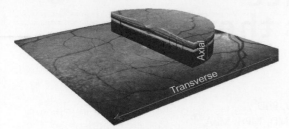

Fig. 1. Transverse versus axial imaging.

The basic principles of OCT technology can be compared with those of ultrasonography, in which the backscatter is used to generate images. In the late 1980s, Fujimoto and colleagues[1] were the pioneers in using light energy to image biological tissues, using femtosecond pulsed lasers to image the cornea with 15 μm resolution. With modification and the use of superluminescent diodes, the technology was then applied to in vivo axial length measures (A-scans) with accuracy of 0.03 mm.[2] However, it was not until 1991 that the first B-scans of human tissue were published using OCT technology.[3] As with ultrasound technology, B-scans are composed of multiple aligned abutting A-scans, used to generate images that now assume a 2-dimensional form similar to the part of the eye imaged.

The first-generation clinical OCT instruments were time domain systems, with scan speeds of up to 400 Hz (A-scans per second) and axial resolution between 7 and 10 μm. However, with advances in technology, most clinical instruments are now spectral/Fourier domain with scan speeds greater than 25,000 Hz and axial resolutions up to 4 μm. The main difference between time domain and spectral domain (SD) systems is the use of a stationary reference arm and spectrometer system that results in faster, higher resolution images with the latter. Using multimodal imaging eye tracking is also available that aids in minimizing eye movement artifact and allows for accurate follow-up scan registration. Overall, with these scan speeds, 3-dimensional volume data of the anterior segment, optic nerve head, and macula regions (Fig. 2) provide important information on the health of the eye. This article describes the current use of posterior segment imaging by OCT technology for the diagnosis and management of neuro-ophthalmic conditions.

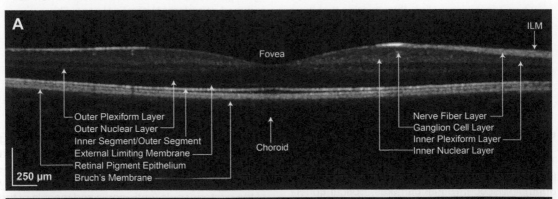

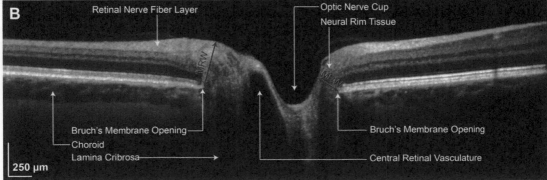

Fig. 2. (A) Retinal OCT centered on the fovea shows the foveal depression and multiple retinal layers seen (see Fig. 3A to see where this section is from). (B) Optic nerve OCT shows a cross-section (see Fig. 3C to see where this section is from).

NORMAL ANATOMY THROUGH THE MACULA AND OPTIC NERVE WITH OPTICAL COHERENCE TOMOGRAPHY

Most commonly OCT is used to image the posterior pole. The posterior pole includes the macula (which subserves 8° of central vision) and the optic nerve. One may choose between 2 types of OCT scans: (1) retinal OCT and (2) optic nerve OCT.

1. The retinal OCT typically can be centered on 2 areas: (a) the fovea and (b) the optic nerve with scans of the peripapillary retina.
    a. The fovea (see **Fig. 2**A; **Fig. 3**A, B).When the retinal OCT is centered on the fovea, it yields a cross-section of the fovea (thinnest point of the retina that has the best central vision and accounts for 20/20 or better vision) and the surrounding retina with a typical scan width of 20°. One concentrates on all

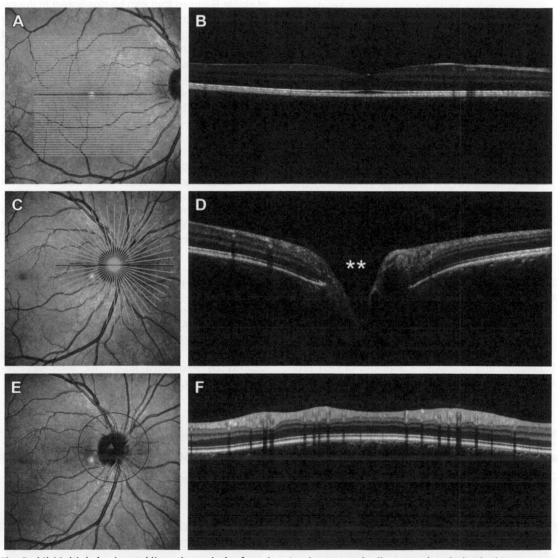

Fig. 3. (A) Multiple horizontal lines through the foveal region (raster scan), all can produce individual B-scans per raster as shown in (B), which is a horizontal raster directly though the center of the fovea (*red line* in 3A). (C) Multiple radial lines through the optic nerve show the morphology of the nerve at each radial line. (D) A radial line horizontally through the optic nerve shows the morphology through that particular section of the optic nerve. *Double asterisk* represents the optic cup depression. (E) The red circle indicates the area in which a 360° cross-section is taken at the retina adjacent to the optic nerve (peripapillary retina). See Fig. 6A–C to see how this protocol translates into the retinal nerve fiber protocol. (F) The image shows the cross-section of peripapillary retina to yield a 360° picture portrayed in a linear fashion, with the far left and far right being the temporal aspect.

the retinal layers in this mode (see **Fig. 2A**). The signal strength along each OCT A-scan depends on tissue reflectivity and the corresponding interference pattern from that location. Resulting B-scans from this technology have a layered appearance representing that of retinal layers. However, the elements of each retinal layer are not homogenous and are represented as intensity changes in OCT scans. Hence, there are additional intensity bands of morphologic information in OCT scans. For accurate correspondence to histology, several studies in various species have reported using both time domain and SD OCT systems. In general, there is good agreement between these studies with similar identification of retinal and optic nerve head features.[4–9]

b. The optic nerve with scans of the peripapillary retina (see **Figs. 3E, F and 6**). The most common scan protocol used to evaluate the health of the optic nerve is a 12° diameter circumpapillary scan that is used to quantify the retinal nerve fiber layer thickness.

2. The optic nerve OCT (see **Figs. 2B and 3C, D**) is centered to take cross-sections of the optic nerve head. The cross-sectional scan shows the morphology of the optic nerve (flat, elevated, or recessed) and the optic cup (see **Fig. 3D**; double asterisk).

Fig. 3 is a comparison of the various protocols used to image the macula (retina) and optic nerve.

QUALITATIVE VERSUS QUANTITATIVE ANALYSIS OF MACULA AND OPTIC NERVE

Qualitative and quantitative analyses of OCT provide useful information in the clinical setting for accurate diagnosis and management of patients. Qualitative scans (see **Figs. 2 and 3; Fig. 4**) provide visualization of the anatomy without distinct numbers or thickness. Quantitative scans provide measurements that make distinction between normal findings and diseases and assist in determining if there are any changes over time.

QUALITATIVE SCANS

Most OCT devices allow for custom scan capture of single B-scans that can be positioned in the regions of interest with specified lengths and tilt. For example, a single line scan through the foveal pit (see **Fig. 2**), with averaging, is often used to determine inner versus outer retinal conditions. In addition, horizontal and vertical scans through the center of the optic nerve head are shown to be beneficial in determining optic nerve head and circumpapillary region changes (see **Fig. 3**).

Line scans can be acquired with or without enhanced depth imaging. To achieve this, instruments have incorporated enhanced depth imaging into their protocol to decrease the time delay of deeper structures with the zero reference.[10] **Fig. 4** shows enhancement in the depths to the choroid compared with **Fig. 2** which does not show depth enhancement.

QUANTITATIVE SCANS
Retina

The macula thickness (see **Fig. 2**) can be quantified in micrometers in various areas. **Fig. 5** shows an example of a patient with macula thickening caused by excessive fluid. The thickness decreases after fluid resorption.

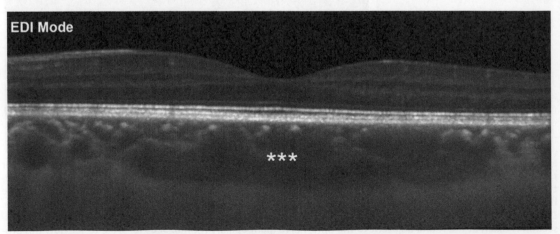

Fig. 4. Enhanced depth imaging of macula OCT shows the detail of deeper structures especially the choroid (*triple asterisk*).

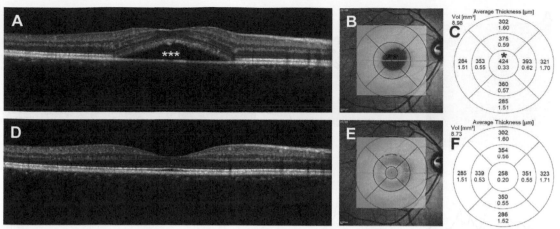

Fig. 5. An example of a serous retinal detachment before resolution (*A–C*) and after resolution (*D–F*). This is a comparison of qualitative imaging on the left (*A* and *D*) and quantitative imaging on the right (*B, C, E,* and *F*). In this case, (*A*) shows serous fluid (black in the middle and deep under the macula [*triple asterisk*]) which is seen as red and yellow (*thickening double asterisk*) in semiquantitative image (*double asterisk* [*B*]), and the exact thickness of 424 μm in the center of the macula (*asterisk* in [*C*]). [*D*] image is obtained after the fluid resolved, the black area in between the retinal layers is no longer visualized, and [*E*] shows the color green in the center, which is thinner and now is in normal range. Note the number for the central thickness lessened from 424 μm to 258 μm.

Optic Nerve

The optic nerve images, as illustrated in **Fig. 3**C–D, have limited automated quantification that includes the cup-to-disc ratio and parameters of the neural rim tissue. Many clinicians will use instrument-based calipers to determine additional parameters including the height and width of the neural rim tissue and the elevation of the Bruch's membrane opening that are monitored in conditions resulting in disc edema.[11] Similarly, the rim tissue at the optic nerve head can be monitored for small changes through measures of the minimum rim width (MRW; see **Fig. 2**B).[12] However the circumpapillary retinal nerve fiber analysis below is an indirect way to quantitatively measure the optic disc swelling and optic atrophy.

CIRCUMPAPILLARY RETINAL NERVE FIBER LAYER ANALYSIS

The optic nerve can appear normal, swollen, or atrophic on OCT. The circumpapillary retinal nerve fiber layer (RNFL) represents the axons of the optic nerve that are adjacent to the optic disc before their entering the nerve. These can indirectly provide useful information about the state of the optic nerve. If the optic nerve is swollen, the RNFL analysis will show thickening, and if the optic nerve is atrophic, the RNFL analysis will show thinning. It may take time for the optic nerve fibers to reflect the damage that occurs acutely; therefore, normal-appearing optic nerve on OCT in the acute phase does not entirely exclude pathologies.

The OCT protocol that measures the thickness of the optic nerve axons (in a healthy eye) can be used as an indirect measurement and determination of optic nerve swelling or atrophy. This is the concept of the circumpapillary retinal nerve fiber layer analysis as shown in **Fig. 6** (see **Fig. 6**A–C, qualitative view, and D–F, quantitative analysis).

The mainstay for the retinal ganglion cell associated nerve fiber layer analysis is a 12° diameter circular scan centered on the optic nerve head (see **Fig. 6**A, green circle) that are shown to have good repeatability.[13–15] This scan shows a nominal circumference of 10.9 mm in the emmetropic eye and samples most of the retinal ganglion cell axons entering the optic nerve. To quantify the RNFL, an instrument-based segmentation algorithm identifies the inner limiting membrane and the junction between the nerve fiber layer and ganglion cell layer. RNFL thickness is traditionally reported as a TSNIT plot (A-scan thickness covering the temporal, superior, nasal, inferior, and back to temporal aspects in order). **Fig. 6**C and D show the view in which the extreme left and right parts of the diagram represent the temporal aspect of the optic nerve (C is qualitative view and D–F is quantitative view).

The retinal ganglion cells are the neurons, which receive the input from the deeper retina (photoreceptors), and they deliver the visual information to the brain. The retinal ganglion cell axons form the retinal nerve fiber layer surrounding the optic disc. These axons migrate toward the optic nerve and bend nearly 90° to enter the nerve. The axons and the supporting cells/tissues (glia,

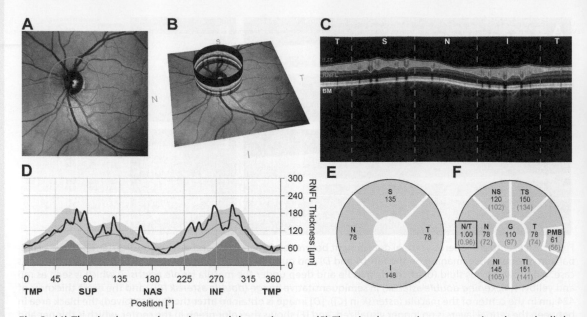

Fig. 6. (A) The circular scan (green) around the optic nerve. (B) The circular scan is a cross-section through all the layers of the retina. (C) Cross-sectional scan presented in a horizontal diagram in which the extreme ends of the diagram represent the temporal retinal nerve fiber. (D) The quantification of the thickness of the retinal ganglion cell axons (this is produced by a segmentation method to analyze the retinal ganglion cell axons only), where white would be above normal, green is within normal range, yellow is borderline, and red is clearly reduced compared with normal. (E) Average measurement in micrometers of the 4 quadrants. (F) More detailed measurements in 6 sections.

oligodendrocytes, myelin, and blood vessels) form the optic nerve. Most of the optic nerve fibers synapse in the lateral geniculate body. Pathologies that affect the optic nerve before the lateral geniculate body will result in atrophy of the retinal nerve fiber layer. Usually, but not always (eg, with transsynaptic degeneration), pathologies that affect the visual pathway beyond the lateral geniculate body (eg, optic radiations and the occipital cortex) do not result in retinal nerve fiber changes, unless present at birth or very longstanding.

Most commonly, as previously stated, a normal average retinal nerve fiber layer (ARNFL) is associated with a normal complement of healthy optic nerve fibers. A normal ARNFL number is approximately 100, and as one ages this number reduces.[16–19] A normal young person may have measurements of 80 to 120. However, a normal examination is not equal to a normal average nerve fiber, as there are several factors that determine if the retinal nerve fiber is normal for a particular person, to include history, prior OCTs, prior optic nerve edema, fundoscopic examination findings, congenital variations, right and left comparisons, and reliability of the study with signal strength.

Because the OCT comes with software that has age-matched normative data regarding the ARNFL, it automatically displays a color-coded analysis. The color code is displayed in a TSNIT plot (see Fig. 6D;

Fig. 7A), which is a graphic representation of the neuroretinal rim and RNFL thickness in micrometers that positions the obtained measurements of the right and left eye among the average normal (green), borderline (yellow), decreased (red), or increased (white) thickness subsets.

Whereas Figs. 6 and 7 show a normal nerve fiber layer, Fig. 8 shows reduced nerve fiber layer in the left eye, which is nonspecific. However, the optic nerve would be expected to be atrophic on the left side, as the average RNFL thickness is 62. Almost any cause of the optic neuropathy can result in a reduced retinal nerve fiber layer (including glaucoma, ischemia, optic neuritis, and infiltrative and compressive lesions). However, in this case the optic cups are large, left greater than right, suggesting the cause of the optic neuropathy in this case may be glaucoma of the left side. Glaucoma on the left side is worse than that on the right side, as there is significant retinal nerve fiber loss on the left. The right side appears to have early loss of the nerve fiber superior temporally (see Fig. 8, in gray RNFL deviation map in the region marked by double asterisk).

Although RNFL thickness measures are fairly robust, several factors including scan quality, scan centration, and refractive status, need to be considered when assessing. For the most reliable measures, signal strength should be within the

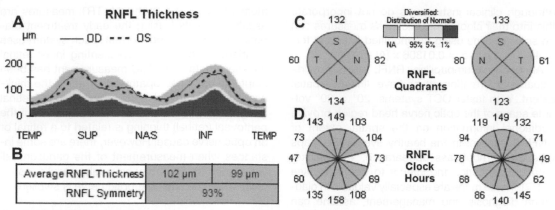

Fig. 7. (A) The TSNIT plot in a normal person. The *continuous line* represents the right eye and the *dashed line* represents the left eye. The nerve fiber layer is totally normal in both eyes (as *lines* are in the green zone). (B) Normal average retinal nerve fiber layer analysis of 102 on the right and 99 on the left. (C) The quadrants of the optic nerve have normal thickness (*green*). (D) The RNFL per clock hour is also normal (*green*) except for the nasal clock hours, which appear mildly thickened (*white*).

range suggested by the instrument manufacturer, which is typically in the upper 70th percentile.[20–22] The effect of suboptimal scan centration, and alignment to the foveal axis is mostly on the distribution of thickness along the TSNIT plot, resulting in measures outside normal limits on sector and quadrant analysis.[23–25] A-scans are acquired through the optics of the eye; ocular magnification needs to be taken into account for scans in which thickness measures change significantly with distance from the optic nerve head rim margin. Specifically, in longer and myopic eyes, the scan path falls further from the rim margin where the nerve fiber thickness measures are less.[26–28]

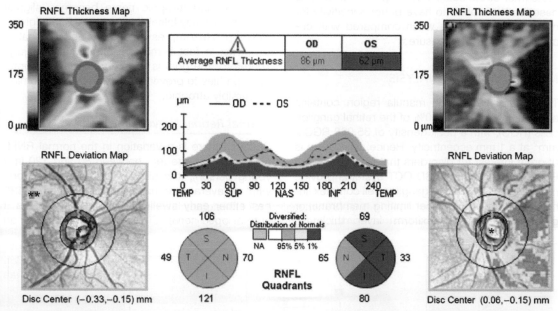

Fig. 8. The right eye has normal retinal nerve fiber layer, although there are a few spots temporally of borderline depression (*double asterisk*). However, the left eye has almost all of the fibers in the red zone except for the nasal region (*green*). The right eye has an average nerve fiber layer thickness of 86, whereas the left eye is depressed with an average nerve fiber layer of 62. The inner red circle of the optic nerve estimates the optic cup, and the left optic cup (*asterisk*) appears to be larger than the right optic cup (*asterisk*). Note that the retinal nerve fiber thickness map represents a semiquantitative map showing the thickness of the nerve fiber layer. Note that the left eye has less thickness semiquantitatively than the right. In this map, yellow and red are thicker than blue. The deviation maps illustrate regions that have less nerve fiber thickness compared with age-matched controls. The TSNIT plot and quadrant plots show the nerve fiber thickness in the circular region, providing additional quantification and probability information.

Although clinical instruments do not incorporate this into their algorithms, thickness measures can be scaled offline using the modified Littmann formula (t = q.p.s, q = 0.01306 x [AL-0.18]).[29]

Although circumpapillary RNFL scans provide valuable information, they have limited spatial extent. With faster OCT systems, 20° × 20° volume scans of the optic nerve head region provide additional information on the spatial extent of RNFL thickness. In the healthy eye, RNFL maps take on an hourglass appearance, with thicker measures superior and inferior to the nerve (see Fig. 7). These maps are especially valuable in glaucoma diagnosis and management, as one can visualize the bundle defect in the region scanned. In fact, RNFL maps are found to be more sensitive than circumpapillary TSNIT analysis in the detection of glaucomatous defects.[30]

Similar to RNFL analysis from volume scans, total retinal thickness (TRT) maps centered on the optic nerve can be used for identifying disease and monitoring disease progression. However, there is a difference in analysis, in that for TRT, measures are often based on early treatment diabetic retinopathy study maps (see Fig. 7). Specifically, average thickness measures are reported for each quadrant for annuli 1, 3, and 5 mm from the center of the scan. TRT (Fig. 9) measures as described are found to have better sensitivity for detecting disc edema when compared with circumpapillary RNFL measures.[31–33]

MACULA VOLUME ANALYSIS

The central 20° of the macula region contains approximately 30% to 40% of the retinal ganglion cells (RGC), with a peak density of 35,000 RGCs/mm^2 at a 1 mm eccentricity. Hence, this region is of great interest for disorders that result in loss of RGCs. Currently, most SD OCT systems provide measures for TRT, either ganglion cell complex (inner plexiform layer to inner limiting membrane) or ganglion cell/inner plexiform layer thickness

measures (Fig. 10). Although TRT measures are usually presented using the early treatment diabetic retinopathy study format, each system uses a different method for representing inner retinal thickness data. The RGC measurement has been helpful in optic neuropathies that affect the thickness of the perifoveal retina by reducing the retinal ganglion cell layer. So there is a way to tell if the perifoveal (retinal) thinning is related to a retinal or an optic nerve cause. However, there are some instances when measurement of the ganglion cell layer (see Fig. 10E) may have false results, especially when the adjacent optic nerve is swollen.

OPTIC NERVE PATHOLOGIES

Optic nerve pathologies are associated with the following circumpapillary retinal nerve fiber layer (RNFL) patterns: (1) normal RNFL, (2) decreased RNFL, and (3) increased RNFL. Acute pathologies can initially have increased RNFL because of acute swelling, and, over time, depending on the cause of the insult, the nerve may return to normal RNFL analysis or the nerve may evolve into optic atrophy, in which case the RNFL will become decreased. Currently we do not have any effective treatment to increase RNFL once the RNFL is lost, suggesting this is a permanent state; however, if a damaged and atrophic nerve becomes slightly swollen, this may falsely increase the RNFL, giving a false-positive impression that the nerve is healthier, when in fact it may be undergoing reinjury. Therefore, the goal is to intervene early in optic neuropathies to prevent the nerve from becoming irreversibly atrophic.

Normal Retinal Nerve Fiber Layer

Because there is a variation in the normal RNFL depending on age (eg, between 80 and 120 in a young person), it is difficult to know if someone with an average retinal nerve fiber layer of 120 has either early swelling or if this represents a normal optic nerve. Similarly, if someone has an

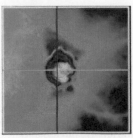
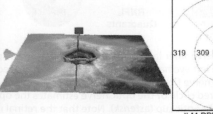
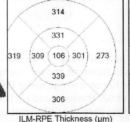
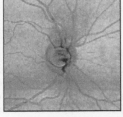

ILM-RPE Thickness (μm)

Fig. 9. A TRT map around the optic nerve measures the total thickness of the peripapillary region without segmentation strategies, and in some instances this may even be more sensitive than the peripapillary nerve fiber layer in detecting disc edema.

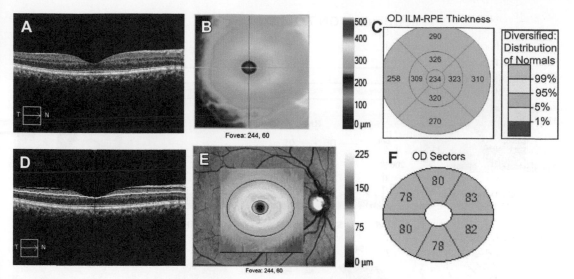

Fig. 10. The perifoveal total retinal thickness (A–C) and ganglion cell inner plexiform layer thickness measured between the yellow and purple lines (D–F), all in the normal range in this case.

average RNFL of 82, although in the normal range, this does not mean it is normal for this patient, as this number may actually be reduced for this particular patient. For example, if this individual had a prior OCT that showed an ARNFL of 112 when there were no symptoms or signs, this would suggest that the current ARNFL of 82 is the result of a substantial loss of retinal nerve fiber by about 30 μm. Also if someone has a normal retinal nerve fiber value of 87, and they now have an average RNFL value of 113, this might suggest there is

likely swelling. These statements are true only if the tests have been taken accurately each time on the same unit.

Several pathologies affecting the optic nerve may cause blindness at onset, and the RNFL may be normal initially (see **Fig. 7**), and only later the nerve undergoes atrophy (**Figs. 11** and **12** OD and **Fig. 13** OU). Depending on the insult, the thinning of the nerve fiber layer can occur in weeks to months. So although having a normal ARNFL analysis is usually a good indicator of a healthy

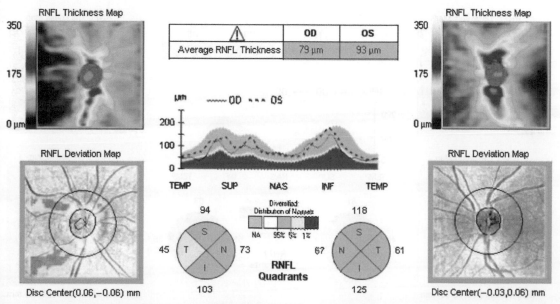

Fig. 11. The right optic nerve is slightly swollen by the gray image, but the nerve fiber layer is slightly reduced.

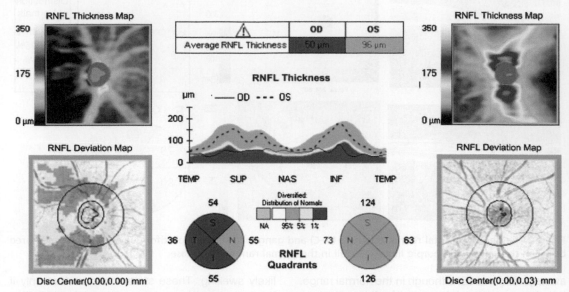

Retrobulbar ON 7/1/2014

Fig. 12. The right optic nerve is no longer swollen (*gray view*), but the nerve fiber layer is extremely atrophic and has become more depressed than it was (50 and 79) in **Fig. 11**, and the sectors are now all red except nasally.

optic nerve, it does not rule out a serious optic nerve condition in evolution in this patient.

Decreased Retinal Nerve Fiber Layer

Many conditions cause decreased nerve fiber layer, and the most common is glaucoma.

Glaucoma is often a progressive disease that is related usually, but not always, to increased intra-ocular pressure, and there is progressive loss of nerve fiber and increase in the optic nerve cupping leading eventually to visual field loss and if not treated successfully can lead to blindness. Neuro-radiologists may not see any pathologic conditions

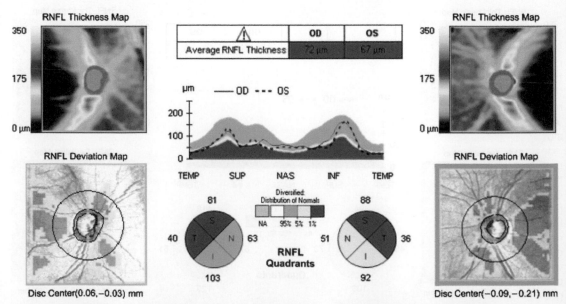

Pituitary tumor

Fig. 13. Bilateral nerve fiber loss owing to a pituitary adenoma with chiasmal compression.

on neuroimaging except that the nerve may become thin on an orbital computed tomography/MR imaging.

The standard clinical OCT scans for glaucoma analysis have been the 12° circumpapillary scan (see **Fig. 6A**).[34] Based on these scans, both trend-based and event-based analyses are used for determining progression.[30] However, measures at the optic nerve head of the neural rim tissue, including the MRW (see **Fig. 2**B), are recently found to have equal or greater sensitivity for detecting glaucoma.[12,35] In addition, analysis of the inner retina in the macula region is shown to be beneficial for disease diagnosis.[36,37] Hence, clinically, both macula inner retinal analysis and optical nerve head (ONH)/RNFL analyses are often used to assess patients at initial presentation and at follow-up visits. When the glaucoma is severe, there is a point that the RNFL analysis is too depressed that it does not really provide definitive information with regard to the progression of the disease. Most optic nerve pathologies, regardless of treatment, may result in a decrease in the normal complement of retinal nerve fibers and manifest as a decrease in the average RNFL. Some optic neuropathies start with normal RNFL and only over time will the nerve become atrophic and show reduced nerve fiber layer. Optic neuritis may be classified into 2 types. In the anterior type (papillitis) the optic nerve is swollen initially and vision is decreased, and over time the optic nerve may become atrophic. In the other type, retrobulbar optic neuritis, the nerve is normal appearing initially on fundoscopic examination and then may become atrophic. **Fig. 11** shows a patient with multiple sclerosis (MS) and right-sided optic neuritis resulting in a reduced RNFL (79). Later the patient experienced another attack of right-sided optic neuritis in previously atrophic optic nerve. So the RNFL is reduced on the right but the nerve is visibly swollen (papillitis) as seen in the gray picture. **Fig. 12** shows there is further reduction of the RNFL after nearly a year, a residual of multiple attacks of optic neuritis on the right side.

In demyelinating diseases that affect the visual pathway, a relationship between contrast sensitivity loss and RNFL thickness measured using circumpapillary scans has been reported.[38,39] The pattern of RNFL loss can be global or greater in the temporal quadrant. Although the loss in neuronal tissue is greatest on the side with clinically symptomatic optic neuritis, MS patients without optic neuritis also have reported decreases in RNFL thickness.[40,41] This finding suggests that there are attacks of clinically silent optic neuritis or there is a progressive RFNL

degeneration over time. Changes in inner retinal thickness of the macula region have also been reported in patients followed up with longitudinally, illustrating the importance of RGC analysis for progression analysis in this patient group.[42,43] In fact, when measured using contrast sensitivity, acuity is better correlated to macula inner retinal thickness (ganglion cell/inner plexiform layer) measures than with circumpapillary RNFL thickness.[43]

In the assessment of MS patients, a qualitative assessment of the retinal anatomy can provide useful information. Reviewing the retinal total thickness analysis is also helpful in patients with MS. This is because one of the drugs that is used in treatment of MS (Gilenya or Fingolimod) can cause cystoid macula edema. Further it has been shown very rarely that a microcystic macular edema and inner nuclear layer thickening, may occur in patients with optic neuritis and thought to be due to an inflammatory or degenerative process.[44]

Just as in MS, patients with optic neuritis from neuromyelitis optica can start out with normal nerve fiber layer and then it lessens over time. In this disease, it occurs quicker than in MS, and the nerve fiber layer is usually more depressed.

Optic atrophy is seen in many conditions resulting in the OCT reflecting thinning of the nerve fiber layer. Glaucoma and MS were discussed here, but optic neuropathies can be caused by a variety of conditions such as optic nerve compressive lesions in the orbit (eg, meningioma, glioma) and parasellar region (eg, pituitary adenoma, craniopharyngioma, aneurysms, meningioma) affecting the visual pathway anterior to the lateral geniculate body. Other optic nerve conditions including infiltrative processes (infectious, granulomatous diseases), ischemia (ischemic optic neuropathy), and inflammatory conditions (optic neuritis) may result in retinal nerve fiber thinning. However, some of these conditions may cause thickening (see later discussion) at the beginning of the insult, then subsequent thinning of the nerve fibers evolves. Sometimes compressive optic neuropathies result in vision loss, but the nerve fiber layer seems normal, and this often helps the neurosurgeon know if there will be recovery of vision after surgery. An example of a compressive optic neuropathy caused by a pituitary adenoma is shown in **Fig. 13**. In this case, there is significant loss of nerve fiber layer; therefore, recovery of vision is less likely after surgery than if this patient had normal retinal nerve fiber preoperatively. However, the patient still may show improvement in vision and visual field testing after surgery but may not be expected to fully recover.

Increased Retinal Nerve Fiber Layer

Generally, increased RNFL usually means there is swelling of the axons rather than more axons than normal. Because the variation of normal nerve fiber layer is considerable, it is often difficult to be certain by using OCT alone if the optic nerve is swollen.

Conditions causing bilateral optic nerve swelling include any causes of increased intracranial pressure (ICP) (eg, brain tumors, hydrocephalus, cerebral venous thrombosis, meningitis, idiopathic intracranial hypertension). If the patient has increased ICP and bilateral optic disc swelling, this represents papilledema. Papilledema typically does not cause vision loss at the beginning; however, if left untreated, in certain cases, progressive vision loss and complete blindness may occur.

OCT has been valuable in assessing disc edema and response to treatment. Initial studies for evaluating disc edema were centered on RNFL analysis using circumpapillary scans, in which total retinal and RNFL thickness were shown to have good correspondence to edema graded on the Frisen scale.[45,46] However, as the circumpapillary scan samples tissue at a distance from the ONH rim margin, recent studies have focused on using volume OCT data to determine changes within and in the adjacent tissues of the optic nerve. Subsequently, total retinal thickness measured at the

ONH is found to be sensitive in detecting subclinical changes.[31–33]

When disc edema is secondary to elevated ICP, quantitative or qualitative assessment of the retinal pigment epithelium angle can be used to assess changes to treatment.[11,47] Specifically, as ICP decreases, there is downward shift in the optic nerve head when compared with the circumpapillary tissue.

RNFL thickness measures are often used as a surrogate for the ganglion cell content in the eye. However, with disc edema, these measures are erroneous. To assess the damage of RGC axons passing through the neural canal, the inner retina of the macula region is often used. This measure also provides a rate of loss if present and potential for vision to return.

Fig. 14 shows an example of a patient with bilateral papilledema. This patient has idiopathic intracranial hypertension (eg, pseudotumor cerebri), but any cause of raised ICP can produce this finding. The patient improved after treatment with weight loss and Diamox. Fig. 15 shows the OCT of the same patient after the papilledema resolved.

Some optic neuropathies may initially present with optic disc swelling (resulting in increased ARNFL) but may develop optic atrophy if the treatment fails. Figs. 16 and 17 show a case of a patient who had anterior ischemic optic neuropathy. In

PAPILLEDEMA

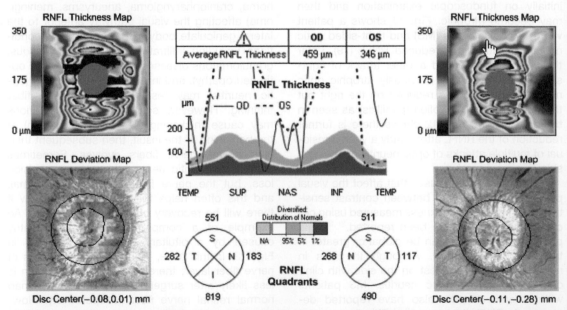

Fig. 14. The right eye average RNFL thickness is 459, whereas the left is 346, which are elevated. All the RNFL quadrants are in the white zone indicating that they are thicker than normal. There is massive disc edema shown in gray photos compared with Fig. 15, when the edema resolved.

RESOLVED PAPILLEDEMA

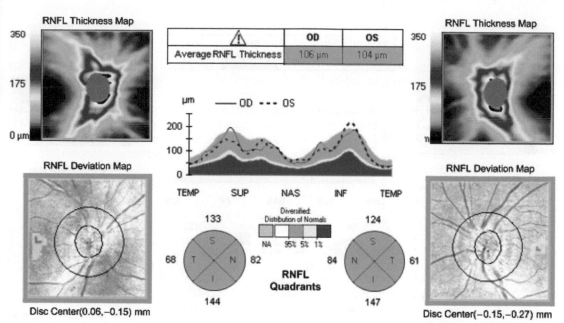

Fig. 15. The right eye average RNFL thickness is 106 (decreased from 459 in **Fig. 14**), whereas the left eye average RNFL thickness is 104 (decreased from 346 in **Fig. 14**). All of the RNFL quadrants are in the green zone, indicating that the thickness is within the normal range. The optic discs in gray photos are unremarkable showing resolution of papilledema. In this case, the patient did not subsequently have disc atrophy, as the insult was corrected rapidly.

NA-AION

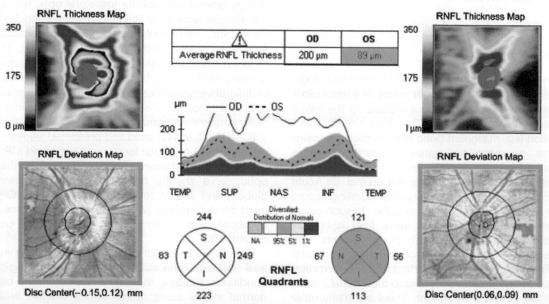

Fig. 16. Swollen right optic nerve caused by anterior ischemic optic neuropathy.

NA-AION

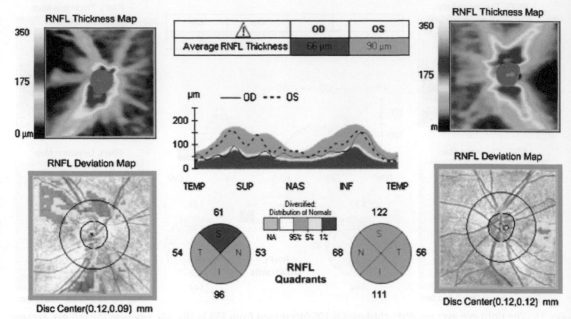

Fig. 17. Optic nerve that was swollen in Fig. 16, has now become atrophic.

Fig. 16, the patient presented with acute vision and visual field loss in the right eye with swollen right optic nerve. Because there was no successful treatment, the patient continued having vision and visual field loss. Fig. 17 shows that the nerve became atrophic and developed irreversible loss of retinal nerve fibers.

PITFALLS OF WHAT APPEARS TO BE A NORMAL AVERAGE RETINAL NERVE FIBER LAYER

The RNFL may appear normal in a few pathologic conditions. (1) In the acute phase of a retrobulbar process, it may take 1 to 4 months for the retinal nerve fiber to be thinned. Therefore, a serious condition (eg, malignant optic chiasm glioma or bilateral neuromyelitis optica) causing blindness cannot be completely ruled out when results of the retinal nerve fiber layer are normal. (2) Acute on top of chronic disease is when swelling occurs in a nerve that is partially atrophic. In such cases the average peripapillary nerve fiber layer may appear falsely normal. (3) Some patients with very high ICP may have normal RNFL. Therefore, clinical correlation is important for OCT interpretation for each patient leading to meaningful impact to the patient's treatment. There are many other pitfalls that we do not address in this article.

BRIEF SUMMARY OF HOW TO USE THE OPTICAL COHERENCE TOMOGRAPHY TO CORRELATE WITH NEUROIMAGING

If the RNFL is reduced, radiologists should look for conditions causing optic nerve atrophy. If only one nerve has reduced RNFL (unilateral optic nerve atrophy), one should look for ipsilateral optic nerve pathologies anterior to the chiasm (ie, intraocular, intraorbital, intracanalicular, and prechiasmatic segments of the optic nerve). If the RNFL is reduced bilaterally, one should look for bilateral orbital conditions (eg, bilateral optic nerve gliomas or infiltrative/compressive lesions) or intracranial optic nerve conditions (eg, tuberculum meningioma, pituitary adenoma).

If the RNFL is thickened and presumed swollen, radiologists should look for signs of increased ICP, which include increased cerebrospinal fluid in the optic nerve sheath, flattening of the posterior globes, and empty sella. The cause of the ICP must be determined (eg, intracranial neoplasms, hydrocephalus, hemorrhage, venous sinus thrombosis).

If the RNFL is normal but the patient is having visual problems, one still has to look for pathologic conditions, realizing that RNFL thickness can be normal in the acute phase of the disease and may eventually become reduced over time.

FUTURE CONSIDERATIONS

The introduction of OCT to clinical practice has enhanced patient care. There have been significant advancements in OCT, and the future instruments will have added features of (1) improved speed and resolution, (2) depth of imaging, and (3) ability for Doppler blood flow imaging. These devices will provide increased flexibility, ability to image from the front to the back of the eye seamlessly, and more accurate quantitative analysis.

REFERENCES

1. Fujimoto JG, De Silvestri S, Ippen EP, et al. Femto-second optical ranging in biological systems. Opt Lett 1986;11(3):150.
2. Fercher AF, Mengedoht K, Werner W. Eye-length measurement by interferometry with partially coherent light. Opt Lett 1988;13(3):186–8.
3. Huang D, Swanson EA, Lin CP, et al. Optical coherence tomography. Science 1991;254(5035):1178–81.
4. Huang Y, Cideciyan AV, Papastergiou GI, et al. Relation of optical coherence tomography to micro-anatomy in normal . and rd chickens. Invest Ophthalmol Vis Sci 1998;39(12):2405–16.
5. Abbott CJ, McBrien NA, Grünert U, et al. Relationship of the optical coherence tomography signal to underlying retinal histology in the tree shrew (Tupaia belangeri). Invest Ophthalmol Vis Sci 2009;50(1):414–23.
6. Anger EM, Unterhuber A, Hermann B, et al. Ultra-high resolution optical coherence tomography of the monkey fovea. Identification of retinal sublayers by correlation with semithin histology sections. Exp Eye Res 2004;78(6):1117–25.
7. Gloesmann M, Hermann B, Schubert C, et al. Histologic correlation of pig retina radial stratification with ultrahigh-resolution optical coherence tomography. Invest Ophthalmol Vis Sci 2003;44(4):1696–703.
8. Strouthidis NG, Yang H, Downs JC, et al. Comparison of clinical and three-dimensional histomorphometric optic disc margin anatomy. Invest Ophthalmol Vis Sci 2009;50(5):2165–74.
9. Strouthidis NG, Yang H, Fortune B, et al. Detection of optic nerve head neural canal opening within histomorphometric and spectral domain optical coherence tomography data sets. Invest Ophthalmol Vis Sci 2009;50(1):214–23.
10. Spaide RF, Koizumi H, Pozzoni MC. Enhanced depth imaging spectral-domain optical coherence tomography. Am J Ophthalmol 2008;146(4):496–500.
11. Kupersmith MJ, Sibony P, Mandel G, et al. Optical coherence tomography of the swollen optic nerve head: deformation of the peripapillary retinal pigment epithelium layer in papilledema. Invest Ophthalmol Vis Sci 2011;52(9):6558–64.
12. Chauhan BC, O'Leary N, Almobarak FA, et al. Enhanced detection of open-angle glaucoma with an anatomically accurate optical coherence tomography-derived neuroretinal rim parameter. Ophthalmology 2013;120(3):535–43.
13. Schuman JS, Hee MR, Puliafito CA, et al. Quantification of nerve fiber layer thickness in normal and glaucomatous eyes using optical coherence tomography. Arch Ophthalmol 1995;113(5):586–96.
14. Blumenthal EZ, Williams JM, Weinreb RN, et al. Reproducibility of nerve fiber layer thickness measurements by use of optical coherence tomography. Ophthalmology 2000;107(12):2278–82.
15. Budenz DL, Fredette MJ, Feuer WJ, et al. Reproducibility of peripapillary retinal nerve fiber thickness measurements with stratus OCT in glaucomatous eyes. Ophthalmology 2008;115(4):661–6.e4.
16. Kanamori A, Escano MF, Eno A, et al. Evaluation of the effect of aging on retinal nerve fiber layer thickness measured by optical coherence tomography. Ophthalmologica 2003;217(4):273–8.
17. Alasil T, Wang K, Keane PA, et al. Analysis of normal retinal nerve fiber layer thickness by age, sex, and race using spectral domain optical coherence tomography. J Glaucoma 2013;22(7):532–41.
18. Leung CK, Yu M, Weinreb RN, et al. Retinal nerve fiber layer imaging with spectral-domain optical coherence tomography: a prospective analysis of age-related loss. Ophthalmology 2012;119(4):731–7.
19. Budenz DL, Anderson DR, Varma R, et al. Determinants of normal retinal nerve fiber layer thickness measured by Stratus OCT. Ophthalmology 2007;114(6):1046–52.
20. Rao HL, Addepalli UK, Yadav RK, et al. Effect of scan quality on diagnostic accuracy of spectral-domain optical coherence tomography in glaucoma. Am J Ophthalmol 2014;157(3):719–27.e1.
21. Sung KR, Wollstein G, Schuman JS, et al. Scan quality effect on glaucoma discrimination by glaucoma imaging devices. Br J Ophthalmol 2009;93(12):1580–4.
22. Vizzeri G, Bowd C, Medeiros FA, et al. Effect of signal strength and improper alignment on the variability of stratus optical coherence tomography retinal nerve fiber layer thickness measurements. Am J Ophthalmol 2009;148(2):249–55.e1.
23. Vizzeri G, Bowd C, Medeiros FA, et al. Effect of improper scan alignment on retinal nerve fiber layer thickness measurements using Stratus optical coherence tomograph. J Glaucoma 2008;17(5):341–9.
24. Gabriele ML, Ishikawa H, Wollstein G, et al. Optical coherence tomography scan circle location and mean retinal nerve fiber layer measurement variability. Invest Ophthalmol Vis Sci 2008;49(6):2315–21.
25. Patel NB, Wheat JL, Rodriguez A, et al. Agreement between retinal nerve fiber layer measures from Spectralis and Cirrus spectral domain OCT. Optom Vis Sci 2012;89(5):E652–66.

26. Kang SH, Hong SW, Im SK, et al. Effect of myopia on the thickness of the retinal nerve fiber layer measured by Cirrus HD optical coherence tomography. Invest Ophthalmol Vis Sci 2010;51(8):4075–83.

27. Savini G, Barboni P, Parisi V, et al. The influence of axial length on retinal nerve fibre layer thickness and optic-disc size measurements by spectral-domain OCT. Br J Ophthalmol 2012;96(1):57–61.

28. Leung CK, Mohamed S, Leung KS, et al. Retinal nerve fiber layer measurements in myopia: an optical coherence tomography study. Invest Ophthalmol Vis Sci 2006;47(12):5171–6.

29. Bennett AG, Rudnicka AR, Edgar DF. Improvements on Littmann's method of determining the size of retinal features by fundus photography. Graefes Arch Clin Exp Ophthalmol 1994;232(6):361–7.

30. Leung CK, Lam S, Weinreb RN, et al. Retinal nerve fiber layer imaging with spectral-domain optical coherence tomography: analysis of the retinal nerve fiber layer map for glaucoma detection. Ophthalmology 2010;117(9):1684–91.

31. Kupersmith MJ. Baseline OCT Measurements in the idiopathic intracranial hypertension treatment trial: part II. Correlations and relationship to clinical features. Invest Ophthalmol Vis Sci 2014;55(12): 8173–9.

32. Vartin CV, Nguyen AM, Balmitgere T, et al. Detection of mild papilloedema using spectral domain optical coherence tomography. Br J Ophthalmol 2012; 96(3):375–9.

33. Wang JK, Kardon RH, Kupersmith MJ, et al. Automated quantification of volumetric optic disc swelling in papilledema using spectral-domain optical coherence tomography. Invest Ophthalmol Vis Sci 2012;53(7):4069–75.

34. Bussel II, Wollstein G, Schuman JS. OCT for glaucoma diagnosis, screening and detection of glaucoma progression. Br J Ophthalmol 2014;98(Suppl 2):ii15–9.

35. Patel NB, Sullivan-Mee M, Harwerth RS. The relationship between retinal nerve fiber layer thickness and optic nerve head neuroretinal rim tissue in glaucoma. Invest Ophthalmol Vis Sci 2014;55(10): 6802–16.

36. Tan O, Chopra V, Lu AT, et al. Detection of macular ganglion cell loss in glaucoma by Fourier-domain optical coherence tomography. Ophthalmology 2009;116(12):2305–14.e1–2.

37. Mwanza JC, Budenz DL, Godfrey DG, et al. Diagnostic performance of optical coherence tomography ganglion cell–inner plexiform layer thickness measurements in early glaucoma. Ophthalmology 2014;121(4):849–54.

38. Laron M, Cheng H, Zhang B, et al. Comparison of multifocal visual evoked potential, standard automated perimetry and optical coherence tomography in assessing visual pathway in multiple sclerosis patients. Mult Scler 2010;16(4):412–26.

39. Cheng H, Laron M, Schiffman JS, et al. The relationship between visual field and retinal nerve fiber layer measurements in patients with multiple sclerosis. Invest Ophthalmol Vis Sci 2007;48(12):5798–805.

40. Sriram P, Wang C, Yiannikas C, et al. Relationship between optical coherence tomography and electrophysiology of the visual pathway in non-optic neuritis eyes of multiple sclerosis patients. PLoS One 2014;9(8):e102546.

41. Talman LS, Bisker ER, Sackel DJ, et al. Longitudinal study of vision and retinal nerve fiber layer thickness in multiple sclerosis. Ann Neurol 2010;67(6):749–60.

42. Narayanan D, Cheng H, Bonem KN, et al. Tracking changes over time in retinal nerve fiber layer and ganglion cell-inner plexiform layer thickness in multiple sclerosis. Mult Scler 2014;20(10):1331–41.

43. Saidha S, Syc SB, Durbin MK, et al. Visual dysfunction in multiple sclerosis correlates better with optical coherence tomography derived estimates of macular ganglion cell layer thickness than peripapillary retinal nerve fiber layer thickness. Mult Scler 2011;17(12):1449–63.

44. Kaufhold F, Zimmermann H, Schneider E, et al. Optic neuritis is associated with inner nuclear layer thickening and microcystic macular edema independently of multiple sclerosis. PLoS One 2013; 8(8):e71145.

45. Scott CJ, Kardon RH, Lee AG, et al. Diagnosis and grading of papilledema in patients with raised intracranial pressure using optical coherence tomography vs clinical expert assessment using a clinical staging scale. Arch Ophthalmol 2010; 128(6):705–11.

46. Menke MN, Feke GT, Trempe CL. OCT measurements in patients with optic disc edema. Invest Ophthalmol Vis Sci 2005;46(10):3807–11.

47. Sibony P, Kupersmith MJ, Honkanen R, et al. Effects of lowering cerebrospinal fluid pressure on the shape of the peripapillary retina in intracranial hypertension. Invest Ophthalmol Vis Sci 2014;55(12): 8223–31.

Advanced MR Imaging of the Visual Pathway

Fang Yu, MD[a],*, Timothy Duong, PhD[b], Bundhit Tantiwongkosi, MD[a,c]

KEYWORDS

- Visual pathway • Retina • Lateral geniculate nucleus • MR imaging • Diffusion tensor imaging
- Diffusion-weighted imaging • Magnetization transfer ratio • Functional imaging
- Retinotopic mapping

KEY POINTS

- MR imaging allows for high-resolution imaging of the retina but remains inferior to optical coherence tomography (OCT) in this aspect. Its primary advantage lies in its ability to characterize anatomic and functional parameters without depth limitation.
- Conventional single-shot echo planar-based diffusion-weighted imaging (DWI) is prone to susceptibility artifacts at tissue interfaces, which can be prominent in the periorbital region.
- Magnetization transfer ratios (MTRs) may play a role in monitoring therapy in demyelinating pathologies, such as multiple sclerosis.
- Diffusion tensor tractography (DTT) may aid in surgical planning of lesions within the vicinity of the optic radiations (ORs).
- Retinotopic mapping using functional MR (fMR) imaging can elucidate the visual cortex and potentially help in surgical planning.

INTRODUCTION

Millions of individuals are afflicted by blindness, and millions more suffer from varying degrees of visual impairment.[1] There are several tools at the clinician's disposal for evaluating this population, including OCT, fluorescein angiography, visual evoked potentials, and high-resolution ultrasonography. However, these techniques have inherent limitations, especially in evaluating the intracranial components of the visual pathway. MR imaging, through its wide selection of sequences, offers an array of structural and functional imaging tools to characterize these otherwise hidden regions. This review describes several advanced MR imaging sequences using an anatomically based approach from the retina to the visual cortex. It also explores their potential clinical applications as well as areas for further development.

RETINAL MR IMAGING

The retina forms the innermost lining of our eyes, measuring between 200 and 250 μm in thickness. It is partitioned into 9 major anatomic layers: the inner limiting membrane, nerve fiber layer, ganglion layer, inner plexiform layer, inner nuclear layer, outer plexiform layer, outer nuclear layer, outer limiting membrane, and the retinal pigment epithelium. Light traverses the cornea, lens, and vitreous before interacting with the retina, where it is then converted into biologic signals in the form of action potentials. These action potentials

The authors have no grants, conflicts of interest, or disclosures to divulge that are applicable to this investigation.
[a] Department of Radiology, University of Texas Health Science Center, 7703 Floyd Curl Drive, Mail Stop 7800, San Antonio, TX 78229-3900, USA; [b] Research Imaging Institute, San Antonio, TX 78229, USA; [c] Imaging Service, South Texas Veterans Health Care System, 7400 Merton Minter, San Antonio, TX 78229, USA
* Corresponding author.
E-mail address: yuf@uthscsa.edu

neuroimaging.theclinics.com

are then transmitted along the optic nerves to the rest of the visual pathway.[2]

Historically, in vivo imaging of the human retina has been confined to the domain of near-infrared light techniques, such as OCT.[3] Recently, high-resolution anatomic MR imaging of the human retina has been performed on 3-T clinical scanners using balanced steady state fast precession (bSSFP) (Fig. 1). To minimize motion artifacts, eye-fixation was used with cued blinking every 4 to 8 seconds. Using a conventional head coil together with a custom-designed eye-shaped receiver coil (to improve signal to noise ratio [SNR]), resolutions of up to 100 × 200 × 2000 µm were achieved.[4] Despite such advances, OCT continues to hold the advantage in terms of spatiotemporal resolution.

MR imaging does offer several advantages including the ability to measure various physiologic as well as functional parameters, such as changes in local blood flow, in a noninvasive manner. The different parameters can be evaluated within a single session without a significant depth limitation (Box 1).[5] For instance, bSSFP-based pseudocontinuous arterial spin labeling (pCASL) has been used to achieve high-resolution blood flow mapping of the human retina. In particular, this sequence is considerably more resistant to susceptibility artifact than many conventional fMR imaging techniques.[6] Similar results have also been achieved using turbo spin echo (TSE)-based pCASL.[7–9] Potential clinical applications include the preclinical and longitudinal evaluation of diabetic retinopathy, glaucoma, and retinal degeneration.[10] Areas for future work include improving the spatiotemporal resolution as well as additional contrasts to better visualize the retinal layers; this can be facilitated through technological advances such as increased field gradients, novel fast acquisition sequences, as well as intravascular contrast agents.

OPTIC NERVE MR IMAGING

The optic nerve (cranial nerve II) transmits visual information from the retina to the brain and comprises retinal ganglion cell axons. It derives from the diencephalon and is considered a part of the central nervous system. Consequently, it is myelinated by oligodendrocytes rather than by Schwann cells. A portion of the optic nerve fibers decussate at the level of the optic chiasm, where most synapse at the lateral geniculate nucleus of the thalamus (Fig. 2 of Imaging of Ocular Motor Pathway). A smaller proportion synapses at other nuclei, including the pretectal nuclei.

DIFFUSION-WEIGHTED IMAGING

DWI is based on the micromovements of extracellular water molecules, which are elucidated by the application of dephasing and rephasing diffusion gradients during the preparatory phase of a sequence (usually spin-echo echo planar imaging

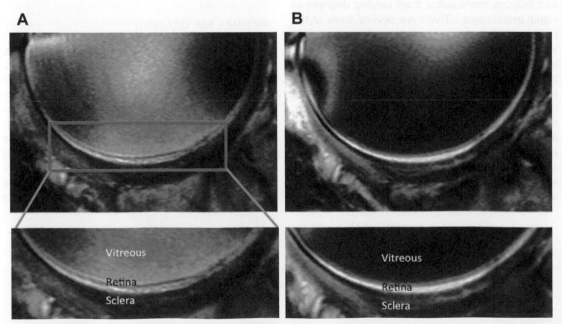

Fig. 1. Precontrast (A) and postcontrast (B) bSSFP anatomic images of the globe at a resolution of 120 × 240 × 2000 µm delineates several retinal layers.

Box 1
Retinal MR imaging

- High-resolution (100 × 200 μm in plane) anatomic images can be obtained using bSSFP as well as turbo spin-echo sequences.

Advantages

- Not depth limited
- Able to characterize different physiologic and functional parameters in a single session

Disadvantages

- Limited spatial resolution compared with optical imaging techniques such as OCT
- May require specialized equipment such as eye-shaped surface receiver coils

---

[EPI]) (**Box 2**). Immobile hydrogen proton molecules (eg, abscesses, stroke) are rephased by the second gradient, whereas those associated with mobile water molecules (eg, cerebrospinal fluid [CSF]) experience a phase shift and generate a weaker signal. The diffusion magnitude is calculated from 3 diffusion images, obtained through the application of the above-mentioned gradients in 3 spatial directions. The degree of diffusion weighting of a sequence is expressed by its b-factor (seconds per square millimeter), which is proportional to the product of the gradient strength squared and the diffusion time interval $(b \sim q^2 \cdot \Delta t)$.[11] An apparent diffusion coefficient (ADC) map can then be generated from 2 diffusion sequences with different b-factors, which is independent of T2:

$$ADC = \frac{-b \cdot \ln DWI}{b_0}$$

DWI is the diffusion-weighted signal intensity for a specific b-value, and b_0 is the reference image.

A variety of conditions may affect the optic nerve, including neoplastic, infectious, ischemic, and autoimmune processes. DWI has been used in the characterization of several of these diseases, including benign and malignant tumors, optic neuritis, and ischemic optic neuropathy (ION).[12–14] ION is typically divided into anterior (AION) and posterior (PION) forms. AION typically presents with sudden painless loss of vision, a relative afferent pupillary defect, and a pale edematous optic disc. It may be further categorized into arteritic (associated with inflammatory causes) and nonarteritic (associated with vasculopathic risk factors) forms.

PION is less common and primarily involves the retrobulbar optic nerve. Its cause is similar to that of nonarteritic AION, with a predominance of systemic vascular diseases, including embolism and thrombosis.[15] Generally, nonarteritic ION has better prognoses than arteritic cases. Like ischemic events in the cerebrum, the optic nerve may demonstrate diffusion restriction during an acute episode, with gradual pseudonormalization. Using ROIs to compare ADC values between the affected regions and normal cerebral white matter may serve as an internal validation. In this regard, MR imaging may be a useful adjunct in diagnosis, as PION is generally normal on fundoscopy.[16] Unfortunately, some diseases that typically present with increased diffusivity, such as optic neuritis (ON), may occasionally demonstrate diffusion restriction. Therefore, other factors (eg, age, cardiovascular risk factors, and clinical presentation) should be taken into consideration when establishing the diagnosis.

From a technical standpoint, several challenges exist to imaging the optic nerves with DWI. For instance, the optic nerves are small structures, and

---

Box 2
Advanced MR imaging of the optic nerve

Diffusion-weighted imaging

- This method uses dephasing and rephasing gradients during the preparatory phase of a sequence to determine the diffusivity of hydrogen protons.
- Diffusion restriction of the optic nerve may be seen in ischemic optic neuropathy, which may help in distinguishing from other causes of acute vision loss.
- Optic nerve imaging can be challenging because of its small size, as well as susceptibility artifacts from the adjacent periorbital structures.

Magnetization transfer contrast

- This method uses an off-resonance saturation pulse to saturate the macromolecular proton population, as seen in lipid-rich myelinated structures, resulting in apparent T1 shortening.
- A useful application is the magnetization ratio, whereby regions of demyelination, as seen in optic neuritis, demonstrate decrease in the ratio.

adjusting parameters such as slice thickness (eg, decreasing from 5 to 3 mm) may be necessary for adequate lesion characterization[17] (Fig. 2). In addition, the typical single-shot EPI-based sequences used for cerebral DWI are sensitive to susceptibility artifact and image distortions, which are prominent at the air-tissue and bone-tissue interfaces surrounding the orbits.[18] Although these artifacts can be decreased to an extent using parallel imaging, they become more pronounced at higher field strengths (3 T and more). Alternative approaches include the implementation of modified multishot EPI sequences, as well as non-EPI-based sequences (which reduce artifacts at the expense of increased scan time). For instance, Porter and Heidemann[19] implemented a readout-segmented EPI with parallel imaging, which combined reduced susceptibility artifact with superior motion correction while only marginally increasing the scan time.[20]

MAGNETIZATION TRANSFER CONTRAST

Magnetization transfer contrast has shown promise in quantifying the extent of demyelination and axonal damage, offering advantages over T1 and T2 mapping in terms of image resolution, acquisition times, and postprocessing requirements. With this technique, an off-resonance saturation pulse is first used to saturate bound macromolecule protons, without affecting the free water proton population, which has a narrow frequency bandwidth (see Box 2).[21] An exchange of longitudinal magnetization then occurs between the free water and macromolecular proton populations, whose longitudinal magnetization has been saturated. This exchange leads to shortening of the apparent longitudinal relaxation time $T_{1\,sat}$, as only the free water protons are visible on clinical MR images. The T_1 shortening is most profound in tissues with a large macromolecule component, such as lipid-rich myelin sheaths (Fig. 3).

A clinically useful parameter is the MTR, which is defined as follows:

$$MTR = 100 \times \frac{M_0 - M_s}{M_0}$$

M_S represents the signal intensity of the free water protons with the off-resonance saturation pulse, and M_0 represents the signal intensity from the free water protons without it. A low MTR corresponds to a decreased exchange of magnetization between free water and macromolecules ($M_s \sim M_0$), as may be seen in CSF, where it approaches 0. In comparison, M_s decreases significantly less than M_0 in normal brain tissues, with MTRs of roughly 40% to 50%.

ON presents as a painful decrease in visual acuity, often with a central scotoma, and may be the initial manifestation of multiple sclerosis.[22] Studies of the prechiasmatic optic nerve in patients with ON generally demonstrate decreases in MTR within the first few months, followed by a gradual increase to near-baseline values.[22,23] These findings suggest that early demyelination occurs, which is then followed by remyelination. However, other studies have demonstrated correlation with measures of axonal damage, such as retinal nerve fiber layer.[24] It is possible that MTR reflects a combination of these biological phenomena, which vary with time.

Clinical application has been limited because of the inherent sensitivity of this technique to small

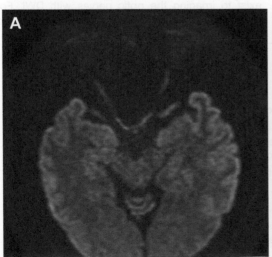
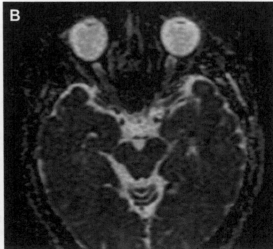

Fig. 2. Axial DWI and ADC images (resolution 1.7 × 1.7 × 3 mm³) at the level of the orbits in a healthy adult man demonstrate the optic nerves with normal signal.

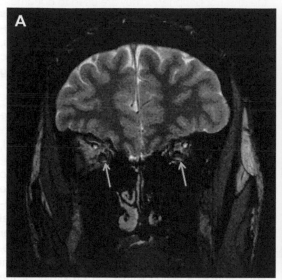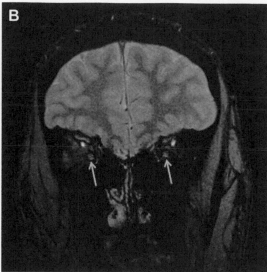

Fig. 3. Coronal gradient echo proton density-weighted images (in-plane resolution 0.7 × 0.7 mm) of a healthy adult man, without (*A*) and with (*B*) off-resonance saturation pulse, demonstrate a relative decrease in signal of the intraorbital optic nerves (*green arrows*) on the magnetization transfer contrast images.

changes in acquisition protocol, as well as other parameters such as the free water relaxation rate. Efforts to improve standardization may help lessen intersubject, interscanner, and intercenter variability. In addition, new techniques have arisen, such as quantitative magnetization transfer, a more comprehensive approach that measures the pool size ratio (ratio of the number of macromolecular protons to free water protons) and thought to be a more direct measure of myelin content.[25] Future work may determine the clinical significance of these techniques.

HIGH-RESOLUTION MR IMAGING OF THE LATERAL GENICULATE NUCLEUS

The lateral geniculate nuclei (LGNs) are a pair of thalamic nuclei involved in relaying visual information between the retina and the visual cortex, located superior to the hippocampus and medial to the ORs (**Box 3**).[26] Each nucleus consists of 2 ventrally oriented magnocellular and 4 dorsally situated parvocellular neuronal layers. These individual layers are retinotopically organized and receive monocular input.[27] Unfortunately, its small size (approximately 5–10 mm) has made in vivo evaluations challenging.[28] However, the development of fast 3-dimensional (3D) sequences, such as magnetization-prepared rapid acquisition gradient echo, have allowed for clinically feasible isometric high-resolution acquisitions of the brain (1 × 1 × 1 mm³ voxels) with high SNRs, which in turn have improved the radiologist's ability to localize and reliably image the LGN (Fig. 2 of Imaging of Ocular Motor Pathway).

Pathology affecting upstream portions of the visual pathway, such as glaucoma and macular degeneration, is associated with atrophy of the

---

Box 3
High-resolution MR imaging of the lateral geniculate nucleus

- The LGNs are a pair of thalamic nuclei located superior to the hippocampus and medial to the optic radiations.
- Upstream lesions (eg, glaucoma and macular degeneration) have been associated with LGN atrophy, although gradual volume loss is also seen in normal aging.
- Magnetization-prepared rapid acquisition gradient echo sequence allows for clinically feasible high-resolution imaging of the LGN (1 × 1 × 1 mm³ voxels).
- Functional mapping using tailored visual stimuli can distinguish between magnocellular and parvocellular LGN layers, which may be applied in the evaluation of psychological and neurodegenerative disorders in the future.

LGN.[29–31] However, postmortem and in vivo MR imaging studies have demonstrated decreasing LGN volume even among otherwise healthy aging adults.[32] Additional research should lead to improved definitions of normal volume ranges.

It is worth noting that the LGN receives a substantial proportion of its input from other regions besides the retina, including cortical regions such as primary visual cortex or V1.[33] Investigations using attention- and perception-related tasks indicate that it is not merely a simple relay but also involved in higher-order visual functions. A promising advance in these efforts has been the addition of noninvasive functional imaging. For instance, Denison and colleagues demonstrated reliable functional mapping of the magnocellular and parvocellular subdivisions through high-resolution fMR imaging (3T and 7T field strength) using a specially designed set of visual stimuli (combination of chromatic, luminance, spatial, and temporal stimulus manipulations). Future work in both healthy and disease populations, including psychological and neurodegenerative disorders, may enhance the understanding of how the LGN and its relationship with other brain regions are affected.[34]

DIFFUSION TENSOR IMAGING OF THE OPTIC RADIATIONS

Certain tissues of the human body, such as myelinated neuronal axons, have an orientation that restricts the diffusion of water along certain directions (Box 4). These tissues are described as anisotropic and are the focus of diffusion tensor imaging (DTI). Like DWI, DTI is usually performed with an EPI-based sequence; however, it requires additional diffusion gradient directions (at least 6 plus a reference image) to generate the diffusion tensors (which are 3×3 matrices characterizing diffusion in 3D space). For high-quality DTT, which demands extensive angular resolution, even more directions are needed.[35] From the diffusion tensors, eigenvalues and eigenvectors can be calculated, which

in turn may be used to determine characteristics such as fractional anisotropy and mean diffusivity.[36] In addition to quantitative DTI analysis, DTT allows the radiologist to visualize the anatomic course of white matter fiber tracts by determining the orientation of maximum diffusion. Various tractography algorithms have been developed (deterministic and statistical methods), which have associated advantages and disadvantages. Nevertheless, DTT shows significant clinical potential, especially as part of preoperative planning.

Visual information is conveyed from the LGN to the primary visual cortex in the occipital lobe through the ORs. Those originating from the inferior retina travel in Meyer loop along the temporal horn of the lateral ventricle, whereas the superior retina signal traverses through the parietal lobe. DTT may be used to determine the optimal approach to a lesion within the proximity of the OR.[35,37] This determination is of particular importance before surgery, as the lesion may displace or involve the OR.[36] If the lesion is determined to infiltrate the OR, visual deficits that may alter treatment planning, decision, and counseling may be unavoidable. Operating room navigational systems are now in wide use, allowing the neurosurgeon real-time visualization of the target lesion superimposed on previously segmented cerebral structures (Fig. 4).

A significant limitation of conventional DTT has been in resolving multiple fiber populations within individual voxels, which is a consequence of the restricted degrees of freedom in the conventional second-order ellipsoid tensor model. These issues may arise in the setting of crossing and highly curved fibers (Fig. 5), as well as areas of altered diffusion, such as tumors.[38] One solution is diffusion spectrum imaging (DSI), which resolves the diffusion probability function by obtaining hundreds of different images with different b-values (from b = 0 to b = 12,000 s/mm^2). Historically, this has been limited secondary to prohibitively lengthy acquisition times. High angular resolution

---

Box 4
Diffusion tensor imaging of the optic radiations

- Structured tissues such as neuronal axons have specific diffusivity orientations, which may be visually represented using DTT.
- DTT may be used for presurgical planning for temporal lobe tumors, potentially altering management and decreasing postoperative visual field defects.
- Spurious results may occur in regions with crossing fibers, sharp angles, and within intratumor segments.
- Diffusion spectroscopy and high angular diffusion imaging may address some of the limitations of conventional DTT but are hindered by increased acquisition times.

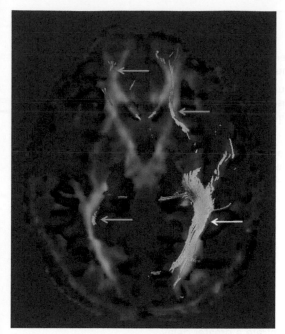

Fig. 4. Axial image of a fractional anisotropy map of the brain, with tractography performed of the left optic radiation (*white arrow*). Spurious tracts (*blue arrows*) are seen in multiple areas.

diffusion imaging (HARDI) is an alternative approach in which the 3D diffusion distribution function is interpolated as the steady function of a sphere. Although it represents a reduction in the number of diffusion-encoding gradients when compared with DSI (60–100 vs 100–500), it remains significantly more time consuming than conventional DTI.[11] To address this limitation, compressed sensing techniques that limit HARDI to a small number of gradients (as few as 20) may be performed, which is on par with modern clinical DTI in terms of scan times. Improvements in MR technology will likely lead to continued advances in this area.

CHARACTERIZATION OF VISUAL ASSOCIATION AREAS WITH FUNCTIONAL MR IMAGING

fMR imaging is a unique technique that has been used in the imaging of brain activity. The underlying principle is known as BOLD (blood oxygenation level dependence) and derives from the relative changes in local cerebral blood flow, blood volume, and oxygen metabolic rate that occur when a certain brain region is activated during a task (**Box 5**). As these parameters increase, so

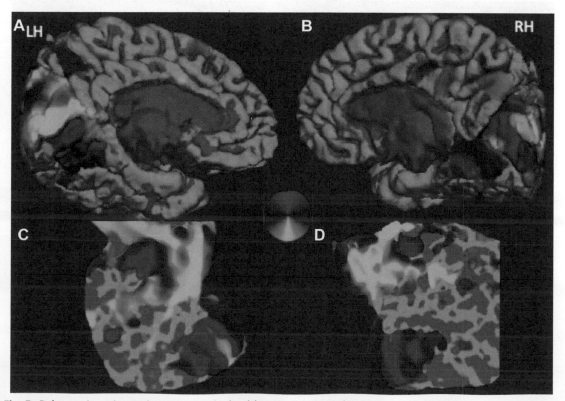

Fig. 5. Polar angle retinotopic mapping of a healthy adult projected onto 3D cortical surface models (*A, B*) and rendered flattened brain images (*C, D*). LH, left hemisphere; RH, right hemisphere.

does the ratio of oxyhemoglobin to deoxyhemoglobin, which is characterized by a detectable increase in T2* signal. Generally, fMR images are obtained using ultrafast gradient echo EPI sequences to achieve high temporal resolution. Acquisitions are repeated multiple times as the patient performs a task.

Traditionally, the stimulus used for cortical mapping of the visual field has been a temporal phase mapping technique (see **Fig. 5**; **Fig. 6**). Eccentricity is mapped using expanding and contracting rings, whereas clockwise and counterclockwise rotating wedges are used for polar angle mapping (**Fig. 7**).[39] The fMR imaging signals produced consist of periodic waveforms, whose corresponding retinotopic locations in the visual cortex can be determined by differences in their temporal phase.[40] Specifically, voxels whose corresponding receptive fields are situated further away from the location of the stimulus demonstrate a greater delay.

Some of the advantages of this technique include its ability to delineate multiple cortical areas associated with vision in a short period. Subsequently, it

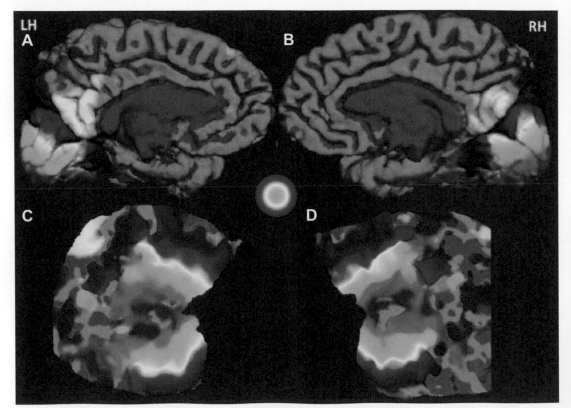

Fig. 6. Eccentricity retinotopic mapping of a healthy adult projected onto 3D cortical surface models (*A, B*) and rendered flattened brain images (*C, D*). LH, left hemisphere; RH, right hemisphere.

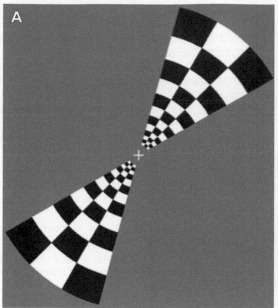 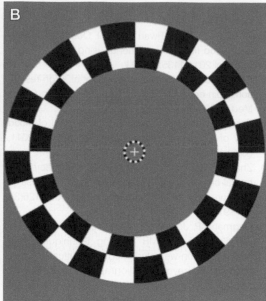

Fig. 7. Examples of visual stimuli used for polar (*A*) and eccentricity (*B*) retinotopic mapping.

has found clinical usage in preoperative planning, as well as in the evaluation of neurodegenerative diseases such as glaucoma and macular degeneration. In addition, altered cortical organization has been demonstrated in the setting of cerebral parenchymal lesions from congenital, ischemic, as well as demyelinating causes.[41]

One limitation to this technique is that the delay inherent to the neurovascular coupling mechanism responsible for the fMR imaging signal also affects the phase change; this can generally be accounted for by having stimuli moving in opposite directions, such as clockwise and counterclockwise rotations. However, the high sensitivity of this method to stimuli timing differences makes it susceptible to even small phase differences caused by noise. Erroneous results may also be encountered within a voxel associated with multiple neurons that have spatially disparate receptive fields (eg, a voxel that spans a sulcus). Newer techniques designed to address this issue, such as multifocal stimulus mapping, may help improve the accuracy of retinotopic mapping in the future.[42]

SUMMARY

Advanced MR imaging sequences offer the ability to characterize pathology involving the visual pathway in a noninvasive manner, providing unique insights that are outside the realm of both clinical examinations and conventional imaging techniques. Familiarity with some of these emerging sequences will allow the radiologist to offer important

information to referring clinicians, which is likely to positively affect patient management.

ACKNOWLEDGMENTS

The authors acknowledge Wei Zhou, BS; Jing Li, PhD; and Eric Muir, PhD, for their expert help in MR image acquisition and editorial assistance.

REFERENCES

1. Resnikoff S, Pascolini D, Etya'ale D, et al. Global data on visual impairment in the year 2002. Bull World Health Organ 2004;82:844–51.
2. Duong TQ. Magnetic resonance imaging of the retina: From mice to men. Magn Reson Med 2013; 71(4):1526–30.
3. Fujimoto JG, Pitris C, Boppart SA, et al. Optical coherence tomography: an emerging technology for biomedical imaging and optical biopsy. Neuoplasia 2000;2(1–2):9–25.
4. Zhang Y, Nateras OSE, Peng Q, et al. Lamina-specific anatomic magnetic resonance imaging of the human retina. Invest Ophthalmol Vis Sci 2011;52: 7232–7.
5. Shen Q, Cheng H, Pardue MT, et al. Magnetic resonance imaging of tissue and vascular layers in the cat retina. J Magn Reson Imaging 2006;23(4): 465–72.
6. Park SH, Wang DJ, Duong TQ. Balanced steady state free precession for arterial spin labeling MRI: initial experience for blood flow mapping in human

brain, retina, and kidney. Magn Reson Imaging 2013;31(7):1044–50.

7. Muir ER, Watts LT, Tiwari YV, et al. Quantitative cerebral blood flow measurements using MRI. Methods Mol Biol 2014;1135:205–11.

8. Duong TQ, Yacoub E, Adriany G, et al. High-resolution, spin-echo BOLD and CBF fMRI. Magn Reson Med 2002;48(4):589–93.

9. Peng Q, Zhang Y, Nateras OS, et al. MRI of blood flow of the human retina. Magn Reson Med 2011; 65(6):1768–75.

10. Zhang Y, Harrison JM, Nateras OS, et al. Decreased retinal-choroidal blood flow in retinitis pigmentosa as measured by MRI. Doc Ophthalmol 2013;126(3): 187–97.

11. Hagmann P, Jonasson L, Maeder P, et al. Understanding diffusion MR imaging techniques: from scalar diffusion-weighted imaging to diffusion tensor imaging and beyond. Radiographics 2006;26(Suppl 1):S205–23.

12. Fatima Z, Ichikawa T, Ishigame K, et al. Orbital masses: the usefulness of diffusion-weighted imaging in lesion categorization. Clin Neuroradiol 2014; 24(2):129–34.

13. Kapur R, Sepahdari AR, Mafee MF, et al. MR imaging of orbital inflammatory syndrome, orbital cellulitis, and orbital lymphoid lesions: the role of diffusion-weighted imaging. AJNR Am J Neuroradiol 2009;30(1):64–70.

14. Al-Shafai LS, Mikulis DJ. Diffusion MR imaging in a case of acute ischemic optic neuropathy. AJNR Am J Neuroradiol 2006;27(2):255–7.

15. Sadda SR, Nee M, Miller NR, et al. Clinical spectrum of posterior ischemic optic neuropathy. Am J Ophthalmol 2001;132(5):743–50.

16. Bender B, Heine C, Danz S, et al. Diffusion restriction of the optic nerve in patients with acute visual deficit. J Magn Reson Imagin 2014;40(2):334–40.

17. Park JY, Lee IH, Song CJ, et al. Diffusion MR imaging of postoperative bilateral acute ischemic optic neuropathy. Korean J Radiol 2012;13(2):237–9.

18. de Graaf P, Pouwels PJ, Rodjan F, et al. Single-shot turbo spin-echo diffusion-weighted imaging for retinoblastoma: initial experience. AJNR Am J Neuroradiol 2012;33(1):110–8.

19. Porter DA, Heidemann RM. High resolution diffusion-weighted imaging using readout-segmented echo-planar imaging, parallel imaging and a two-dimensional navigator-based reacquisition. Magn Reson Med 2009;62(2):468–75.

20. Morelli J, Porter D, Ai F, et al. Clinical evaluation of single-shot and readout-segmented diffusion-weighted imaging in stroke patients at 3 T. Acta Radiol 2013;54(3):299–306.

21. Grossman RI, Gomori JM, Ramer KN, et al. Magnetization transfer: theory and clinical applications in neuroradiology. Radiographics 1994;14(2):279–90.

22. Wang Y, van der Walt A, Paine M, et al. Optic nerve magnetisation transfer ratio after acute optic neuritis predicts axonal and visual outcomes. PLoS One 2012;7(12):e52291.

23. Hickman SJ, Toosy AT, Jones SJ, et al. Serial magnetization transfer imaging in acute optic neuritis. Brain 2004;127:692–700.

24. Klistorner A, Chaganti J, Garrick R, et al. Magnetisation transfer ratio in optic neuritis is associated with axonal loss, but not with demyelination. Neuroimage 2011;56(1):21–6.

25. Ou X, Sun SW, Liang HF, et al. Quantitative magnetization transfer measured pool size ratio reflects optic nerve myelin content in ex vivo mice. Magn Reson Med 2009;61(2):364–71.

26. Lee JY, Jeong HJ, Lee JH, et al. An investigation of lateral geniculate nucleus volume in patients with primary open-angle glaucoma using 7 tesla magnetic resonance imaging. Invest Ophthalmol Vis Sci 2014;55(6):3468–76.

27. Schneider KA, Richter MC, Kastner S. Retinotopic organization and functional subdivisions of the human lateral geniculate nucleus: a high-resolution functional magnetic resonance imaging study. J Neurosci 2004;24(41):8975–85.

28. Andrews TJ, Halpern SD, Purves D. Correlated size variations in human visual cortex, lateral geniculate nucleus, and optic tract. J Neurosci 1997;17(8): 2859–68.

29. Gupta N, Greenberg G, de Tilly LN, et al. Atrophy of the lateral geniculate nucleus in human glaucoma detected by magnetic resonance imaging. Br J Ophthalmol 2009;93(1):56–60.

30. Hernowo AT, Prins D, Baseler HA, et al. Morphometric analyses of the visual pathways in macular degeneration. Cortex 2013;45:99–110.

31. Chen Z, Wang J, Lin F, et al. Correlation between lateral geniculate nucleus atrophy and damage to the optic disc in glaucoma. J Neuroradiol 2013; 40(4):281–7.

32. Li M, He HG, Shi W, et al. Quantification of the human lateral geniculate nucleus in vivo using MR imaging based on morphometry: volume loss with age. AJNR Am J Neuroradiol 2012;33(5):915–21.

33. Denison RN, Vu AT, Yacoub E, et al. Functional mapping of the magnocellular and parvocellular subdivisions of human LGN. Neuroimage 2014;102:358–69.

34. Núñez D, Rauch J, Herwig K, et al. Evidence for a magnocellular disadvantage in early-onset schizophrenic patients: a source analysis of the N80 visual-evoked component. Schizophr Res 2013; 144(1–3):16–23.

35. Winston GP, Yogarajah M, Symms MR. Diffusion tensor imaging tractography to visualize the relationship of the optic radiation to epileptogenic lesions prior to neurosurgery. Epilepsia 2011;52(8): 1430–8.

36. Zhang Y, Wan SH, Wu GJ, et al. Magnetic resonance diffusion tensor imaging and diffusion tensor tractography of human visual pathway. Int J Ophthalmol 2012;5(4):452–8.

37. de Blank PM, Berman JI, Liu GT, et al. Fractional anisotropy of the optic radiations is associated with visual acuity loss in optic pathway gliomas of neurofibromatosis type 1. Neuro Oncol 2013;15(8):1088–95.

38. Kuhnt D, Bauer MH, Sommer J, et al. Optic radiation fiber tractography in glioma patients based on high angular resolution diffusion imaging with compressed sensing compared with diffusion tensor imaging - initial experience. PLoS One 2013;8(7): e70793.

39. Warnking J, Dojat M, Guerin-Duque A, et al. fMRI retinotopic mapping - step by step. NeuroImage 2002;17(4):1665–83.

40. Ma Y, Ward BD, Ropella KM, et al. Comparison of randomized multifocal mapping and temporal phase mapping of visual cortex for clinical use. Neuroimage Clin 2013;3:143–54.

41. Reitsma DC, Mathis J, Ulmer JL, et al. Atypical retinotopic organization of visual cortex in patients with central brain damage: congenital and adult onset. J Neurosci 2013;33(32):13010–24.

42. Ward BD, Janik J, Mazaheri Y, et al. Adaptive Kalman filtering for real-time mapping of the visual field. NeuroImage 2012;59(4):3533–47.

Imaging of Optic Neuropathy and Chiasmal Syndromes

Bundhit Tantiwongkosi, MD[a,b,c],*, Mahmood F. Mafee, MD[d]

KEYWORDS

• Vision loss • MR imaging • Optic neuropathy • Chiasm • Visual field defect

KEY POINTS

• When clinical presentations of optic neuropathy and chiasm disorders are nonspecific, imaging plays a critical role in detecting, localizing, and differentiating the wide variety of causes.
• Some key imaging features are characteristic, leading to appropriate treatment and preventing unnecessary tissue biopsies.
• The following entities have characteristic imaging findings: optic neuritis, optic nerve sheath meningioma, optic nerve glioma, pituitary adenoma, aneurysm, etc.

INTRODUCTION

Optic neuropathy is characterized by loss of visual acuity, color vision (dyschromatopsia), and visual field defect. Fundoscopic examination may reveal a swollen, pale, anomalous, or normal optic disc.[1] Chiasmal disorders classically present with gradual onset of vision loss, bitemporal hemianopsia, and occasionally, endocrinopathy if the pituitary gland and/or hypothalamus are the causes or are involved.[2]

NORMAL ANATOMY
Optic Nerve

Retinal ganglion cell axons form the optic nerves, which are myelinated by oligodendrocytes and supported by astrocytes.[3] The optic nerve is divided into 4 segments: intraocular, intraorbital, intracanalicular, and intracranial (Fig. 1).[4] The optic nerve is isointense to cerebral white matter on T1-weighted and T2-weighted images. The optic nerve is surrounded by the optic nerve sheath, which contains pia, cerebrospinal fluid, arachnoid, and dura.[1]

Optic Chiasm

The nasal retinal fibers of the optic nerve cross at the optic chiasm, whereas the temporal fibers remain uncrossed (Fig. 2). The chiasm is surrounded by multiple critical structures including the pituitary gland inferiorly, infundibulum posteriorly, third ventricle and hypothalamus superiorly, inferior frontal lobe anteriorly, and supraclinoid internal carotid artery laterally.[2] The chiasm (Fig. 3) is typically located directly above the pituitary gland; in a minority of cases, it may be in prefixed (above the tuberculum sella) or postfixed positions (above the dorsum sella).[5] Mass lesions of the pituitary gland typically compress the central portion of chiasm resulting in classic bitemporal hemianopsia, which may not present in cases of prefixed or postfixed chiasms.[2]

Disclosures: None.
[a] Division of Neuroradiology, Department of Radiology, University of Texas Health Science Center at San Antonio, 7703 Floyd Curl Drive, Mail Code 7800, San Antonio, TX 78229, USA; [b] Department of Otolaryngology–Head Neck Surgery, University of Texas Health Science Center at San Antonio, 7703 Floyd Curl Drive, Mail Code 7800, San Antonio, TX 78229, USA; [c] Imaging Service, South Texas Veterans, 7400 Merton Minter, San Antonio, TX 78229, USA; [d] Division of Neuroradiology, Department of Radiology, University of California, San Diego, 200 West Arbor Drive, San Diego, CA 92103, USA
* Corresponding author. Division of Neuroradiology, Department of Radiology, University of Texas Health Science Center at San Antonio, 7703 Floyd Curl Drive, Mail Code 7800, San Antonio, TX 78229.
E-mail address: tantiwongkos@uthscsa.edu

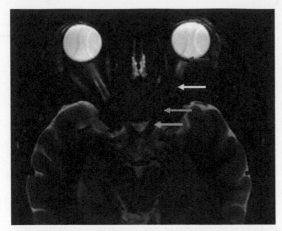

Fig. 1. The 4 segments of optic nerves. Axial T2-weighted image shows intraocular (*red arrow*), intraorbital (*yellow arrow*), intracanalicular (*orange arrow*), and intracranial (*green arrow*) segments.

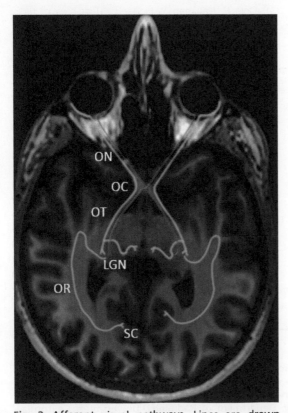

Fig. 2. Afferent visual pathways. Lines are drawn superimposed on an axial T1-weighted image showing expected location of the optic nerves (ON), optic chiasm (OC), optic tract (OT), lateral geniculate nucleus (LGN), optic radiation (OR), and striate cortex (SC).

IMAGING PROTOCOL
Computed Tomography Versus MR Imaging

Computed tomography (CT) and MR imaging are complementary to each other in identifying anatomy and pathology of optic nerve and chiasm.[6] MR imaging provides exquisite details of optic nerve and chiasm because of high tissue contrast differentiation.[7] CT is valuable in the evaluation of bony structures (optic canals), calcified lesions, and metallic foreign bodies when MR imaging is contraindicated.[6]

MR Imaging Protocol

Optic nerve and sella MR imaging protocols are suggested in **Box 1**. Fat saturation sequences with intravenous gadolinium are helpful in detecting optic neuritis, neoplasms, postoperative changes, and optic nerve infarction.[8,9]

PATHOLOGY
Optic Neuropathy

Optic neuritis
Optic neuritis is a clinical diagnosis of optic nerve inflammation secondary to demyelination. A typical clinical scenario is a young white woman presenting with rapid onset of painful vision loss with optic disc swelling seen on fundoscopy.[1] In cases with typical presentations, MR imaging does not aid in the diagnosis and does not alter the clinical course, management, or final visual outcome.[10] If performed, MR imaging may show enlargement and enhancement of the nerve with hyperintensity on T2-weighted images in over 90% of cases (**Fig. 4**A–D).[11] The findings are often similar to those of other inflammatory (eg, sarcoidosis) and infectious causes of optic neuropathy. However, involvement of the optic nerve, optic nerve sheath, and ciliary body favors the diagnosis of sarcoidosis over optic neuritis associated with multiple sclerosis (MS). Visual outcome is worse with longitudinally extensive lesions and with involvement of the intracanalicular segment (rigid bony canal).[12] Eye pain correlates with intraorbital segment involvement, which is the most common segment to be involved.[12] Enhancement suggests active disease, while resolution of enhancement is seen in the recovery phase.[1]

Patients with optic neuritis are at increased risk for developing MS; it can occur as the first presentation of MS or develop later on.[13] The presence of abnormal cerebral white matter lesions on MR imaging is the most important predictor for the development of MS in the future.[1] It was found that 60% to 90% of patients with optic neuritis with abnormal cerebral white matter eventually develop MS. Only 20% to 25% of patients with normal-appearing MR

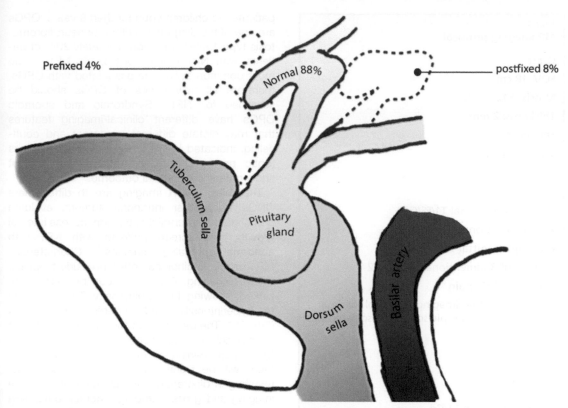

Fig. 3. Variation of optic chiasm position. Diagram of the sella (sagittal view) demonstrates normal position of the chiasm (above the pituitary gland: 88% of population), prefixed position (above the tuberculum sella: 4%), and postfixed position (above the dorsum sella: 8%).

images developed MS.[14,15] If there are typical brain lesions (T2-hyperintense periventricular and juxtacortical white matter lesions, see **Fig. 4**C), the administration of high-dose intravenous steroids has been found to decrease the incidence of MS development if given within 2 years.[16] Therefore detection of brain lesions in patients with optic neuritis is a crucial task of radiologists.

Neuromyelitis optica (Devic disease)

Neuromyelitis optica (NMO) is a distinct severe autoimmune demyelinating disease mainly affecting the optic nerves and spinal cord.[17] Acute optic neuritis in NMO is typically bilateral and severe (see **Fig. 4**E–H). Longitudinally extensive lesions (≥3 vertebral segments), which may occupy the entire cross section of the cord, characterize spinal cord involvement.[18] Brain lesions can be found in locations similar to those of MS as well as in atypical areas including hypothalamus, periaqueductal gray, and area postrema.[19] Most patients test positive for aquaporin-4 antibody.[20] Prognosis is poor, and treatment is different from that of MS.[21]

Optic perineuritis

Optic perineuritis occurs when there is inflammation of the optic nerve sheath. The nerve itself is not involved. MR imaging shows enhancement and enlargement of optic nerve sheath, which may mimic a meningioma (**Fig. 5**).[22] Optic perineuritis can be idiopathic; however, it may be associated with some conditions such as inflammatory orbital syndrome, sarcoidosis, syphilis, Lyme disease, and tuberculosis.[1] Coexisting intracranial leptomeningeal enhancement suggests an infection or neoplasm (leptomeningeal carcinomatosis [from breast or lung carcinomas] or lymphomatosis [from lymphoma]) as the cause.

Ischemic optic neuropathy

Acute interruption of the blood flow to the optic nerve can cause ischemic optic neuropathy (ION), typically presenting as acute painless vision loss in the elderly. ION is classified as anterior (intraocular segment) and posterior (retrobulbar segment) types. Anterior ischemic optic neuropathy (AION) is further classified as arteritic AION (A-AION) and nonarteritic AION (NA-AION).[23] The distinction between A-AION and NA-AION is shown in **Table 1**.

Posterior ischemic optic neuropathy (PION) is relatively rare. The optic nerve head is normal on fundoscopy.[1] MR imaging may show restricted diffusion of the retrobulbar optic nerve in the early

Box 1
MR imaging protocol

Orbit

FOV: 18 cm

Matrix: 512 × 512

Thickness: 2 mm

Sequences

- Axial T1 TSE
- Axial T2 TSE/FS
- Coronal T2/FS
- Axial and coronal T1/FS/Gd
- Axial or coronal DWI
- Oblique sagittal T1/FS/Gd
- Thin-cut 3-dimensional heavily T2
- Axial T2 TSE brain
- Full brain MR imaging protocol with and without Gd (multiple-sclerosis-associated optic neuritis)

Sella

FOV 15 cm

Sequences

- Sagittal T1 and T1/Gd
- Coronal T1 and T1/Gd
- Coronal T2
- Axial T2 brain

Abbreviations: DWI, diffusion-weighted imaging; FOV, field of view; FS, fat saturation; Gd, gadolinium; TSE, turbo spin echo.

phase (**Fig. 6**) with atrophy seen after 6 to 12 weeks.[24] The posterior segment of the optic nerve, especially the central portion, is more vulnerable to ischemia than the anterior segment because of less vascular supply (the anterior segment has dual arterial supplies from the central retinal and posterior ciliary arteries). PION can be seen in patients with giant cell arteritis, perioperative hypotension, vasculopathic risk factors, infection (varicella zoster, herpes), systemic inflammation (lupus, polyarteritis nodosa), and compressive optic neuropathy.[1,24,25]

Optic Nerve and Optic Nerve Sheath Neoplasms

Optic nerve gliomas

Optic nerve gliomas (ONGs), as a part of the optic pathway gliomas (OPGs), are slowly growing low-grade astrocytomas, and not hamartomas.[26] Most

patients are children younger than 8 years. OPGs are one of the diagnostic criteria of neurofibromatosis type 1 (NF1) with approximately 20% of patients with NF1 having OPGs.[27,28] NF1 is the most common syndrome associated with OPGs, therefore all new cases of OPGs should be screened for NF1.[1] Syndromic and sporadic OPGs have different clinical/imaging features that may dictate different treatment and counseling, indicated in **Table 2**. Locations of tumors (optic nerve, chiasm, or retrochiasm) do not show difference in visual outcome.[29]

The roles of MR imaging are to differentiate ONGs from other intraconal tumors, evaluate orbital apex/intracranial extension, assess interval growth, and screen patients with NF1 with abnormal ophthalmic findings.[28] Characteristic MR imaging findings can often preclude biopsies. On MR imaging, the tumors can be fusiform or kinked, showing T1 hypointensity, T2 isointensity to hyperintensity, and variable enhancement (**Fig. 7**).[30] The periphery of the tumor may appear T2 hyperintense, representing arachnoidal gliomatosis (leptomeningeal involvement).[28] At times there will be significant arachnoid hyperplasia, resulting in discrepancy in size measurement on imaging and gross pathology (actual tumor size on pathology is smaller). Some ONGs may not enhance and look like cystic lesions.

ONGs associated with NF1 tend to be bilateral, enlarged, kinked, and tortuous with or without chiasm involvement. In patients without NF1, the tumors appear fusiform.[30] Even though they are benign, the tumors can invade surrounding structures and grow significantly.[26] Fortunately, the tumors usually do not undergo malignant transformation, and they can regress spontaneously with uncertain incidence and mechanisms.[26] Although cases of spontaneous regression were reported, the authors have not seen such cases in their 35-year experiences. It is important for the radiologists to detect tumor progression because chemotherapy and radiation can effectively halt tumor growth and improve visual outcome.[31]

Optic nerve sheath meningiomas

Optic nerve sheath meningiomas (ONSMs) are rare benign neoplasms arising from the optic nerve sheath, accounting for 2% of all intraorbital neoplasms.[32] The intraorbital tumors may extend intracranially, or vice versa. Most ONSMs are unilateral and extend from an intracranial origin (90%) with a minority primarily originating within the orbit (10%).[32,33] However, the authors' experiences are different. Most of their cases are isolated intraorbital ONSMs. There is a female predilection with a mean age of 40.8 years.[32]

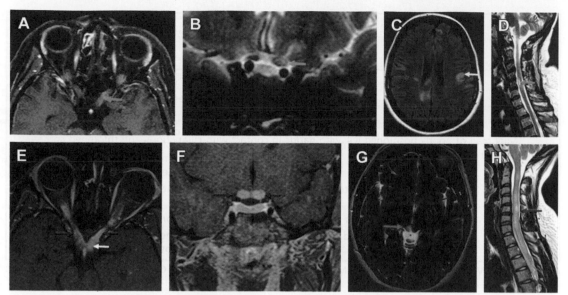

Fig. 4. Multiple sclerosis (MS) versus neuromyelitis optica (NMO). In this patient with MS, there is unilateral optic neuritis seen as left optic nerve enhancement (*blue arrow* in *A*) and nerve enlargement with T2 hyperintensity (*blue arrow* in *B*) when compared with normal temporal lobe white matter. Multiple brain lesions are seen in the periventricular (*red arrow* in *C*) and juxtacortical white matter (*yellow arrow* in *C*). Typical cord lesions are small and in peripheral location (*green arrow* in *D*). In NMO, optic neuritis is typically more severe and bilateral (*purple arrows* in *E* and *F*) and may extend to involve optic chiasm (*white arrow* in *E*). Brain lesions may be seen in atypical locations for MS such as periaqueductal gray (*orange arrow* in *G*). Longitudinally extensive cord lesions may be seen (*pink arrow* in *H*).

Younger patients with bilateral tumors may have neurofibromatosis type II.[34,35] The tumors vary in morphology ranging from tubular, fusiform (mimicking ONGs), globular, to focal.[36] On imaging, the tumors show concentric enlargement of the avidly enhancing calcified optic nerve sheath, sparing the optic nerve, referred to as the tram track sign (**Fig. 8**).[37] Biopsy may be avoided when the imaging findings are characteristic and the patients present with the classic clinical triad of progressive vision loss, optic nerve atrophy, and visualization of optociliary shunts on fundoscopy.[1,38] Enlargement of the adjacent sphenoid and posterior ethmoid sinuses can be seen but is not specific for ONSMs (also known as sinus blistering).[39]

Compressive optic neuropathy

The optic nerves can be compressed by various pathologies. Compression initially leads to venous occlusion, nerve fiber edema, and partial vision

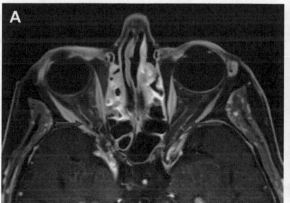
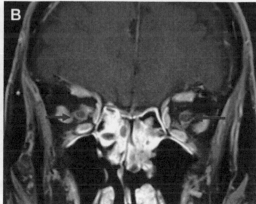

Fig. 5. Optic perineuritis. Axial (*A*) and coronal (*B*) T1-weighted images of the orbits show thin and smooth enhancement of the bilateral optic nerve sheaths (*red arrows*) in a 76-year-old man who presented with bilateral eye pain.

Table 1
Distinctions between NA-AION and A-AION

Features	A-AION	NA-AION
Age (y)	>60	>55
Sex	Females > males	Females = males
Vision loss	Severe	Less severe
Risk factors/ association	Giant cell arteritis (headache, scalp tenderness, jaw claudication)	Disc with small central cup, hypertension, hypercholesterolemia, diabetes mellitus, nocturnal systemic hypotension, obstructive sleep apnea, anemia, etc.
Fundoscopic finding	Pale edematous disc cotton wool spots	Hyperemic edematous disc
MR imagine	Restricted diffusion with enhancement	Restricted diffusion without enhancement
Treatment	Immediate corticosteroid	No specific treatment, risk factor modification, steroid is controversial

Data from Addis VM, DeVore HK, Summerfield ME. Acute visual changes in the elderly. Clin Geriatr Med 2013;29(l):165–80.

loss that are potentially reversible with early surgical decompression. Prolonged pressure can cause arterial occlusion, optic nerve infarction, and permanent vision loss.[40] Typically, patients present with subacute to chronic vision loss with optic nerve atrophy. Patients tend to present early when the lesions involve the optic canal. Contrast-enhanced MR imaging is the modality of choice to evaluate the underlying cause (**Fig. 9**). Common causes of compressive neuropathy are discussed below.

Thyroid-associated ophthalmopathy (TAO) is an autoimmune inflammatory disease secondary to excessive thyroid-stimulating hormone receptor antibodies, which cross-react with extraocular muscles and retrobulbar soft tissue.[41] TAO may occur before, during, or after

hyperthyroidism.[42] Occasionally, patients with euthyroid may also be affected. CT and MR imaging are valuable in the diagnosis and treatment assessment. On imaging, eyelids, lacrimal glands, and bellies of the extraocular muscles (inferior > medial > superior > lateral recti) are swollen with sparing of the tendinous insertion.[43] Rarely, the disease involves only a single muscle or primarily involves the lateral rectus.[1] There is increase in the volume of retrobulbar fat, resulting in proptosis.[44] The enlarged muscles can compress the optic nerve at the orbital apex, causing compressive optic neuropathy, which can present in patients with only mild proptosis.[44] Intensity of the most affected muscle measured on short tau inversion recovery sequence correlates with clinical disease activity.[45] Hypodensity

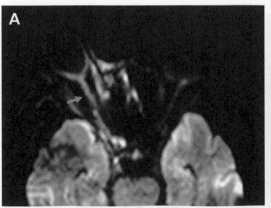
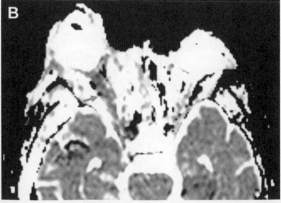

Fig. 6. PION. Diffusion-weighted (*A*) and apparent diffusion coefficient (*B*) images show restricted diffusion of the right intraorbital optic nerve in a diabetic patient who has invasive sinonasal mucomycosis with orbital involvement. Invasion of blood supplies to the optic nerve results in PION.

Table 2
Differences in clinical and imaging features of syndromic (NF1-associated) and sporadic OPGs

Features	Syndromic	Sporadic
Age	Younger children	Older children
Location	Optic nerve with or without chiasm	Chiasm and retrochiasm
Morphology	Tubular, kinked	Fusiform
Bilaterality	More common	Less common
Behavior	Indolent, progress slower, asymptomatic, incidentally found during screening	More invasive, progress faster, symptomatic
Visual loss	Less common	More common
Proptosis	More pronounced	Less pronounced
Increased intracranial pressure and hydrocephalus	Less common	More common

Data from Shamji MF, Benoit BG. Syndromic and sporadic pediatric optic pathway gliomas: review of clinical and histopathological differences and treatment implications. Neurosurg Focus 2007;23(5):E3.

in the muscle bellies seen on CT represents glycoaminoglycans or lymphocyte infiltration (**Fig. 10**).[1] Later the muscles are replaced by fat.

The intracranial optic nerve is in close proximity to the supraclinoid internal carotid artery, anterior cerebral artery, and anterior communicating artery.[1] The intraorbital segment is in close relation to the ophthalmic artery. Aneurysms of these arteries can directly compress or rupture into the nerve (**Fig. 11**).[46,47] Vision loss can fluctuate because of changes in size of the aneurysm.[1] Acute monocular vision loss with severe headache and neck stiffness strongly suggest aneurysm rupture, prompting emergent neuroimaging and intervention.[47]

The lateral walls of the sphenoid or posterior ethmoid sinuses (Onodi cell) form the medial wall of the orbit and the optic canal. Mucoceles of these air cells can directly compress the optic nerve.[48] The presence of active infection in the

mucocele and initial poor vision are important prognostic factors for visual outcome regardless of the origin of the mucoceles.[48] Infection can directly spread to involve the optic nerve through a dehiscent wall and nutrient foramina, resulting in optic nerve ischemia.[49] Presence of vision loss in patients with sphenoid/ethmoid sinus mucocele mandates early surgical drainage.[48] Sinus expansion and wall erosion are common in allergic fungal sinusitis (AFS), which may lead to optic nerve compression (**Fig. 12**). Direct invasion of fungus in AFS into the optic nerve is found in a series of case studies.[40]

Chiasmal Disorders

Pituitary macroadenomas

The most common cause of chiasm disorder in adults is extrinsic compression from pituitary macroadenomas.[50] The tumors initially compress the

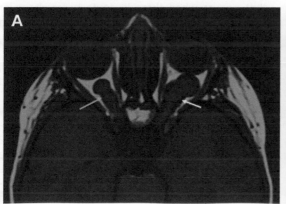
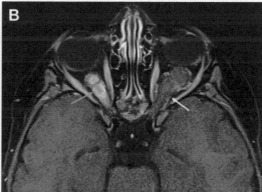

Fig. 7. ONGs. Axial precontrast (*A*) and postcontrast (*B*) T1-weighted images of the orbits show enlargement and tortuosity of the bilateral optic nerves. The right optic nerve (*blue arrows*) is intensely enhancing. The left optic nerve (*yellow arrows*) is mildly enhancing.

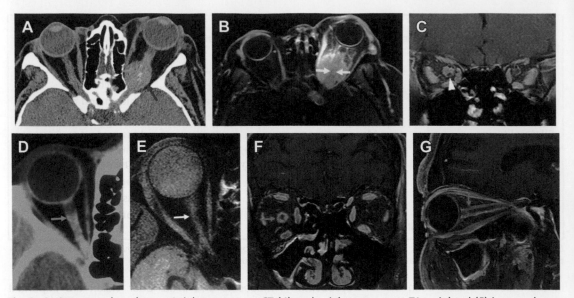

Fig. 8. ONSM versus lymphoma. Axial noncontrast CT (*A*) and axial postcontrast T1-weighted (*B*) images show a fusiform meningioma (*red arrow* in *A* and *B*) of the left optic nerve sheath with tram track calcifications (*blue arrow* in *A*). The optic nerve is normal in size without tortuosity (*yellow arrows* in *B*). In long-standing cases, the optic nerve can be atrophic and the tumor tends to be eccentric (*arrowhead* in *C*). Tumor microcalcifications may be detected only on CT (*green arrow* in *D*) and the optic nerve sheath may appear unremarkable on MR imaging (*white arrow* in *E*). Lymphomas may present with enhancing optic nerve sheath (*orange arrow* in *F* and *G*), simulating meningiomas.

inferior aspect of the chiasm where the superior nasal retinal fibers are located, resulting in superior bitemporal defects. The tumors tend to grow slowly and eventually compress the whole central portion of chiasm, causing classic bitemporal hemianopsia.[1] MR imaging is the modality of choice for imaging chiasm compression (**Fig. 13**) and cavernous sinus invasion and for preoperative evaluation for endoscopic transsphenoidal hypophysectomy. It is important to inform the surgeons regarding the size and components of the tumors because of the high failure rate of chiasm decompression in tumors larger than 4 cm in craniocaudal dimension and those that contain solid fibrotic components, which may show T2 hypointensity and restricted diffusion. Cystic/necrotic (T2 hyperintense, non–rim enhancing/rim enhancing) and hemorrhagic (signal depends on stages of blood products) tumors are easier to evacuate and correlate with successful chiasm decompression.[51] CT is valuable to evaluate bony structure before surgery.

Bromocriptine and cabergoline have been used to treat macroprolactinomas successfully, measured objectively by decreasing serum prolactin levels and improved visual field defect. Rapid shrinkage of the tumors may cause cerebrospinal fluid rhinorrhea or an increasingly recognized optic

chiasm herniation into the enlarged partial empty sella (**Fig. 14**). If the latter complication occurs, the patients may develop secondary worsening visual field defect, which can be alleviated by decreasing medication dose. Sellar MR imaging is mandatory to evaluate secondary deterioration of vision from other causes including tumor regrowth or pituitary apoplexy.[52,53]

Pituitary apoplexy
Pituitary apoplexy is a life-threatening condition that occurs when there is acute hemorrhage or infarction within pituitary mass lesions leading to acute headache, vision loss, ophthalmoplegia, altered mental status, and hypopituitarism.[54] Known risk factors include pituitary adenomas, bromocriptine therapy, closed head injury, blood pressure fluctuation, radiation, and pregnancy.[55] MR imaging is the modality of choice and may show a pituitary mass and blood products depending on the stages of hemorrhage with T2 gradient recalled echo (GRE) as the most sensitive sequence (**Fig. 15**).[56] It is important for radiologists to assess the size, underlying mass lesions, presence of hemorrhage/infarction, and compression on cavernous sinuses/optic chiasm. Patients with chiasm and cavernous sinus compression may require timely surgery.[57]

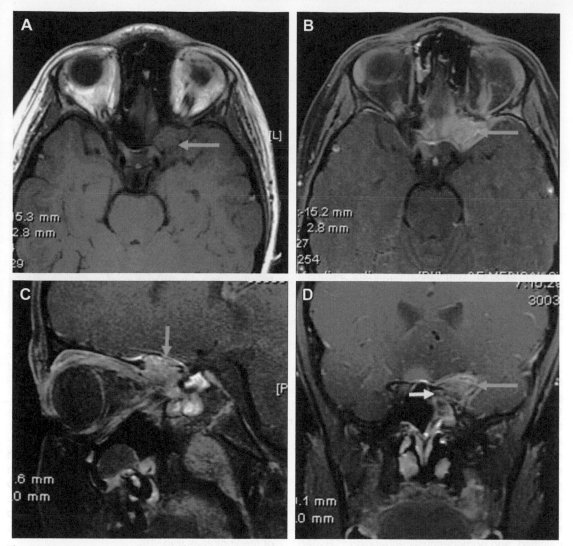

Fig. 9. Compressive optic neuropathy due to Langerhans cell histiocytosis in a 12-year-old boy who presented with left vision loss. Axial precontrast (*A*) and axial (*B*), sagittal (*C*), and coronal (*D*) postcontrast T1-weighted images of the orbits show an enhancing mass (*blue arrows*) compressing the intracanalicular segment of the left optic nerve (*yellow arrow*).

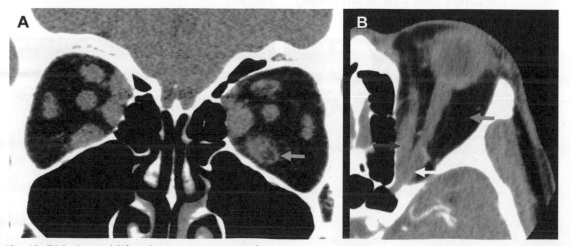

Fig. 10. TAO. Coronal (*A*) and axial (*B*) CT images show diffuse enlargement of the extraocular muscles relatively sparing the lateral rectus muscle. Hypodensity with the left inferior rectus (*blue arrow*) represents presence of glycoaminoglycans. The left optic nerve (*white arrow*) is stretched by increased intraorbital fat (*green arrow*) and compressed by the enlarged medial rectus (*red arrow*).

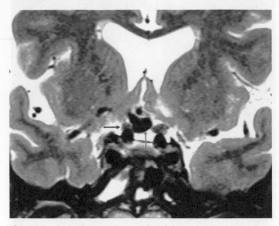

Fig. 11. Anterior communicating artery aneurysm causing compressive optic neuropathy. Coronal T2-weighted image shows compression of the right prechiasmatic optic nerve (*red arrow*) by the anterior communicating artery aneurysm (*blue arrow*).

Meningiomas

Meningiomas are the second most common neoplasms in the sellar/parasellar regions after pituitary adenomas.[58] Meningiomas can compress the optic chiasm causing progressive vision loss and optic atrophy because of their slow growth rate. Large anterior skull base meningiomas near the optic canal can compress the ipsilateral optic nerve leading to optic nerve atrophy and contralateral papilledema because of increased intracranial pressure (Foster Kennedy syndrome).[2] On CT, meningiomas are typically hyperdense, partially calcified, and homogenously enhancing.[59] Hyperostosis of the adjacent bone, dural tail sign, and pneumosinus dilatans (hyperpneumatized paranasal sinus) can also be seen but are not specific.[60,61] The tumors have variable MR imaging

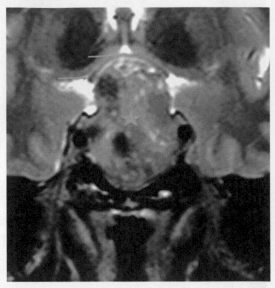

Fig. 13. Pituitary macroadenomas. Coronal T2-weighted imaging of the sella demonstrated a pituitary macroadenoma (*star*) causing elevation and stretching of the chiasm (*blue arrows*), resulting in bitemporal hemianopsia.

signal with homogenous enhancement.[60] MR imaging is very helpful for evaluating optic chiasm compression and cerebral edema. Even though imaging findings of meningiomas may overlap with those of macroadenomas, separation of the tumors from the normal-appearing pituitary gland by the diaphragma sella suggests the diagnosis of meningiomas (Fig. 16).

Meningiomas also tend to have serrated margins, whereas macroadenomas, lymphocytic hypophysitis, and sarcoidosis have variable smooth margin.

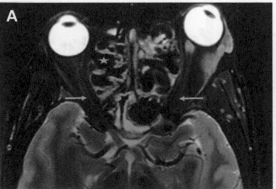
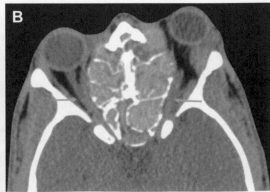

Fig. 12. AFS causing compressive optic neuropathy. Axial fat-suppressed T2-weighted (*A*) and axial noncontrast CT (*B*) images demonstrate AFS of the ethmoid and sphenoid sinuses with sinus expansion compressing on the bilateral optic nerves (*blue arrows*). The sinuses are filled with hyperdense material seen on CT and signal void on T2-weighted image (*star*), a characteristic imaging finding of AFS.

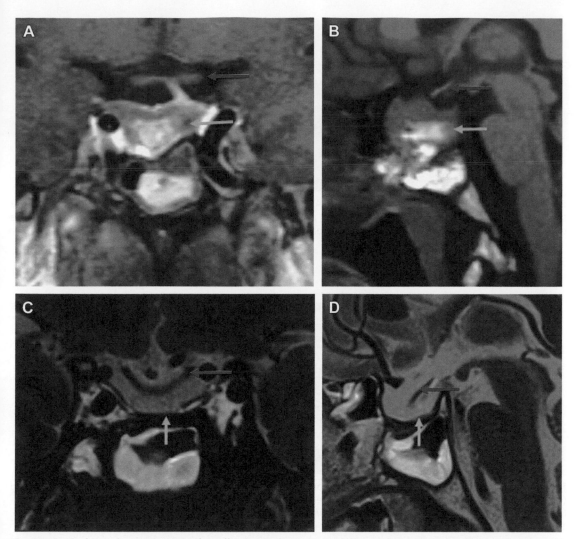

Fig. 14. Optic chiasm herniation into the sella. Coronal postcontrast T1-weighted (*A*) and sagittal precontrast T1-weighted (*B*) images of the sella show a pituitary prolactinoma (*blue arrow*) after surgery with chiasm (*red arrow*) in a normal location. Three years after bromocriptine therapy, coronal (*C*) and sagittal (*D*) T2-weighted images revealed that the tumor is markedly decreased in size with only a small amount of tissue evident along the sellar floor (*blue arrow*). The chiasm (*red arrow*) was herniated inferiorly into the enlarged partially empty sella.

Aneurysms

Large or giant (>2.5 cm) aneurysms of the cavernous/ophthalmic/supraclinoid internal carotid arteries can compress the optic chiasm.[62] With superomedial growth of the aneurysms, the anterolateral aspect of the chiasm is a common location to be affected, leading to asymmetric visual field defects.[2] Fluctuation of symptoms, rapid progression, or improvement suggest aneurysms as the cause rather than other mass lesions.[63] On MR imaging, the aneurysms typically show flow void with pulsation artifacts along the phase-

encoding direction (**Fig. 17**). Partially thrombosed aneurysms may demonstrate heterogeneous signal on T1- and T2-weighted images depending on stages of blood components. Rim calcifications can be seen along the aneurysmal walls.

Craniopharyngiomas

Craniopharyngiomas are locally invasive benign epithelial tumors arising from the Rathke pouch remnants.[64] Typically the tumors grow from the suprasellar region and then extend to the sella. Visual field defects are secondary to compression or

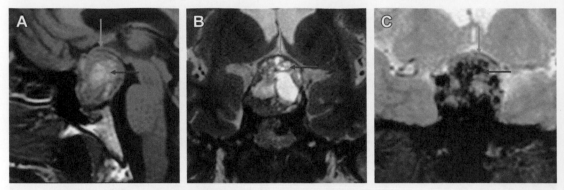

Fig. 15. Pituitary apoplexy. Sagittal T1-weighted (*A*), coronal T2-weighted (*B*), and coronal GRE (*C*) images of the sella show subacute hemorrhage (*red arrows*) in a pituitary macroadenoma with elevation and stretching of the chiasm (*blue arrows*). The hemorrhage is hypointense on GRE sequence (*C*).

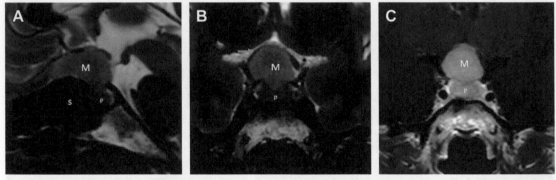

Fig. 16. Meningioma. Sagittal T2-weighted (*A*), coronal T2-weighted (*B*), and coronal postcontrast T1-weighted (*C*) images of the sella show a planum sphenoidale meningioma (M) with pneumosinus dilatans (S) and suprasellar extension causing mass effect on the chiasm (*blue arrow*) resulting in bitemporal homonymous hemianopsia. The normal-appearing pituitary gland (P) is separated from the tumor by the diaphragma sella (*red arrow*).

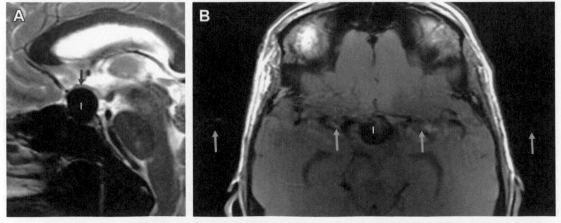

Fig. 17. Internal carotid aneurysm. Sagittal T2-weighted (*A*) and axial T1-weighted (*B*) images of the brain show a supraclinoid internal carotid aneurysm (I) with characteristic signal void and pulsation artifacts (*blue arrows*) in the phase-encoding direction. The chiasm (*red arrow*) is elevated.

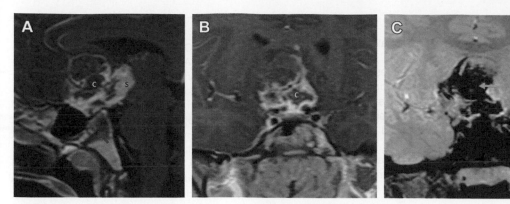

Fig. 18. Craniopharyngioma. Postcontrast sagittal (*A*), coronal (*B*) T1-weighted, and coronal GRE (*C*) images of the sella show a complex suprasellar mass containing enhancing solid (S), nonenhancing cystic (C), and hemorrhagic (*blue arrow*) components in an adolescent boy (open sphenooccipital synchondrosis [*red arrow*]).

invasion of the chiasms.[2] The tumors have bimodal peaks of incidence: second and sixth decades. The adamantinomatous type tends to occur in children, whereas the squamous papillary type is seen in adults.[65] Imaging findings are characteristic and reflective of the tumor components (**Fig. 18**). The cystic parts may show T1 hyperintensity because of machine-oil-appearing fluid, proteins, cholesterol, and blood products.[66] Solid components are variably enhancing. Calcifications are T2/GRE hypointense and dense on CT. Recurrence is common because of adherence of tumors to the surrounding structures.

Chiasmal-hypothalamic gliomas

Chiasmal-hypothalamic gliomas have a worse clinical course and prognosis than isolated ONGs because of associated endocrine/hypothalamic dysfunction.[2] Involvement of the third ventricle can lead to hydrocephalus. Size, growth, extension, and location of the tumors may not correlate with visual impairment.[67] On imaging, the tumors are best evaluated on the coronal view. The tumors are typically hyperintense on T2-weighted images, isointense to hypointense on T1-weighted images, and may enhance (**Fig. 19**). Extension into the optic nerve and tracts may be seen.[68]

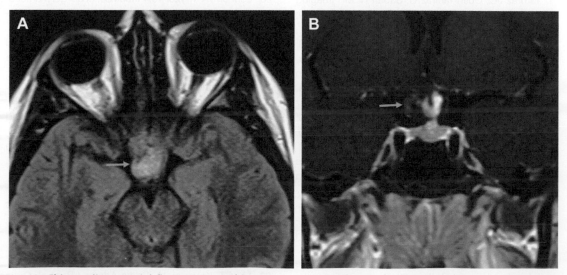

Fig. 19. Chiasm glioma. Axial fluid-attenuated inversion recovery (*A*) and postcontrast coronal T1-weighted (*B*) images show enlargement and partially enhancing mass (*blue arrows*) of the chiasm in a patient who has chronic painless vision loss without neurofibromatosis.

SUMMARY

Advance in neuroimaging, especially MR imaging, can reveal pathologic conditions previously detected only clinically. Some entities have imaging characteristics leading to appropriate treatment without the need for tissue biopsies. These entities include acute optic neuritis, ischemic optic neuropathy, OPGs, aneurysms, and pituitary adenomas, among others. Imaging also provides disease surveillance and posttreatment assessment, with CT and MR imaging being complementary to each other.

ACKNOWLEDGMENTS

The authors would love to acknowledge the diligent help of Dr Fang Yu for editorial assistance and diagram preparation and Dr Achint Singh for some images.

REFERENCES

1. Liu GT, Volpe NJ, Galetta SL. Visual loss: optic neuropathies. In: Liu GT, Volpe NJ, Galetta SL, editors. Neuro-ophthalmology diagnosis and management. 2nd edition. New York: Saunders Elsevier; 2010. p. 103–98.

2. Liu GT, Volpe NJ, Galetta SL. Visual loss: disorders of the chiasm. In: Liu GT, Volpe NJ, Galetta SL, editors. Neuro-ophthalmology diagnosis and management. 2nd edition. New York: Saunders Elsevier; 2010. p. 237–91.

3. Kupfer C, Chumbley L, Downer JC. Quantitative histology of optic nerve, optic tract and lateral geniculate nucleus of man. J Anat 1967;101(Pt 3):393–401.

4. Tamraz JC, Outin-Tamraz C, Saban R. MR imaging of the optic pathways. Radiol Clin North Am 1999; 37(1):1–36.

5. Griessenauer CJ, Raborn J, Mortazavi MM, et al. Relationship between the pituitary stalk angle in prefixed, normal, and postfixed optic chiasmata: an anatomic study with microsurgical application. Acta Neurochir (Wien) 2014;156(1):147–51.

6. McCollough CH, Zink FE. Performance evaluation of a multi-slice CT system. Med Phys 1999;26(11): 2223–30.

7. Bilaniuk LT, Atlas SW, Zimmerman RA. Magnetic resonance imaging of the orbit. Radiol Clin North Am 1987;25(3):509–28.

8. Hendrix LE, Kneeland JB, Haughton VM. MR imaging of optic nerve lesions: value of gadopentetate dimeglumine and fat suppression technique. AJNR Am J Neuroradiol 1990;11:749–54.

9. Mathur S, Karimi A, Mafee MF. Acute optic nerve infarction demonstrated by diffusion-weighted imaging in a case of rhinocerebral mucormycosis. Am J Neuroradiol 2007;28(3):489–90.

10. The clinical profile of optic neuritis. Experience of the Optic Neuritis Treatment Trial. Optic, Neuritis Study Group. Arch Ophthalmol 1991;109(12):1673–8.

11. Rizzo JF 3rd, Andreoli CM, Rabinov JD. Use of magnetic resonance imaging to differentiate optic neuritis and nonarteritic anterior ischemic optic neuropathy. Ophthalmology 2002;109(9):1679–84.

12. Dunker S, Wiegand W. Prognostic value of magnetic resonance imaging in monosymptomatic optic neuritis. Ophthalmology 1996;103(11):1768–73.

13. Optic Neuritis Study Group. Multiple sclerosis risk after optic neuritis: final optic neuritis treatment trial follow-up. Arch Neurol 2008;65(6):727–32.

14. Optic Neuritis Study Group. High- and low-risk profiles for the development of multiple sclerosis within 10 years after optic neuritis: experience of the optic neuritis treatment trial. Arch Ophthalmol 2003; 121(7):944–9.

15. Brex PA, Ciccarelli O, O'Riordan JI, et al. A longitudinal study of abnormalities on MRI and disability from multiple sclerosis. N Engl J Med 2002;17(346):3.

16. Beck RW, Cleary PA, Trobe JD, et al. The effect of corticosteroids for acute optic neuritis on the subsequent development of multiple sclerosis. The Optic Neuritis Study Group. N Engl J Med 1993;9(329):1764–9.

17. Wingerchuk DM, Lennon VA, Pittock SJ, et al. Revised diagnostic criteria for neuromyelitis optica. Neurology 2006;66(10):1485–9.

18. Wingerchuk DM, Lennon VA, Pittock SJ, et al. Revised diagnostic criteria for neuromyelitis optica. Neurology 2006;23(10):1485–9.

19. Tackley G, Kuker W, Palace J. Magnetic resonance imaging in neuromyelitis optica. Mult Scler 2014; 20(9):1153–64.

20. Lennon VA, Kryzer TJ, Pittock SJ, et al. IgG marker of optic-spinal multiple sclerosis binds to the aquaporin-4 water channel. J Exp Med 2005;202(4):473–7.

21. Sato DK, Lana-Peixoto MA, Fujihara K, et al. Clinical spectrum and treatment of neuromyelitis optica spectrum disorders: evolution and current status. Brain Pathol 2013;23(6):647–60.

22. Pakdaman MN, Sepahdari AR, Elkhamary SM. Orbital inflammatory disease: pictorial review and differential diagnosis. World J Radiol 2014;28(6):4.

23. Hayreh SS. Ischemic optic neuropathies-where are we now? Graefes Arch Clin Exp Ophthalmol 2013; 251(8):1873–84.

24. Bhatt NP, Morales RE, Mathews MK. MRI findings in post-operative bilateral posterior ischemic optic neuropathy. Open J Ophthalmol 2013;3:51–3.

25. Nickels TJ, Manlapaz MR, Farag E. Perioperative visual loss after spine surgery. World J Orthop 2014; 18(5):100–6.

26. Liu GT, Katowitz JA, Rorke-Adams LB, et al. Optic pathway gliomas: neoplasms, not hamartomas. JAMA Ophthalmol 2013;131(5):646–50.

27. Housepian EM, Chi TL. Neurofibromatosis and optic pathways gliomas. J Neurooncol 1993;15(1):51–5.

28. Avery RA, Fisher MJ, Liu GT. Optic pathway gliomas. J Neuroophthalmol 2011;31(3):269–78.

29. Segal L, Darvish-Zargar M, Dilenge ME, et al. Optic pathway gliomas in patients with neurofibromatosis type 1: follow-up of 44 patients. J AAPOS 2010; 14(2):155–8.

30. Tailor TD, Gupta D, Dalley RW, et al. Orbital neoplasms in adults: clinical, radiologic, and pathologic review. Radiographics 2013;33(6):1739–58.

31. Nair AG, Pathak RS, Iyer VR, et al. Optic nerve glioma: an update. Int Ophthalmol 2014;34(4): 999–1005.

32. Dutton JJ. Optic nerve sheath meningiomas. Surv Ophthalmol 1992;37:167–83.

33. Wright JE, McNab AA, McDonald WI. Primary optic nerve sheath meningioma. Br J Ophthalmol 1989; 73:960–6.

34. Cunliffe IA, Moffat DA, Hardy DG, et al. Bilateral optic nerve sheath meningiomas in a patient with neurofibromatosis type 2. Br J Ophthalmol 1992; 76(5):310–2.

35. Harold Lee HB, Garrity JA, Cameron JD, et al. Primary optic nerve sheath meningioma in children. Surv Ophthalmol 2008;53(6):543–58.

36. Schick U, Dott U, Hassler W. Surgical management of meningiomas involving the optic nerve sheath. J Neurosurg 2004;101:951–9.

37. Zimmerman CF, Schatz NJ, Glaser JS. Magnetic resonance imaging of optic nerve meningiomas. Enhancement with gadolinium-DTPA. Ophthalmology 1990;97(5):585–91.

38. Berman D, Miller NR. New concepts in the management of optic nerve sheath meningiomas. Ann Acad Med Singap 2006;35(3):168–74.

39. Mafee MF, Goodwin J, Dorodi S. Optic nerve sheath meningiomas. Role of MR imaging. Radiol Clin North Am 1999;37(1):37–58.

40. Thakar A, Lal P, Dhiwakar M, et al. Optic nerve compression in allergic fungal sinusitis. J Laryngol Otol 2011;125(4):381–5.

41. Bahn RS. Graves' ophthalmopathy. N Engl J Med 2010;362:726–38.

42. Wiersinga WM, Smit T, van der Gaag R, et al. Temporal relationship between onset of Graves' ophthalmopathy and onset of thyroidal Graves' disease. J Endocrinol Invest 1988;11:615–9.

43. Kahaly GJ. Imaging in thyroid-associated orbitopathy. Eur J Endocrinol 2001;145:107–18.

44. Melcescu E, Horton WB, Kim D, et al. Graves orbitopathy: update on diagnosis and therapy. Southampt Med J 2014;107(1):34–43.

45. Mayer EJ, Fox DL, Herdman G, et al. Signal intensity, clinical activity and cross-sectional areas on MRI scans in thyroid eye disease. Eur J Radiol 2005; 56:20–4.

46. Chang JH, Lee DK, Kim BT, et al. Computed tomographic angiogram of an anterior communicating artery aneurysm causing acute retrobulbar optic neuropathy: a case report. Korean J Ophthalmol 2011;25(5):366–8.

47. Chan JW, Hoyt WF, Ellis WG, et al. Pathogenesis of acute monocular blindness from leaking anterior communicating artery aneurysms: report of six cases. Neurology 1997;48(3):680–3.

48. Kim YS, Kim K, Lee JG, et al. Paranasal sinus mucoceles with ophthalmologic manifestations: a 17-year review of 96 cases. Am J Rhinol Allergy 2011;25(4):272.

49. Rothstein J, Maisel RH, Berlinger NT, et al. Relationship of optic neuritis to disease of the paranasal sinuses. Laryngoscope 1984;94:1501–8.

50. Abboud CF, Laws EJ. Diagnosis of pituitary tumors. Endocrinol Metab Clin North Am 1988;17: 241–80.

51. Boxerman JL, Rogg JM, Donahue JE, et al. Preoperative MRI evaluation of pituitary macroadenoma: imaging features predictive of successful transsphenoidal surgery. AJR Am J Roentgenol 2010;195(3): 720–8.

52. Raverot G, Jacob M, Jouanneau E, et al. Secondary deterioration of visual field during cabergoline treatment for macroprolactinoma. Clin Endocrinol (Oxf) 2009;70(4):588–92.

53. Jones SE, James RA, Hall K, et al. Optic chiasmal herniation-an under recognized complication of dopamine agonist therapy for macroprolactinoma. Clin Endocrinol (Oxf) 2000;53(4):529–34.

54. Murad-Kejbou S, Eggenberger E. Pituitary apoplexy: evaluation, management, and prognosis. Curr Opin Ophthalmol 2009;20(6):456–61.

55. Nawa R, AbdelMannan D, Selman W, et al. Pituitary tumor apoplexy: a review. J Intensive Care Med 2008;23:75–90.

56. Tosaka M, Sato N, Hirato J, et al. Assessment of hemorrhage in pituitary macroadenoma by T2-weighted gradient echo MR imaging. AJNR Am J Neuroradiol 2007;28:2023–9.

57. Jho DH, Biller BM, Agarwalla PK, et al. Pituitary apoplexy: large surgical series with grading syste. World Neurosurg 2014;82(5):781–90.

58. Johnsen DE, Woodruff WW, Allen IS. MR imaging of the sellar and juxtasellar regions. Radiographics 1991;11:727–58.

59. Zee C, Go J, Kim P, et al. Imaging of the pituitary and parasellar region. Neurosurg Clin N Am 2003; 14:55–80.

60. Pisaneschi M, Kapoor G. Imaging the sella and parasellar region. Neuroimaging Clin N Am 2005;15(1): 203–19.

61. Miller NR, Golnik KC, Zeidman SM, et al. Pneumosinus dilatans: a sign of intracranial meningioma. Surg Neurol 1996;46(5):471–4.

62. Kasner SE, Liu GT, Galetta ST. Neuro-ophthalmo-logic aspects of aneurysms. Neuroimaging Clin N Am 1997;7:679–92.

63. Kupersmith MJ. Aneurysms involving the motor and sensory visual pathways. In: Kupersmith MJ, editor. Neurovascular neuroophthalmology. Berlin: Springer-Verlag; 1993. p. 239–99.

64. Prabhu VC, Brown HG. The pathogenesis of cra-niopharyngiomas. Childs Nerv Syst 2005;21(8–9): 622–7.

65. Adamson TE, Wiestler OD, Kleihues P, et al. Correla-tion of clinical and pathological features in surgically

66. Elster AD. Modern imaging of the pituitary. Radi-ology 1993;187:1–14.

67. Fletcher WA, Imes RK, Hoyt WF. Chiasmal gliomas: appearance and long-term changes demonstrated by computerized tomography. J Neurosurg 1986; 65:154–9.

68. Kumar J, Kumar A, Sharma R, et al. Magnetic reso-nance imaging of sellar and suprasellar pathology: a pictorial review. Curr Probl Diagn Radiol 2007;36(6): 227–36.

Imaging of Retrochiasmal and Higher Cortical Visual Disorders

Bundhit Tantiwongkosi, MD[a,b,c,*],
Noriko Salamon, MD, PhD[d]

KEYWORDS

- MR imaging • Optic tract • Optic radiation • Lateral geniculate nucleus • Striate cortex
- Visual cortex • Visual association areas

KEY POINTS

- Retrochiasmal visual pathways include optic tracts, lateral geniculate nuclei, optic radiations, and striate cortex.
- Homonymous hemianopsia and field defect variants with relatively normal visual acuity suggest that the lesions are in retrochiasmatic areas.
- Higher visual association areas (VAA) interpret visual information from the primary visual cortex, resulting in perception of objects, faces, colors, and orientation.
- Each VAA has a specific function.
- Lesions involving VAA produce impairment of the specific abnormal visual perception despite normal visual fields.

INTRODUCTION

The retrochiasmal (or retrochiasmatic) visual pathways consist of the optic tracts, lateral geniculate nuclei (LGN), optic radiations (ORs), and striate cortex (primary visual cortex). Diseases involving the retrochiasmal visual pathway typically result in contralateral homonymous hemianopsia with relatively intact visual acuity.[1] The primary visual cortex (V1) projects information to the higher visual cortex or visual association areas (V2, V3, and so forth), where more complex visual perceptions are processed.[2] Patients suffering from higher cortical dysfunction may have specific visual perception abnormalities including achromatopsia, prosopagnosia, and Balint syndrome, despite normal visual acuity and fields.[3] This article elucidates the anatomy and pathology of diseases affecting these particular visual pathways, focusing on imaging and clinical correlation.

NORMAL ANATOMY
Optic Tract

Each optic tract is composed of ipsilateral temporal fibers and contralateral nasal fibers; therefore, it corresponds to the contralateral visual hemi-field (ie, the left optic tract corresponds to the right

Disclosures: None.
[a] Division of Neuroradiology, Department of Radiology, University of Texas Health Science Center San Antonio, 7703 Floyd Curl Drive, Mail Code 7800, San Antonio, TX 78229, USA; [b] Division of Neuroradiology, Department of Otolaryngology Head Neck Surgery, University of Texas Health Science Center San Antonio, 7703 Floyd Curl Drive, Mail Code 7800, San Antonio, TX 78229, USA; [c] Imaging Service, South Texas Veterans, 7400 Merton Minter, San Antonio, TX 78229, USA; [d] Division of Neuroradiology, Department of Radiology, University of California Los Angeles, 757 Westwood Plaza, Suite 1621D, Los Angeles, CA 90095, USA
* Corresponding author. 7703 Floyd Curl Drive, Mail Code 7800, San Antonio, TX 78229.
E-mail address: tantiwongkos@uthscsa.edu

Neuroimag Clin N Am 25 (2015) 411–424
http://dx.doi.org/10.1016/j.nic.2015.05.005
1052-5149/15/$ – see front matter Published by Elsevier Inc.

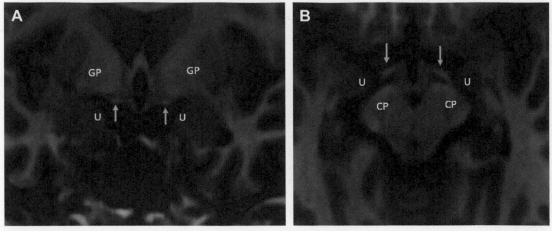

Fig. 1. Optic tract anatomy. Coronal (*A*) and axial (*B*) T1-weighted images show anatomy of the optic tracts (*blue arrows*). Optic tracts are ventral to globus pallidus (GP), medial to the uncus (U), and anterior to the cerebral peduncles (CP).

visual field and vice versa).[1] The optic tract projects posterolaterally. It is ventral to the rostral midbrain, globus pallidus, and thalamus; anterior to the cerebral peduncle; and medial to the uncus (**Fig. 1**).[1,4] Most of the fibers terminate in the LGN with some synapsing at the pretectal nuclei, which is responsible for the pupillary light reflex.[1]

Lateral Geniculate Nucleus

LGN is one of the thalamic nuclei and contains six neuronal layers that receive visual input from the optic tracts. Layers 2, 3, and 5 receive input from the ipsilateral eye, and layers 1, 4, and 6 receive input from the contralateral eye. Visual information

is projected to the striate cortex via OR. The LGN has characteristic anatomy on MR imaging, best visualized on coronal thin-cut three-dimensional T1-weighted images, showing it located superior to the ambient cistern and superomedial to the hippocampal body (**Fig. 2**).[5,6]

Optic Radiations

ORs (see Fig. 4 of Advanced MR Imaging of the Visual Pathway) are white matter tracts connecting LGN and striate cortex. Each OR contains three bundles: (1) dorsal, (2) central, and (3) anterior (Meyer loop).[7] The dorsal bundle is located in the parietal lobe, carrying information from the

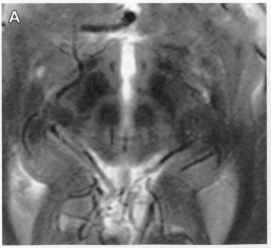
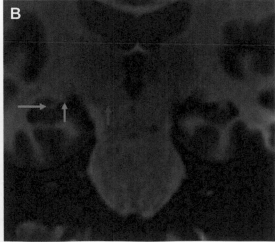

Fig. 2. LGN (*blue arrow*). Axial T2-weighted (*A*) and coronal T1-weighted (*B*) images show characteristic appearance and location of LGN. It is a small bulging gray matter located superomedial to the hippocampal body (*green arrow*) at the level of red nucleus (*red arrow*).

lower visual field, and terminates in the striate cortex superior to the calcarine sulcus. The central bundle and Meyer loop are found in the temporal lobe, carrying information from the superior visual field to the striate cortex, inferior to the calcarine sulcus.[7] Meyer loop is prone to damage from anterior temporal lobectomies because of its course along the anterior aspect of the temporal horn.[8]

Striate Cortex

The striate cortex is located in the medial aspect of the occipital lobe (Fig. 3), serving as the primary visual area (Brodmann area 17 or V1). It demonstrates retinotopic organization, with each retinal ganglion cell having a specific projection on striate cortex, preserving point-to-point mapping.[2] The occipital tip corresponds to central (macular) vision, whereas the more anterior regions correspond to peripheral vision.[9] The peripheral visual areas are supplied by the posterior cerebral arteries (PCA), whereas the central visual area (occipital tip) has a dual arterial supply from the PCA and middle cerebral arteries (MCA).[1]

Visual Association Areas

Area V1 receives basic visual information from the retina via geniculostriate pathways. Complex visual analysis occurs in visual association areas, which initially receive input from area V1.[10] Areas V2 (Brodmann area 18) and V3 (Brodmann area 19) are situated immediately anterior to V1.[11] Higher visual cortical processing is complex with extensive connections, and can be simplified as ventral occipitotemporal and dorsal occipitoparietal pathways (Fig. 4).[10]

The ventral pathway is located in the inferior aspect of the occipitotemporal lobes and contains area V4 (fusiform and lingual gyri). The ventral stream through area V4 represents color, shape, pattern, facial, and object recognition ("what" pathway).[12] The dorsal stream is located in the lateral surface of the occipitotemporal lobes (area V5) and parietal lobes, and is responsible for spatial orientation, motion, and visual attention ("where" pathway).[12,13] Another important aspect of higher visual analysis is the ability to precisely perceive multiple stimuli presented in sequential orders, to plan, and to react to

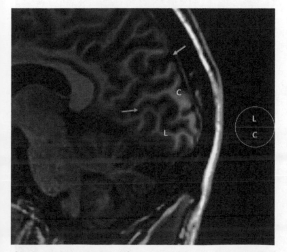

Fig. 3. Striate cortex. The striate cortex is separated from the parietal lobe by the parieto-occipital sulcus (*blue arrow*) and is divided into cuneus (C) and lingual cortex (L) by the calcarine sulcus (*green arrow*) as demonstrated on this sagittal T1-weighted image. The cuneus corresponds to the lower hemifield, whereas the lingual cortex corresponds to the upper hemifield as indicated in the *white circle*.

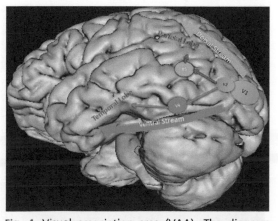

Fig. 4. Visual association area (VAA). The diagram represents dorsal and ventral streams of the higher visual cortical function. The ventral steam or "what" pathway is located in the inferior aspect of the occipitotemporal lobe and receives primary visual input from V1 and V2 via V4. The dorsal stream or "where" pathway is located in the parietal lobe and receives primary visual input from V1 and V2 via V5. (*Data from* Girkin CA, Miller NR. Central disorders of vision in humans. Surv Ophthalmol 2001;45:379–495.)

potential threats, a so-called "when" pathway. Recently, researchers have found areas in the right parietal lobe, temporoparietal junction, and area V5 to be responsible for this crucial temporal discrimination role.[14–17]

PATHOLOGY
Optic Tract

Isolated diseases of the optic tract are rare, and most lesions are contiguous with the optic chiasm including chiasmal neuritis, sarcoidosis, and

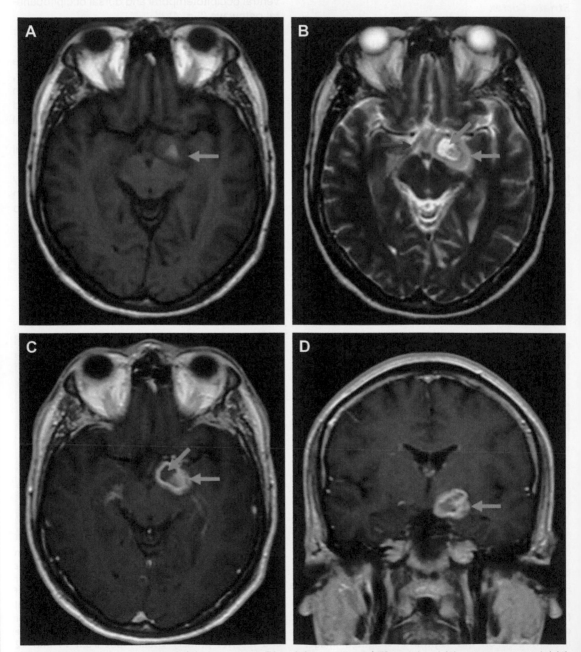

Fig. 5. Optic tract astrocytoma. Axial noncontrast T1-weighted (*A*), axial T2-weighted (*B*), postcontrast axial (*C*), and coronal (*D*) T1-weighted images show an enhancing mass (*green arrow*) involving the left optic tract. Internal nonenhancing T2 hyperintense area represents necrosis (*blue arrow*). The right optic tract (*red arrow*) is normal.

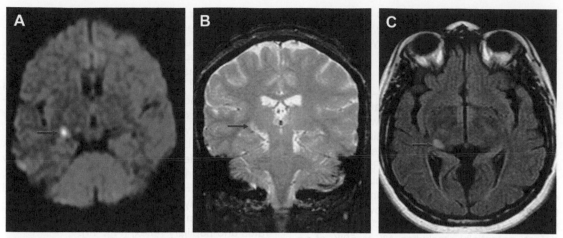

Fig. 6. Lateral geniculate nucleus infarction. Axial diffusion-weighted image (DWI) (*A*), coronal T2-gradient recalled echo (*B*), and axial fluid attenuated inversion recovery (FLAIR) (*C*) images of the brain show restricted diffusion with T2 and FLAIR hyperintensity of the right lateral geniculate nucleus (*pink arrow*).

glioma.[18] Optic tract infarction is unusual because optic tract receives dual arterial supply from the anterior choroidal and posterior communicating arteries.[19] Other neoplasms of optic tracts have been reported, including astrocytomas (**Fig 5**) and gangliogliomas.[20] Craniopharyngiomas[21] and dolichoectatic basilar artery[22] may compress the optic tracts.

Optic Tract Localization and Deep Brain Stimulation

Deep brain stimulation and pallidotomy are surgical treatment options for Parkinson disease. The target of deep brain stimulation and pallidotomy is the globus pallidus interna, which is situated immediately superior to the optic tracts. The use of MR imaging and neurophysiologic monitoring for stereotactic guidance allows for precise localization of the target and prevents damage to the optic tract.[4,23]

Lateral Geniculate Nucleus

A lesion involving only the LGN is very uncommon. However, a spectrum of diseases may involve LGN and produces contralateral homonymous

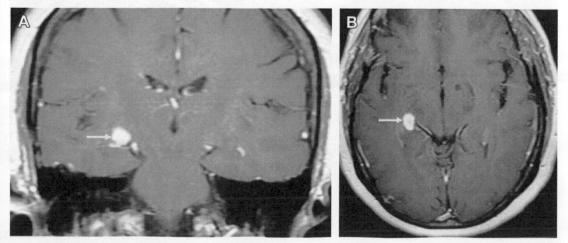

Fig. 7. Lateral geniculate nucleus astrocytoma. Postcontrast coronal (*A*) and axial (*B*) T1-weighted images of the brain demonstrate a vividly enhancing solid mass (*yellow arrow*) in the right lateral geniculate nucleus in a patient who was found to have left homonymous hemianopsia.

hemianopsia with characteristic sectoranopia. These include infarction (Fig. 6), astrocytomas (Fig. 7), metastasis, osmotic myelinolysis, and arteriovenous malformation.[24–28]

Optic Radiation

The most common pathology affecting OR is stroke of MCA distribution, followed by hemorrhage, neoplasm (Fig. 8), herpes simplex encephalitis, and postsurgical injury.[2,18] Lesions involving the parietal and temporal lobe ORs may result in inferior and superior quadrantanopia, respectively. Anterior temporal lobectomy is an effective surgery for temporal lobe epilepsy; however, damage of Meyer loop may lead to a "pie-in-the-sky" defect, potentially precluding 4% to 50% of patients from driving (Fig. 9).[8]

Striate Cortex

Strokes in the PCA distribution are the most common cause of occipital lobe hemianopia in

adults.[2] Other etiologies include hemorrhage, neoplasm, infection, trauma, progressive multifocal leukoencephalopathy, and posterior reversible encephalopathy syndrome.[18,29] For pediatric patients, trauma and neoplasm are the most common lesions.[29] Other less common causes include adrenoleukodystrophy, acute disseminated encephalomyelopathy, and periventricular leukomalacia, which have other associated clinical features.[2] Lesions involving the striate cortex superior or inferior to the calcarine sulcus may result in inferior or superior quadrantanopia, respectively (Fig. 10). Bilateral occipital lobe and OR lesions may lead to cortical or cerebral blindness (ie, vision loss despite normal optic apparatus and pupillary reflex) (Fig. 11).[2,29]

Higher Cortical Visual Disorders

Cerebral hemiachromatopsia

Damages of the ventromedial aspect of the occipitotemporal cortex (posterior fusiform and

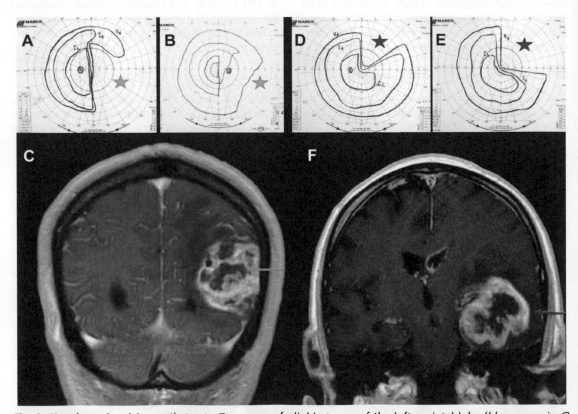

Fig. 8. Neoplasms involving optic tracts. Two cases of glioblastomas of the left parietal lobe (*blue arrow* in *C*) causing right incongruous inferior quadrantanopia (*blue star* in *A* and *B*) and left temporal lobe (*red arrow* in *F*) causing right incongruous superior quadrantanopia (*red star* in *D* and *E*). *A, B, D,* and *E* are visual field maps; *C* and *F* are postcontrast coronal T1-weighed images of the brain.

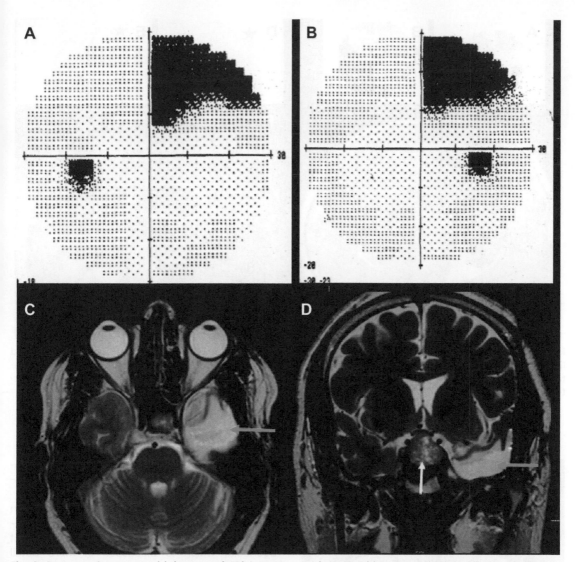

Fig. 9. Post anterior temporal lobectomy (ATL) in patient with intractable temporal lobe epilepsy. The patient developed contralateral "pie-in-the-sky" visual field defects as demonstrated in Humphrey visual field maps (*A*, left; *B*, right). Axial (*C*) and coronal (*D*) T2-weighted images of the brain show a resection cavity post ATL (*blue arrow*). There is an incidental pituitary macroadenoma (*yellow arrow*) that does not cause this type of visual field defect.

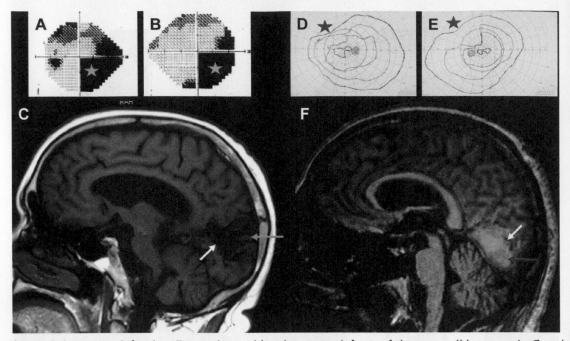

Fig. 10. Striate cortex infarction. Two patients with striate cortex infarcts of the cuneus (*blue arrow* in *C*) and lingual cortex (*red arrow* in *F*) causing inferior (*blue star* in *A* and *B*) and superior (*red star* in *D* and *E*) quadrantanopsia. The *white arrow* points to the calcarine sulcus that divides cuneus and lingual cortex of the striate cortex. *A, B, D,* and *E* are visual field maps. *C* and *D* are sagittal T1-weighted images.

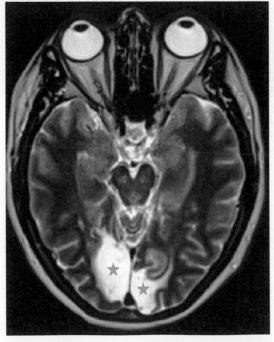

Fig. 11. Cortical blindness. Axial T2-weighted image of the brain shows remote infarcts of bilateral striate cortex (*stars*) resulting in cortical blindness. Optic apparatus and pupillary reflex are normal.

lingual gyri: area V4 complex) may result in deficits of color perception of the contralateral hemifield or hemiachromatosia.[30]

Many patients also have other visual perception symptoms (eg, homonymous superior quadrantanopia, pure alexia, prosopagnosia, and object agonosia, which is discussed in more detail later).[3,31,32] Severity varies from fading to completely devoid of colors ("black-and-white" pictures).[3] Infarction in the PCA territory is the most common cause (**Fig. 12**), followed by trauma, hemorrhage, neoplasms, encephalitis, arteriovenous malformation, posterior cortical atrophy, migraine, postictal status, and vertebrobasilar insufficiency.[33–36]

Prosopagnosia
Patients with prosopagnosia suffer from loss of recognition of familial faces, with either a defect in perception (apperceptive prosopagnosia) caused by damage in fusiform gyrus (**Fig. 12**) or an inability to match the perceived face with the stored memory (associative variant) because of damage in anterior temporal lobe.[37,38] The defect tends to be more severe in the setting of bilateral lesions. Again, most patients have associated homonymous hemianopia and hemiachromatopsia.

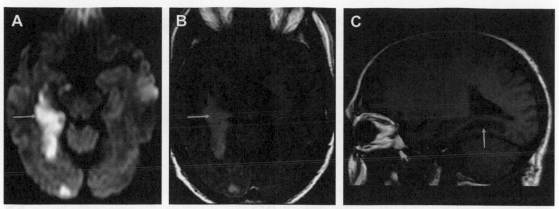

Fig. 12. Cerebral hemiachromatopsia and prosopagnosia. Axial DWI (*A*), FLAIR (*B*), and sagittal T1-weighted (*C*) images of the brain show acute infarction (*blue arrow*) of the ventromedial aspect of the temporal lobe (posterior fusiform gyrus) resulting in hemiachromatopsia and prosopagnosia.

Acquired etiologies are similar to those causing hemiachromatopsia. In the developmental form, there is no gross structural damage; instead it is thought to be secondary to neural and behavioral impairment.[39,40]

Balint syndrome

Balint syndrome consists of simultanagnosia (inability to interpret the full meaning of a complex scene despite intact ability to grasp individual components), optic ataxia (inability to reach for objects precisely because of visual-motor disconnection), and ocular apraxia (impairment of voluntary saccades despite normal involuntary saccadic reflex).[41–43] Lesions are localized to the bilateral occipitoparietal lobes (**Fig. 13**) caused by various pathologies including watershed cerebral infarction, Creutzfeldt-Jakob disease, reversible cerebral vasoconstriction syndrome, and Alzheimer disease.[2,43–45]

Visual hemi-inattention

Multiple areas of the brain are responsible for visual attention, such as the parietal lobe, frontal lobe, superior temporal gyrus, cingulate gyrus, basal ganglia, thalamus, and cerebellum with right-sided dominance.[2,46,47] The patient ignores stimuli of the affected hemifield despite a normal visual field. Potential causes include MCA territory infarction (**Fig. 14**), trauma, neoplasm, and progressive multifocal leukoencephalopathy.[2]

Pure alexia (alexia without agraphia)

Pure alexic patients suffer from an inability to read despite intact writing and lexical recognition.[3] The reading center resides in the left angular gyrus, which receives visual information from the bilateral striate cortex, via the splenium of the corpus callosum if the input comes from the right side.[48] The most common cause is a left PCA distribution infarction involving the left occipital lobe and left splenium of the corpus callosum, preventing transmission of visual input from the right occipital lobe to the left language cortex (including angular gyrus) (**Fig. 15**).

Posterior cortical atrophy

Posterior cortical atrophy is a rare neurodegenerative disorder affecting the posterior aspect of the cerebral cortex and connecting white matter, resulting in impairment of ventral and dorsal visual perception pathways, which typically precedes memory and executive impairment.[49] Alzheimer disease is the most common cause of posterior

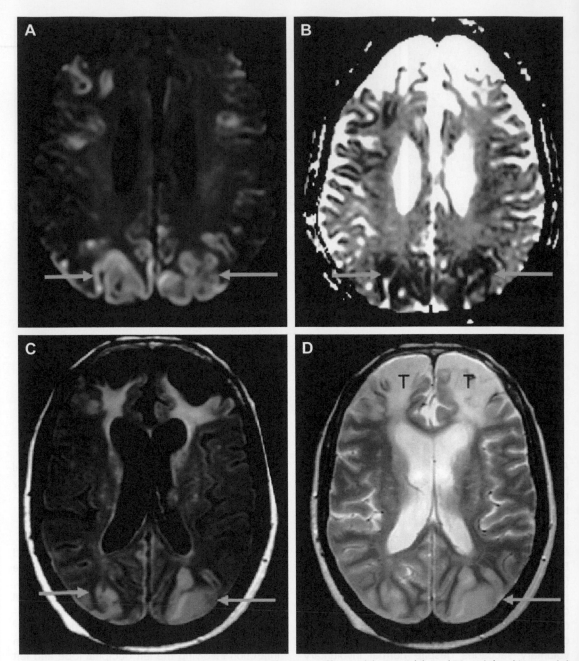

Fig. 13. Balint syndrome. Axial DWI (*A*), apparent diffusion coefficient (*B*), FLAIR (*C*), and T2-weighted images (*D*) of the brain show restricted diffusion with T2/FLAIR hyperintensity representing acute infarction of the bilateral parieto-occipital cortex (*blue arrows*) resulting in Balint syndrome in a patient who had cardiac arrest. Bifrontal encephlomalacia is secondary to remote traumatic brain injury (T).

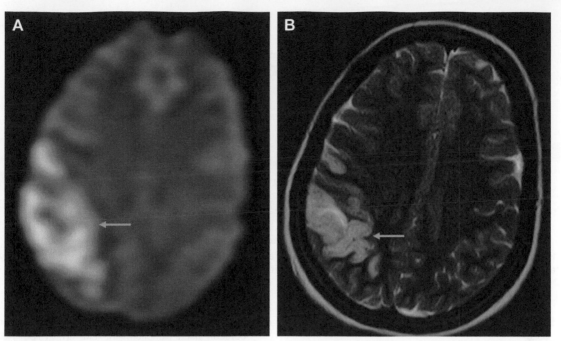

Fig. 14. Visual hemineglect. Axial DWI (A) and T2-weighted (B) images of the brain demonstrate restricted diffusion and T2 hyperintensity representing acute infarction of the right parietal lobe (*blue arrows*) resulting in left-sided visual neglect.

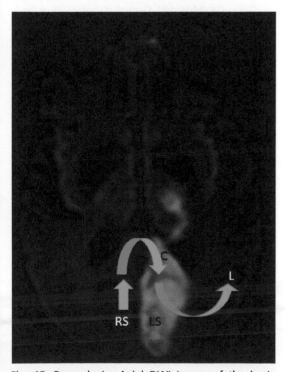

Fig. 15. Pure alexia. Axial DWI image of the brain shows restricted diffusion representing acute infarction of the left striate cortex (LS) and splenium of corpus callosum (C). Visual input from the right striate cortex (RS) is prevented from arriving at the language network of the left hemisphere (L) because of insult of the splenium of the corpus callosum. The patient was not able to read when a newspaper was presented in the left hemifield. His writing ability is intact (without agraphia).

cortical atrophy, and patients with posterior cortical atrophy are usually younger than patients with Alzheimer disease.[50,51] Visual perception defects of the ventral and dorsal pathways include visual agnosia, achromatopsia, alexia, simultanagnosia, and visual inattention.[52,53] The posterior portions of the cerebral cortex are atrophic (Fig. 16) with reduced integrity of the corresponding white matter tracts (inferior longitudinal fasciculus for ventral stream and superior longitudinal fasciculus for the dorsal stream) on diffusion tensor imaging.[54]

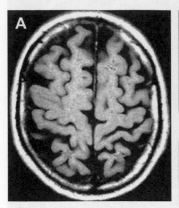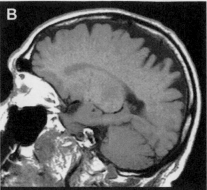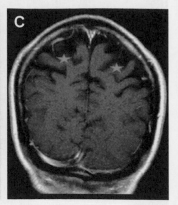

Fig. 16. Posterior cortical atrophy. Axial (A), sagittal (B), and coronal (C) T1-weighted images of the brain show atrophy of bilateral posterior parietal lobes (*blue stars*) in a patient who has visual neglect and dementia.

SUMMARY

Radiologists must scrutinize the contralateral retrochiasmal areas in patients presenting with homonymous hemianopsia. The optic tracts and LGN are typically involved by larger lesions from adjacent structures. The LGN is a small structure and difficult to identify on axial images; coronal thin-cut T1- and T2-weighted images are helpful in identifying the LGN based on its characteristic location. Common diseases involving the ORs and striated cortex are ischemic stroke, hemorrhage, neoplasms, and trauma.

The ventral or "what" pathway resides in the occipitotemporal lobes and is primarily responsible for color, shape, pattern, face, and object recognition. Damage to the ventral stream results in visual object agnosia, prosopagnosia, and achromatopsia. Spatial orientation and attention are controlled by the dorsal or "where" pathway in the occipitoparietal lobes. Balint syndrome, visual inattention, and pure alexia are examples of dorsal stream disorders. Posterior cortical atrophy can involve ventral and dorsal streams, often preceding dementia.

ACKNOWLEDGMENTS

The authors acknowledge the diligent help of Dr Fang Yu for editorial assistance and diagram preparation.

REFERENCES

1. Liu GT, Volpe NJ, Galetta SL. Retrochiasmal disorders. In: Liu GT, Volpe NJ, Galetta SL, editors. Neuro-ophthalmology diagnosis and management. 2nd edition. New York: Saunders Elsevier; 2010. p. 293–337.

2. Liu GT, Volpe NJ, Galetta SL. Disorders of higher cortical visual function. In: Liu GT, Volpe NJ, Galetta SL, editors. Neuro-ophthalmology diagnosis and management. 2nd edition. New York: Saunders Elsevier; 2010. p. 339–62.

3. Girkin CA, Miller NR. Central disorders of vision in humans. Surv Ophthalmol 2001;45:379–495.

4. Landi A, Pirillo D, Cilia R, et al. Cortical visual evoked potentials recorded after optic tract near field stimulation during GPi-DBS in non-cooperative patients. Clin Neurol Neurosurg 2011;113(2):119–22.

5. Horton JC, Landau K, Maeder P, et al. Magnetic resonance imaging of the human lateral geniculate body. Arch Neurol 1990;47:1201–6.

6. Fujita N, Tanaka H, Takanashi M, et al. Lateral geniculate nucleus. Anatomic and functional identification by use of MR imaging. Am J Neuroradiol 2001;22:1719–26.

7. Mandelstam SA. Challenges of the anatomy and diffusion tensor tractography of the Meyer loop. Am J Neuroradiol 2012;33(7):1204–10.

8. Winston GP. Epilepsy surgery, vision, and driving: what has surgery taught us and could modern imaging reduce the risk of visual deficits? Epilepsia 2013;54(11):1877–88.

9. Horton JC, Hoyt WF. The representation of the visual field in human striate cortex. A revision of the classic Holmes map. Arch Ophthalmol 1991;109:816–24.

10. Zeki S. The visual association cortex. Curr Opin Neurobiol 1993;3:155–9.

11. Zeki SM. The secondary visual areas of the monkey. Brain Res 1969;13:197–226.

12. Callaway EM. Structure and function of parallel pathways in the primate early visual system. J Physiol 2005;566:13–9.

13. De Renzi E. Disorders of spatial orientation. In: Vinken PJ, Bruyn GW, Klawans HL, editors. Handbook of clinical neurology. Amsterdam: Elsevier; 1985. p. 405–22.

14. Battelli L, Walsh V, Pascual-Leone A, et al. The 'when' parietal pathway explored by lesion studies. Curr Opin Neurobiol 2008;18(2):120–6.

15. Davis B, Christie J, Rorden C. Temporal order judgments activate temporal parietal junction. J Neurosci 2009;29(10):3182–8.

16. Spierer L, Bernasconi F, Grivel J. The temporoparietal junction as a part of the "when" pathway. J Neurosci 2009;29(27):8630–2.

17. Battelli L, Pascual-Leone A, Cavanagh P. The 'when' pathway of the right parietal lobe. Trends Cogn Sci 2007;11(5):204–10.

18. Zhang X, Kedar S, Lynn MJ. Homonymous hemianopias. Clinical-anatomic correlations in 904 cases. Neurology 2006;66:906–10.

19. Kupersmith MJ. Circulation of the eye, orbit, cranial nerves, and brain. In: Kupersmith MJ, editor. Neurovascular neuro-ophthalmology. Berlin: Springer-Verlag; 1993. p. 1–67.

20. Albayrak R, Albayram S, Port J, et al. Ganglioglioma of the right optic tract: case report and review of the literature. Magn Reson Imaging 2004;22(7):1047–51.

21. Nagahata M, Hosoya T, Kayama T, et al. Edema along the optic tract: a useful MR finding for the diagnosis of craniopharyngiomas. Am J Neuroradiol 1998;19(9):1753–7.

22. Guirgis MF, Lam BL, Falcone SF. Optic tract compression from dolichoectatic basilar artery. Am J Ophthalmol 2001;132(2):283–6.

23. Bulluss KJ, Pereira EA, Joint C, et al. Pallidotomy after chronic deep brain stimulation. Neurosurg Focus 2013;35(5):E5.

24. Shacklett DE, O'Connor PS, Dorwart RH, et al. Congruous and incongruous sectoral visual field defects with lesions of the lateral geniculate nucleus. Am J Ophthalmol 1984;98(3):283–90.

25. Goldman JE, Horoupian DS. Demyelination of the lateral geniculate nucleus in central pontine myelinolysis. Ann Neurol 1981;9(2):185–9.

26. Mulholland C, Best J, Rennie I, et al. Bilateral sectoranopia caused by bilateral geniculate body infarction in a 14-year-old boy with inflammatory bowel disease. J AAPOS 2010;14(5):435–7.

27. Wong SH, Briggs MC, Enevoldson TP. Quadruple sectoranopia due to lateral geniculate nucleus infarct. Pract Neurol 2010;10(3):167–8.

28. Grabe HM, Bapuraj JR, Wesolowski JR, et al. Homonymous hemianopia from infarction of the optic tract and lateral geniculate nucleus in deep cerebral venous thrombosis. J Neuroophthalmol 2012;32(1):38–41.

29. Kedar S, Zhang X, Lynn MJ, et al. Pediatric homonymous hemianopia. J AAPOS 2006;10(3):249–52.

30. Zeki S. A century of cerebral achromatopsia. Brain 1990;113:1721–77.

31. Freedman L, Costa L. Pure alexia and right hemiachromatopsia in posterior dementia. J Neurol Neurosurg Psychiatry 1992;55:500–2.

32. Damasio A, Yamada T, Damasio H, et al. Central achromatopsia. Behavioral, anatomic, and physiologic aspects. Neurology 1980;30:1064–71.

33. Paulson HL, Galetta SL, Grossman M, et al. Hemiachromatopsia of unilateral occipitotemporal infarcts. Am J Ophthalmol 1994;118:518–23.

34. Green GJ, Lessell S. Acquired cerebral dyschromatopsia. Arch Ophthalmol 1977;95:121–8.

35. Lapresle J, Metreau R, Annabi A. Transient achromatopsia in vertebrobasilar insufficiency. J Neurol 1977;215:155–8.

36. Lawden MC, Cleland PG. Achromatopsia in the aura of migraine. J Neurol Neurosurg Psychiatr 1993;56:708–9.

37. Davies-Thompson J, Pancaroglu R, Barton J. Acquired prosopagnosia: structural basis and processing impairments. Front Biosci (Elite Ed) 2014;5:159–74.

38. Barton JJ. Structure and function in acquired prosopagnosia: lessons from a series of 10 patients with brain damage. J Neuropsychol 2008;2(Pt):197–225.

39. Németh K, Zimmer M, Schweinberger SR, et al. The background of reduced face specificity of n170 in congenital prosopagnosia. PLoS One 2014;9(7):e101393.

40. Avidan G, Behrmann M. Impairment of the face processing network in congenital prosopagnosia. Front Biosci (Elite Ed) 2014;6:236–57.

41. Hausser CO, Robert F, Giard N. Balint's syndrome. Can J Neurol Sci 1980;7:157–61.

42. Balint R. Seelenlähmung des Schauens, optische Ataxie, räumliche Strörung der Aufmerksamkeit. Monatsschr Psychiatr Neurol 1909;25:51–81.

43. Walsh RD, Floyd JP, Eidelman BH, et al. Bálint syndrome and visual allochiria in a patient with reversible cerebral vasoconstriction syndrome. J Neuroophthalmol 2012;32(4):302–6.

44. Graff-Radford NR, Bolling JP, Earnest F IV, et al. Simultanagnosia as the initial sign of degenerative dementia. Mayo Clin Proc 1993;68(10):955–64.

45. Ances BM, Ellenbogen JM, Herman ST, et al. Balint syndrome due to Creutzfeldt–Jakob disease. Neurology 2004;63:395.

46. Hildebrandt H, Spang K, Ebke M. Visuospatial hemiinattention following cerebellar/brain stem bleeding. Neurocase 2002;8(4):323–9.

47. Weintraub S, Mesulam MM. Right cerebral dominance in spatial attention. Further evidence based on ipsilateral neglect. Arch Neurol 1987;44:621–5.

48. Petersen SE, Fox PT, Posner MI, et al. Positron emission tomographic studies of the cortical anatomy of single- word processing. Nature 1988;331:585–9.

49. Benson DF, Davis RJ, Snyder BD. Posterior cortical atrophy. Arch Neurol 1988;45:789–93.

50. Renner JA, Burns JM, Hou CE, et al. Progressive posterior cortical dysfunction: a clinicopathologic series. Neurology 2004;63:1175–80.

51. Migliaccio R, Agosta F, Rascovsky K, et al. Clinical syndromes associated with posterior atrophy: early age at onset AD spectrum. Neurology 2009;73: 1571–8.

52. Mendez MF. Visuospatial deficits with preserved reading ability in a patient with posterior cortical atrophy. Cortex 2001;37:535–43.

53. Ross SJ, Graham N, Stuart-Green L, et al. Progressive biparietal atrophy: an atypical presentation of Alzheimer's disease. J Neurol Neurosurg Psychiatry 1996;61:388–95.

54. Migliaccio R, Agosta F, Scola E, et al. Ventral and dorsal visual streams in posterior cortical atrophy: a DT MRI study. Neurobiol Aging 2012;33(11):2572–84.

Imaging of Ocular Motor Pathway

Bundhit Tantiwongkosi, MD[a,b,c,*], John R. Hesselink, MD[d]

KEYWORDS

- Eye movement • Diplopia • Ocular motor • Oculomotor nerve • Trochlear nerve • Abducens nerve

KEY POINTS

- Eye movement is controlled by cortical eye centers, brainstem nuclei, and ocular motor nerves that innervate the extra ocular muscles.
- Lesions in certain locations, such as the dorsal brainstem, cavernous sinuses, and superior orbital fissures, may produce localizing signs, which are very helpful for radiologists to focus on those anatomic regions.
- Some conditions are life threatening and require urgent or emergent imaging, including pupil-involving oculomotor palsy caused by posterior communicating artery aneurysms, cavernous sinus thrombosis, brainstem stroke, severe trauma, and so forth.

INTRODUCTION

To be able to follow a visual target in either vertical or horizontal directions in a slow or rapid manner (pursuit or saccade), both eyes need to move in a conjugate fashion. This movement is controlled by the cerebral cortex, vestibular system, multiple brainstem nuclei, and cranial nerves (CNs) that finally innervate the extraocular muscles, constituting ocular motor pathways. The diseases affecting these pathways may cause diplopia, ocular misalignment, nystagmus, eye movement restriction, and so forth. Clinical presentations can be highly localizing and help alert the radiologist to search for subtle lesions in specific locations. Some of these lesions have imaging characteristics that may help preclude unnecessary biopsies.

NORMAL ANATOMY
Oculomotor Nerve (Cranial Nerve III)

Oculomotor nuclear complex contains individual motor subnuclei and parasympathetic Edinger–

Westphal nuclei (EWN).[1] The motor nuclei are located in the dorsal aspect of the midbrain, ventral to the periaqueductal gray at the level of the superior colliculi (**Fig. 1**). The EWN are dorsomedial to the motor nuclei.[2] The nerve fascicles pass ventrally through the red nuclei and exit the midbrain at the medial aspect of the cerebral peduncles. The cisternal segments of the nerves are located in the interpeduncular/prepontine cisterns, between the posterior cerebral arteries (PCA) and superior cerebellar arteries (SCA). The nerves then pass medially to the uncus. The parasympathetic fibers are located in the periphery of the nerves; therefore, external compression (eg, posterior communicating aneurysms or uncal herniation) often cause pupil-involving CN III palsy. The short and variable dural cave segments are also surrounded by cerebrospinal fluid (CSF) before the nerves pierce the dura to become the interdural segments in the cavernous sinuses. Within the cavernous sinus, the nerves lie within the lateral walls, superior to CN IV.[3–5] The nerves

Disclosures: None.
[a] Division of Neuroradiology, Department of Radiology, University of Texas Health Science Center at San Antonio, 7703 Floyd Curl Drive, Mail Code 7800, San Antonio, TX 78229, USA; [b] Division of Neuroradiology, Department of Otolaryngology Head Neck Surgery, University of Texas Health Science Center at San Antonio, 7703 Floyd Curl Drive, Mail Code 7800, San Antonio, TX 78229, USA; [c] Imaging Service, South Texas Veterans, 7400 Merton Minter, San Antonio, TX 78229, USA; [d] Division of Neuroradiology, Department of Radiology, UCSD Medical Center, 200 West Arbor Drive, San Diego, CA 92103-8749, USA
* Corresponding author. 7703 Floyd Curl Drive, Mail Code 7800, San Antonio, TX 78229.
E-mail address: tantiwongkos@uthscsa.edu

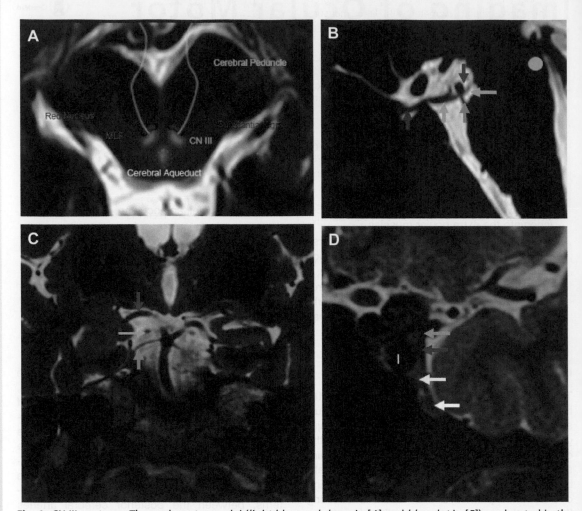

Fig. 1. CN III anatomy. The oculomotor nuclei (*light blue oval shape* in [A] and *blue dot* in [B]) are located in the dorsomedial aspect of the midbrain tegmentum at the level of superior colliculi and dorsal to the medial longitudinal fasciculus (MLF). The CN III fascicles (*blue line* in [A]) pass ventrally through the red nuclei. (*C*) The cisternal segments (*blue arrow*) are between the superior cerebellar (*green arrow*) and posterior cerebral (*pink arrow*) arteries. The dural cave segment (*brown arrow* in [B]) is distal to the posterior margin of the clivus and surrounded by CSF. (*D*) The cavernous segments of CN III (*orange arrow*), IV (*red arrow*), ophthalmic division of the trigeminal nerve or V1 (*yellow arrow*), and maxillary division of the trigeminal nerve or V2 (*white arrow*) lie lateral to the cavernous internal carotid artery (I), within the lateral wall of the cavernous sinus.

then exit anteriorly to enter the superior orbital fissures as foraminal segments. The extraforaminal segments enter the orbits and stay within the annulus of Zinn and intraconal spaces, where they divide into superior and inferior divisions to supply the extra-ocular muscles.[6,7]

Trochlear Nerve (Cranial Nerve IV)

CN IV is the smallest of the 3 ocular motor nerves, which poses challenges for neuroimaging. The trochlear nuclei are located in the dorsal midbrain, ventral to the periaqueductal gray at the level of the inferior colliculi (**Fig. 2**). The nerve

fascicles decussate within the superior medullary velum and exit the midbrain dorsally.[8] The long cisternal segments course within the quadrigeminal and ambient cisterns, inferior to the tentorial cerebelli free edge.[9] The dural cave segments are typically not visible on imaging.[6] Similar to CN III, the interdural segments (see **Fig. 1**D) are within the lateral walls of the cavernous sinuses, between CN III and ophthalmic division of the trigeminal nerve (CN V1). CN IV exits the cavernous sinuses to enter the superior aspect of the superior orbital fissures as the foraminal segments, before reaching the orbit superior to the annulus of Zinn.[6,7]

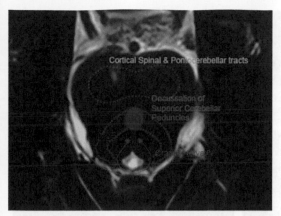

Fig. 2. CN IV anatomy. The trochlear nuclei (*orange dots*) are located in the dorsomedial aspect of the midbrain tegmentum at the level of inferior colliculi and dorsal to the medial longitudinal fasciculus (MLF). The fascicles (*orange line*) decussate dorsally and exit the midbrain as the cisternal segments (*orange line*) within the perimesencephalic cisterns.

Abducens Nerve (Cranial Nerve VI)

The abducens nuclei are located in the dorsomedial aspect of the caudal pons at the level of the facial colliculi, where the fascicular facial nerves loop around to the abducens nuclei (**Fig. 3**). The CN VI fascicles pass ventrally to exit the pons at the pontomedullary junction.[10] The cisternal segments ascend within the prepontine cistern before entering the dural cave where the nerves remain surrounded by CSF.[6,11] The interdural segments are divided into 2 subsegments, including the proximal petroclival and distal cavernous subsegments, where the nerves are surrounded by venous channels.[6] The cavernous segments (see **Fig. 1D**) are inferolateral to the cavernous internal carotid arteries and medial to the CN V1.[5]

Horizontal Conjugate Gaze

To be able to rapidly follow a visual target to the left side (leftward saccade), the right cortical eye fields (frontal, parietal, and supplementary eye fields) control the left omnipause neurons and the paramedian pontine reticular formation (PPRF). The latter activates the left abducens nucleus and the left lateral rectus via the left CN VI. The left abducens nucleus activates the right medial rectus subnucleus via the crossing medial longitudinal fasciculus (MLF) (**Fig. 4**). This activation results in simultaneous contraction of the left lateral rectus and the right medial rectus, leading to left conjugate saccade. Therefore, the left abducens nucleus controls the left lateral rectus and the right medial rectus. Lesions of the abducens nucleus cause ipsilateral conjugate gaze palsies,

whereas lesions of the MLF result in internuclear ophthalmoplegia (ie, inability to adduct the ipsilateral eye).[12]

Vertical Conjugate Gaze

The pretectal area (area in the midbrain rostral to the red nucleus) houses the vertical conjugate gaze center, which consists mainly of the interstitial nucleus of Cajal (INC), rostral interstitial nucleus of the MLF (riMLF), and the posterior commissure (**Fig. 5**). For downward gaze, the contralateral INC and the ipsilateral riMLF activate the inferior rectus subnucleus and the trochlear nucleus. Upward gaze occurs when each riMLF activates bilateral INC and ocular motor complex (superior rectus and inferior oblique subnuclei).[12]

IMAGING TECHNIQUE AND PROTOCOL

MR imaging is the technique of choice for depicting the anatomy and disease of the ocular motor pathways.[13] The nuclear and fascicular segments are not typically visualized discretely with 3-T MR imaging but can be localized in the expected location of the brainstem.[13] The cisternal and dural cave segments can be demonstrated on steady-state free precession (SSFP) imaging (eg, constructive interference in the steady state [CISS] or fast imaging employing steady-state acquisition [FIESTA] sequence), which yields heavily T2-weighted images. Acquiring images using thin-cut high-resolution 3-dimensional isotropic sequences enable reconstruction in multiple planes. It is reported that the interdural segment is better demonstrated on contrast-enhanced SSFP. In this sequence, the nonenhancing ocular motor nerves are seen within the lateral wall or inside of the enhancing cavernous sinuses.[14] Computed tomography (CT) and MR imaging are complementary in evaluating the foraminal segments, with CT being valuable in delineating the osseous margins of the foramina, skull base, and orbital walls.[15] Contrast-enhanced T1-weighted MR images help depict pathologic enhancement of the nerves.[6,13]

PATHOLOGY
Nuclear and Fascicular

The CN nuclei and fascicles reside in the midbrain and pons; therefore, they can be involved by diseases of the brainstem, including ischemia, neoplasms, demyelination, rhombencephalitis, trauma, neurodegenerative diseases, and metabolic disorders.[16] Because of the close proximity with other brainstem structures, patients typically present with associated brainstem dysfunctions that may produce highly localizing clinical

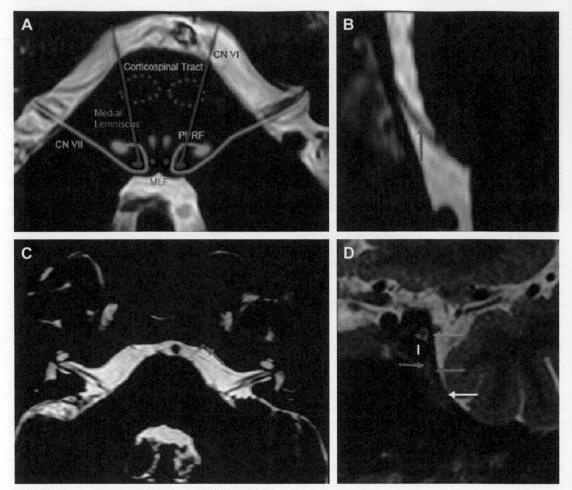

Fig. 3. CN VI anatomy. (A) The abducens nuclei (*pink dot*) are located in the dorsomedial aspect of the caudal pons, lateral to the medial longitudinal fasciculus (MLF) and the paramedian pontine reticular formation (PPRF). The fascicles (*pink line*) pass ventrally to exit the pons and become the cisternal segments (*pink arrow* in [B]), which ascend within the prepontine cistern. The dural cave segment is in the Dorello canal (*pink arrow* in [C]). Within the cavernous sinus proper, the CN VI (*pink arrow* in [D]) is inferolateral to the internal carotid artery (I) and surrounded by venous blood. (D) The CN V1 (*orange arrow*) is superior to CN V2 (*white arrow*) and inferior to CN III (*green arrow*).

syndromes, such as Weber syndrome (**Fig. 6**), one-and-a-half syndrome (**Fig. 7**), and so forth.[17]

Ischemia

Approximately 10% of ischemic strokes involve the brainstem, with the pons more commonly effected than the medulla and midbrain.[18,19] Isolated midbrain stroke is very rare, but ophthalmoplegia is the second most common symptom after ataxia.[16] Similar to ischemia in other parts of the brain, MR imaging is more sensitive than CT in early detection, showing restricted diffusion (see **Fig. 6**).[20] Pontine infarctions typically do not cross the midline, which follow the distribution of paramedian penetrating branches of the basilar artery (BA). Patients typically present with horizontal

gaze palsy. In contrast, infarcts of the midbrain may cross the midline because the arterial supply is not limited to paramedian distribution; patients may present with more complex eye movement disorders.[19] Infarcts of the midbrain can be divided into anteromedial, anterolateral, lateral, and dorsal infarction according to differences in arterial supplies.[19]

Neoplasms

Brainstem gliomas are the most common primary brainstem neoplasms and are more prevalent in pediatric patients than adult patients. The tumors are classified by MR imaging findings into 4 types: (1) diffusely infiltrative low-grade gliomas (**Fig. 8A**, B), (2) enhancing focal malignant gliomas (see

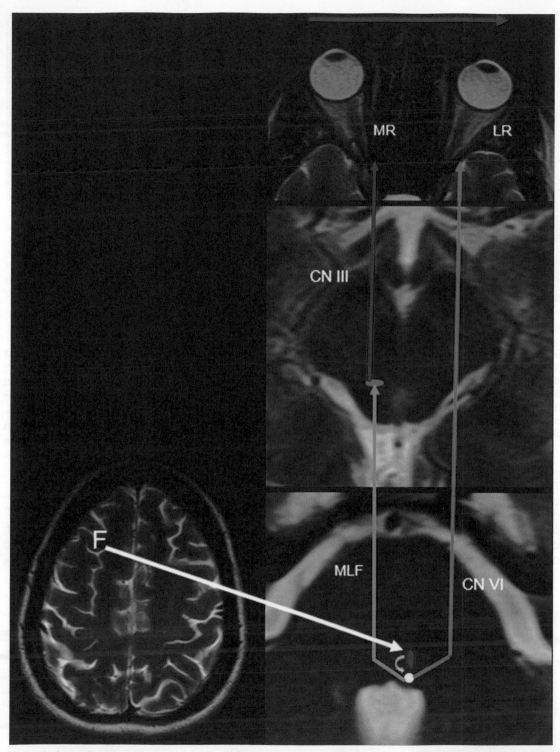

Fig. 4. Horizontal conjugate gaze pathway (*leftward gaze, pink arrow*). The right frontal eye field (F) activates the left PPRF (*red dot*). The left PPRF activates the left abducens nucleus (*yellow dot*), which stimulates the left lateral rectus (LR) via the left CN VI (*blue arrow*). The left abducens nucleus activates the right oculomotor nucleus (*blue dot*) via the crossing MLF (*green arrow*). The right CN III (*red arrow*) activates the right medial rectus (MR). Simultaneous contraction of the right MR and left LR results in leftward conjugate saccade.

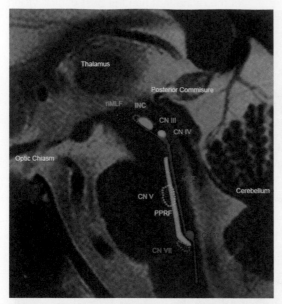

Fig. 5. Vertical conjugate center. The pretectal area houses the center for vertical conjugate gaze, which contains the INC (*small dotted green circle*), riMLF (*dotted pink circle*), and posterior commissure. The pons and remaining part of the midbrain control the horizontal conjugate gaze via the CN III (*solid blue dot*), CN IV (*solid yellow dot*), CN VI, MLF (*pink line*), and PPRF (*yellow line*). The expected locations of the CN V nucleus and CN VII nucleus are demonstrated in green and blue dotted circles.

Fig. 8C, D), (3) tectal gliomas, and (4) exophytic gliomas.[21] Approximately 36% of adults with the diffusely infiltrative type present with CN VI palsy.[22] Most patients also have other brainstem dysfunction including weakness, dizziness, ataxia, dysphagia, and so forth.[22]

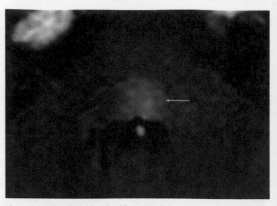

Fig. 7. One-and-a-half syndrome. Axial fluid-attenuated inversion recovery (FLAIR) image of the brain shows an ill-defined area of FLAIR hyperintensity of the dorsal pons (a multiple sclerosis plaque, *green arrow*) at the expected location of the left MLF, abducens nucleus, and PPRF. The patient has left internuclear ophthalmoplegia and leftward conjugate gaze paralysis.

Multiple sclerosis

A variety of abnormal eye movements are caused by multiple sclerosis, which may manifest as internuclear ophthalmoplegia (Fig. 9), one-and-a-half syndrome, nystagmus, ocular motor palsy, ocular misalignment, and so forth.[23] Eye movement abnormalities may predict overall disabilities in some patients.[24] MR imaging may show multiple oval, small, T2 hyperintense subcortical and periventricular white matter lesions, oriented perpendicular to the lateral ventricles.

Infection

Brainstem encephalitis has been associated with multiple infections, which include (in decreasing frequency) listeria monocytogenes, enterovirus,

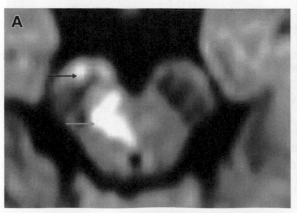
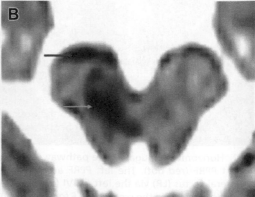

Fig. 6. Weber syndrome. Axial diffusion-weighted image (*A*) and apparent diffusion coefficient (*B*) show restricted diffusion of the right cerebral peduncle (*red arrow*) and the expected location of the fascicular CN III in the midbrain (*green arrow*), resulting in ipsilateral CN III palsy and contralateral hemiparesis.

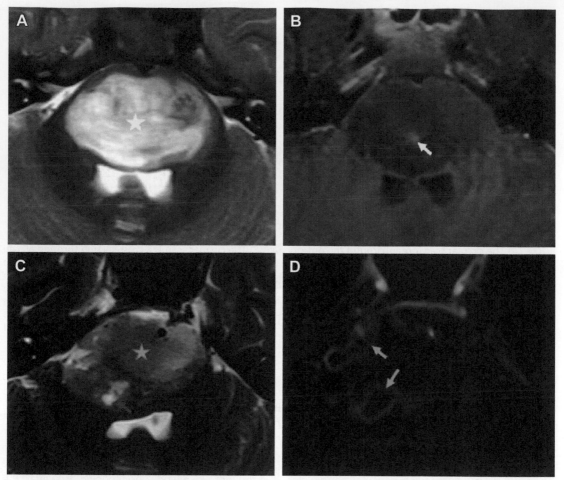

Fig. 8. Pontine gliomas. Two patients with pontine gliomas. A diffusely infiltrative low-grade tumor (*yellow star* in [*A*]: T2-weighted image) shows minimal enhancement (*yellow arrow* in [*B*]: postcontrast T1-weighted image). On the other hand, the malignant glioma is more heterogeneous and contains both solid (*blue star* in [*C*]) and necrotic (*red arrow* in [*C*]) components with focal enhancement (*blue arrows* in [*D*]: postcontrast T1-weighted image). Both patients had CN VI palsy, limb weakness, and ataxia.

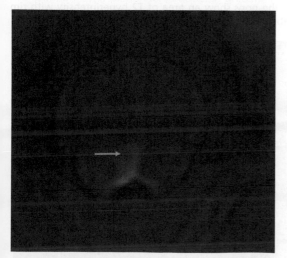

Fig. 9. Multiple sclerosis involving MLF. Axial fluid-attenuated inversion recovery (FLAIR) image at the level of the rostral pons shows a FLAIR hyperintense demyelination plaque involving the right MLF (*blue arrow*), resulting in internuclear ophthalmoplegia.

herpes simplex virus, Epstein-Barr virus, and human herpesvirus 6.[25] Patients may present with fever, ataxia, areflexia, and ophthalmoplegia.[26] On MR imaging, the brainstem may be swollen, demonstrating T2 hyperintensity with enhancement.[26] Restricted diffusion and rim enhancement suggest abscess formation (**Fig. 10**).

Wernicke encephalopathy
Wernicke encephalopathy is caused by thiamine deficiency and can be seen in patients with alcoholism, cancer, malabsorption, and so forth.[27] Ophthalmoplegia is a part of the clinical triad (ophthalmoplegia, ataxia, and encephalopathy) and may be the only presentation leading to the diagnosis of this potentially reversible disease (if treated early).[28] Typical MR imaging findings include symmetric T2 hyperintensity of the medial thalami, midbrain, and periaqueductal gray with atrophy of the mammillary bodies (**Fig. 11**). Enhancement of the mammillary bodies may be the only imaging finding.[29]

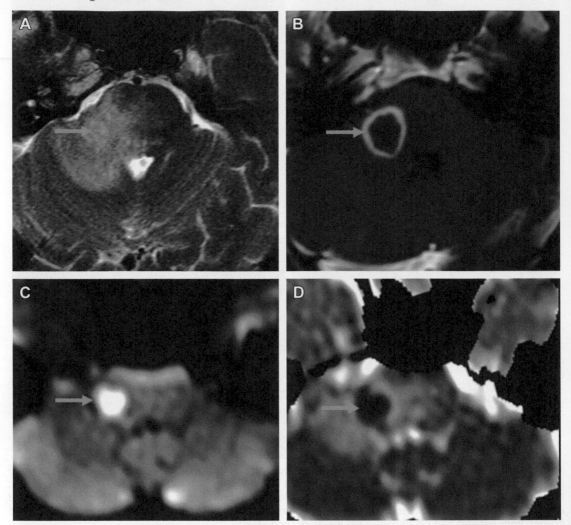

Fig. 10. Pontine abscess. Axial T2-weighted (*A*), postcontrast T1-weighted (*B*), diffusion-weighted image (*C*), and apparent diffusion coefficient (*D*) images at the level of the pons show an area of T2 hyperintensity with rim enhancement and restricted diffusion, representing an abscess (*blue arrows*).

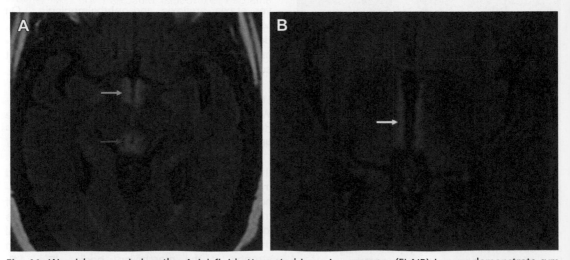

Fig. 11. Wernicke encephalopathy. Axial fluid-attenuated inversion recovery (FLAIR) images demonstrate symmetric FLAIR hyperintensity of the (*A*) hypothalamus (*blue arrow*) and periaqueductal gray matter (*red arrow*) and (*B*) medial thalami (*yellow arrow*).

Cisternal and Dural

Microvascular ischemia

Ischemia of ocular motor nerves can lead to acute ocular motor mononeuropathy. Most patients are greater than 50 years of age with vasculopathic risk factors (eg, hypertension, diabetes, hyperlipidemia, and so forth).[30] Even though MR imaging may not reveal CN abnormalities, a recent study supports obtaining neuroimaging in patients presenting with isolated CN III, IV, or VI palsies presumed to have microvascular ischemia, because up to 16.5% were found to have other identifiable causes that altered management.[31]

Neurovascular conflicts

Neurovascular conflicts occur when the CNs are compressed by nearby vessels in the subarachnoid space. This compression may result in denervation atrophy or abnormal contraction of the muscles supplied by the nerves, especially when compression occurs at the root exit zone (REZ) (ie, the transitional segment between central and peripheral myelination). CN VI is the most common ocular motor nerve to be affected and may be compressed by the basilar (**Fig. 12**), vertebral, and persistent trigeminal arteries.[32,33] CN III can be compressed by the PCA and SCA.[34,35] CN IV is reported to be affected by the SCA.[36] Because it is common to have normal contacts between the CNs and vasculature, it is important to search for other causes of cranial neuropathy when normal contact outside the REZ is seen.[35]

Aneurysm

CN III can be compressed by aneurysms arising from posterior communicating (PCOM) artery,

PCA, SCA, anterior choroidal artery, and BA.[37] The pupillomotor fibers are located in the superomedial aspect of the nerve and prone to compression by inferolaterally oriented PCOM aneurysms (**Fig. 13**), resulting in pupillary dilatation and ophthalmoplegia. These clinical features may be the only presentations of impending aneurysmal rupture.[38] Magnetic resonance angiography (MRA) or CT angiography (CTA) is urgently indicated to exclude and localize the aneurysm in cases of isolated pupil-involving CN III palsy; proper urgent treatment can be done.[39,40] CN IV and VI are less frequently affected but can be compressed by SCA/PCA and vertebral artery (VA)/BA, respectively.[41]

Infection and inflammation

Both aseptic and infectious meningitis can affect the cisternal segments of the ocular motor nerves (CN III>VI>IV).[42,43] Detection of CN involvement in bacterial meningitis suggests poor outcome.[44] Guillain-Barre syndrome (GBS) and Miller Fisher syndrome (MFS, variant of GBS) are characterized by inflammatory demyelination of peripheral nerves and can affect the ocular motor nerves (**Fig. 14**).[45] Ophthalmoplegia is a prominent feature of MFS and part of the clinical triad (ataxia, ophthalmoplegia, areflexia).[46] Gradenigo syndrome (petrous apicitis, facial pain, and lateral rectus palsy) affects the ipsilateral CN V and dural cave segment of CN VI, which are in close proximity to the petrous apex (**Fig. 15**).[47] Regardless of cause, the inflamed CNs may show smooth enhancement.

Neoplasms

Isolated schwannomas of ocular motor nerves occurring without neurofibromatosis are

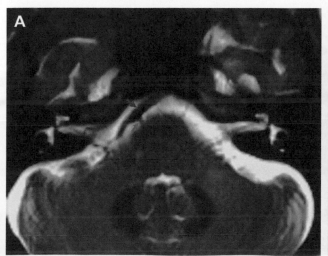
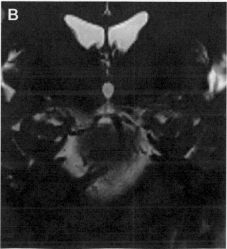

Fig. 12. Neurovascular conflicts. Axial (*A*) and coronal (*B*) T2-weighted images of the brain shows a dolichoectatic basilar artery (*red arrow*) compressing on the REZ of the right CN VI cisternal segment (*blue arrow*), resulting in right CN VI palsy.

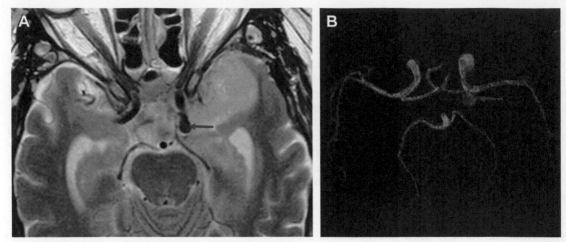

Fig. 13. PCOM artery aneurysm. Axial T2-weighted image (*A*) and time-of-flight magnetic resonance angiography image of circle of Willis (*B*) show a saccular aneurysm of the left PCOM artery (*red arrows*). The patient presented with pupil-involving left CN III palsy.

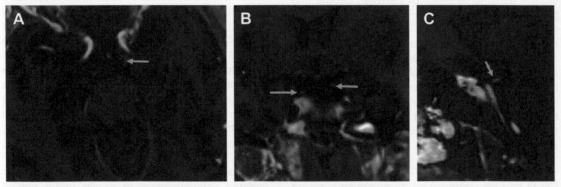

Fig. 14. GBS. Postcontrast axial (*A*), coronal (*B*), and sagittal (*C*) T1-weighted images of the brain show abnormal smooth enhancement of the cisternal segment of bilateral CN III (*blue arrows*).

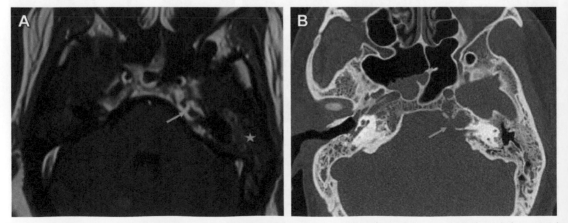

Fig. 15. Gradenigo syndrome. Postcontrast axial T1-weighted image (*A*) and CT of the head (*B*) show left mastoiditis (*blue stars*). The infection spread medially to involve the petrous apex, seen as bony destruction (*blue arrow* in [*B*]) and rim enhancement or abscess (*blue arrow* in [*A*]). The patient had left CN VI palsy and facial pain.

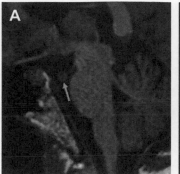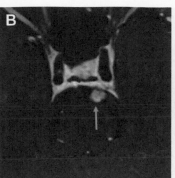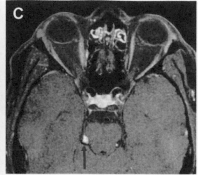

Fig. 16. Schwannomas. Sagittal (*A*) and postcontrast axial (*B*) T1-weighted images show a well-defined enhancing mass (*blue arrows*) arising from the left CN III. Postcontrast axial T1-weight (*C*) image of another patient reveals an enhancing mass (*red arrow*) in the expected location of the CN IV. Schwannomas are the presumed diagnosis of both cases. The patients were asymptomatic.

exceedingly rare. With widespread use of MR imaging, more incidental cases are reported, with some given a presumed diagnosis because of the lack of confirmatory pathology. Tumor size is variable and may not correlate with clinical severity.[48] On MR imaging, the lesions are well defined with variable appearance on T1- and T2-weighted images as well as variable enhancement patterns depending on the tumor components (**Fig. 16**).[16] Apart from diagnosis, MR imaging also plays a critical role in surgical planning in symptomatic cases and follow-up in asymptomatic patients with small lesions.[49] Other tumors affecting cisternal ocular motor nerves may arise from the skull base (eg, retroclival meningiomas or clival chordomas can compress CN VI

[**Fig. 17**]) or a distant origin via leptomeningeal metastasis (**Fig. 18**).[50]

Interdural (Cavernous Sinus) and Foraminal (Superior Orbital Fissure)

Cavernous sinus thrombosis/thrombophlebitis
Spread of bacterial or fungal infections from maxillofacial and sinonasal sources via draining veins or direct extension into cavernous sinuses is a life-threatening condition, especially in immunocompromised patients. Total ophthalmoplegia caused by involvement of all ocular motor nerves, fever, proptosis, pain/paresthesia along the distribution of CN V1/V2, and Horner syndrome are classic clinical features.[51] Contrasted MR imaging is the

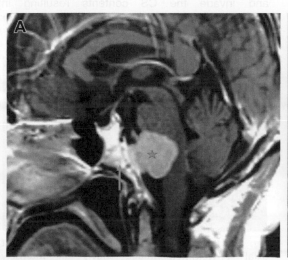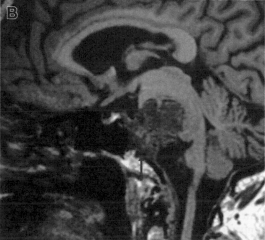

Fig. 17. Retroclival meningioma and clival chordoma. Postcontrast (*A*) and noncontrast (*B*) sagittal T1-weighted images show intense enhancement of the meningioma (*blue star* in [*A*]) without clival destruction (*blue arrow*), whereas the chordoma (*red star* in [*B*]) destroys the clivus (*red arrow*). Both patients had CN VI palsy.

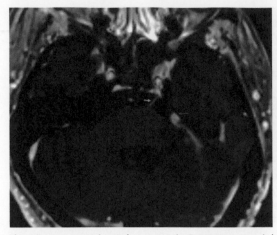

Fig. 18. Leptomeningeal metastasis. Postcontrast axial T1-weighted image of the brain shows enhancement of the cisternal segment of the left CN V (*red arrow*) and CN VI (*blue arrow*) in a patient with metastatic melanoma. The patient had CN VI palsy without facial pain.

imaging modality of choice and may show enlargement and filling defects in the cavernous sinuses (**Fig. 19**).

Tolosa-Hunt syndrome
Tolosa-Hunt syndrome (THS) is a clinical syndrome characterized by painful ophthalmoplegia

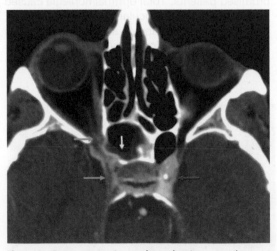

Fig. 19. Cavernous sinus thrombosis secondary to sphenoid sinus mucormycosis. A poorly controlled diabetic patient presented with fever, headache, acute right-sided vision loss, and ophthalmoplegia. Postcontrast axial CT image shows markedly hypoenhancement of the right cavernous sinus (*blue arrow*) as compared with the left side (*red arrow*) representing right cavernous sinus thrombosis. The infection arose from the right sphenoid sinus (*yellow arrow*) and spread into the superior orbital fissure and orbital apex (*green arrow*).

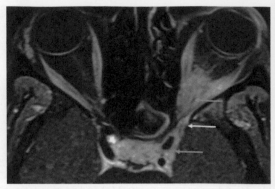

Fig. 20. THS. Postcontrast axial T1-weighted image of the orbit shows enhancement of the left CS (*blue arrow*) extending into the superior orbital fissure (*yellow arrow*) and orbital apex (*green arrow*).

(CN III>VI>IV) secondary to self-limited steroid-responsive granulomatous inflammation in the cavernous sinus (CS) that may extend into the superior orbital fissure and orbital apex.[52] MR imaging is valuable to exclude other causes of ophthalmoplegia and to detect findings that may support the diagnosis, such as enlargement and abnormal enhancement of the CS (**Fig. 20**). It is important to emphasize that THS is a clinical diagnosis and MR imaging can be subtle or even normal.[53]

Meningiomas
Meningiomas account for 41% of CS neoplasms.[54] They can be divided into 2 groups: intracavernous and extracavernous types. Intracavernous meningiomas (**Fig. 21**) arise from the endosteal layer of the dura, tend to grow medially, and invade the CS contents resulting in ophthalmoplegia, facial paresthesia, Horner

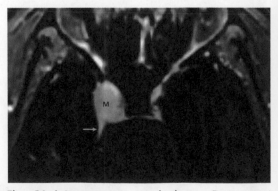

Fig. 21. Intracavernous meningioma. Postcontrast axial T1-weighted image shows an intensely enhancing mass (M) in the right cavernous sinus. Enhancement of the tentorium (dural tail sign [*blue arrow*]) is seen.

syndrome, and internal carotid artery occlusion. Primary treatment is radiotherapy. Extracavernous meningiomas arise from the meningeal layer of the dura, tend to grow laterally, and are less likely to invade CS. Primary treatment is surgery.[55]

SUMMARY

Eye movement is controlled by ocular motor pathways that encompass supranuclear, nuclear, and infranuclear levels. Lesions affecting certain locations may produce localizing signs that help radiologists focus on specific anatomic regions, such as the superior orbital fissures, cavernous sinuses, or brainstem. Some pathologic conditions, such as aneurysms and meningiomas, have unique imaging characteristics that may preclude unnecessary biopsies. MR imaging is the imaging of choice in evaluation of ocular motor palsy, with MRA or CTA indicated in cases of suspected aneurysms or neurovascular conflicts.

ACKNOWLEDGMENTS

The authors would love to acknowledge the diligent help of Dr Fang Yu for editorial assistance and diagram preparation and Dr Carlos Bazan III and Dr Achint Singh for some images.

REFERENCES

1. Donzelli R, Marinkovic S, Brigante L, et al. The oculomotor nuclear complex in humans. Microanatomy and clinical significance. Surg Radiol Anat 1998; 20:7–12.

2. Miller MJ, Mark LP, Ho KC, et al. Anatomic relationship of the oculomotor nuclear complex and medial longitudinal fasciculus in the midbrain. AJNR Am J Neuroradiol 1997;18(1):111–3.

3. Inoue T, Rhoton AL Jr, Theele D, et al. Surgical approaches to the cavernous sinus: a microsurgical study. Neurosurgery 1990;26(6):903–32.

4. Martins C, Yasuda A, Campero A, et al. Microsurgical anatomy of the oculomotor cistern. Neurosurgery 2006;58(4):220–7.

5. Harris FS, Rhoton AL. Anatomy of the cavernous sinus, a microsurgical study. J Neurosurgery 1976;45: 169–80.

6. Blitz AM, Macedo LL, Chonka ZD, et al. High-resolution CISS MR imaging with and without contrast for evaluation of the upper cranial nerves: segmental anatomy and selected pathologic conditions of the cisternal through extraforaminal segments. Neuroimaging Clin N Am 2014;24(1):17–34.

7. Morard M, Tcherekayev V, de Tribolet N. The superior orbital fissure: a microanatomical study. Neurosurgery 1994;35(6):1087–93.

8. Ferreira T, Verbist B, van Buchem M, et al. Imaging the ocular motor nerves. Eur J Radiol 2010;74(2):214–22.

9. Tubbs RS, Oakes WJ. Relationships of the cisternal segment of the trochlear nerve. J Neurosurg 1998; 89(6):1015–9.

10. Marinkovic SV, Gibo H, Stimec B, et al. The neurovascular relationships and the blood supply of the abducent nerve: surgical anatomy of its cisternal segment. Neurosurgery 1994;34(6):1017–26.

11. Yousry I, Camelio S, Wiesmann M, et al. Detailed magnetic resonance imaging anatomy of the cisternal segment of the abducent nerve: Dorello's canal and neurovascular relationships and landmarks. J Neurosurg 1999;91(2):276–83.

12. Liu GT, Volpe NJ, Galetta SL. Eye movement disorders: conjugate gaze abnormalities. In: Liu GT, Volpe NJ, Galetta SL, editors. Neuro-ophthalmology diagnosis and management. 2nd edition. New York: Saunders Elsevier; 2010. p. 551–86.

13. Blitz AM, Choudhri AF, Chonka ZD, et al. Anatomic considerations, nomenclature, and advanced cross-sectional imaging techniques for visualization of the cranial nerve segments by MR imaging. Neuroimaging Clin N Am 2014;24(1):1–15.

14. Yagi A, Sato N, Taketomi A, et al. Normal cranial nerves in the cavernous sinuses: contrast-enhanced three-dimensional constructive interference in the steady state MR imaging. AJNR Am J Neuroradiol 2005;26(4):946–50.

15. Koskas P, Héran F. Towards understanding ocular motility: III, IV and VI. Diagn Interv Imaging 2013; 94(10):1017–31.

16. Adams ME, Linn J, Yousry I. Pathology of the ocular motor nerves III, IV, and VI. Neuroimaging Clin N Am 2008;18(2):261–82.

17. Bennett JL, Pelak VS. Palsies of the third, fourth, and sixth cranial nerves. Ophthalmol Clin North Am 2001;14(1):169–85.

18. Burger KM, Tuhrim S, Naidich P. Brainstem vascular stroke anatomy. Neuroimaging Clin N Am 2005;15: 297–324.

19. Ortiz de Mendivil A, Alcalá-Galiano A, Ochoa M, et al. Brainstem stroke: anatomy, clinical and radiological findings. Semin Ultrasound CT MR 2013; 34(2):131–41.

20. Kuker W, Weise J, Krapf H, et al. MRI characteristics of acute and subacute brainstem and thalamic infarctions: value of T2-and diffusion- weighted sequences. J Neurol 2002;249:33–42.

21. Guillamo JS, Monjour A, Taillandier L, et al. Brainstem gliomas in adults: prognostic factors and classification. Brain 2001;124:2528–39.

22. Reyes-Botero G, Mokhtari K, Martin-Duverneuil N, et al. Adult brainstem gliomas. Oncologist 2012; 17(3):388–97.

23. Prasad S, Galetta SL. Eye movement abnormalities in multiple sclerosis. Neurol Clin 2010;28(3):641–55.

24. Derwenskus J, Rucker JC, Serra A, et al. Abnormal eye movements predict disability in MS: two-year follow-up. Ann N Y Acad Sci 2005;1039:521–3.

25. Jubelt B, Mihai C, Li TM, et al. Rhombencephalitis/brainstem encephalitis. Curr Neurol Neurosci Rep 2011;11(6):543–52.

26. Wasenko JJ, Park BJ, Jubelt B, et al. Magnetic resonance imaging of mesenrhombencephalitis. Clin Imaging 2002;26(4):237–42.

27. Reuler JB, Girard DE, Cooney TG. Wernicke encephalopathy. N Engl J Med 1985;312:1035–9.

28. Kesler A, Stolovitch C, Hoffmann C, et al. Acute ophthalmoplegia and nystagmus in infants fed a thiamine-deficient formula: an epidemic of Wernicke encephalopathy. J Neuroophthalmol 2005;25(3):169–72.

29. Zuccoli G, Pipitone N. Neuroimaging findings in acute Wernicke's encephalopathy: review of the literature. Am J Roentgenol 2009;192:501–8.

30. Richards BW, Jones FR Jr, Younge BR. Causes and prognosis in 4,278 cases of paralysis of the oculomotor, trochlear, and abducens cranial nerves. Am J Ophthalmol 1992;113:489–96.

31. Tamhankar MA, Biousse V, Ying GS, et al. Isolated third, fourth, and sixth cranial nerve palsies from presumed microvascular versus other causes: a prospective study. Ophthalmology 2013;120(11):2264–9.

32. Nakamagoe K, Mamada N, Shiigai M, et al. Recurrent isolated abducens nerve paresis associated with persistent trigeminal artery variant. Intern Med 2012;51(16):2213–6.

33. Narai H, Manabe Y, Deguchi K, et al. Isolated abducens nerve palsy caused by vascular compression. Neurology 2000;55(3):453–4.

34. Albayram S, Ozer H, Sarici A, et al. Unilateral mydriasis without ophthalmoplegia-a sign of neurovascular compression? Case report. Neurosurgery 2006;58(3):582–3.

35. Tsai TH, Demer JL. Nonaneurysmal cranial nerve compression as cause of neuropathic strabismus: evidence from high-resolution magnetic resonance imaging. Am J Ophthalmol 2011;152(6):1067–73.

36. Marinkovic S, Gibo H, Zelic O, et al. The neurovascular relationships and the blood supply of the trochlear nerve: surgical anatomy of its cisternal segment. Neurosurgery 1996;38:161–9.

37. Fujiwara S, Fujii K, Nishio S, et al. Oculomotor nerve palsy in patients with cerebral aneurysms. Neurosurgery 1989;12:23–32.

38. Kasner SE, Liu GT, Galetta SL. Neuro-ophthalmologic aspects of aneurysms. Neuroimaging Clin N Am 1997;7(4):679–92.

39. Inamasu J, Nakamura Y, Saito R, et al. Early resolution of third nerve palsy following endovascular treatment of a posterior communicating artery aneurysm. J Neuroophthalmol 2002;22:12–4.

40. Wardlaw JM, White PM. The detection and management of unruptured intracranial aneurysms. Brain 2001;123:205–21.

41. Zhu Y, Thulborn K, Curnyn K, et al. Sixth cranial nerve palsy caused by compression from a dolichoectatic vertebral artery. J Neuroophthalmol 2005;25(2):134–5.

42. Wright SE, Shaikh ZH, Castillo-Lugo JA, et al. Aseptic meningitis and abducens nerve palsy as a serious side effect of high dose intravenous immunoglobulin used in a patient with renal transplantation. Transpl Infect Dis 2008;10(4):294–7.

43. Di Comite G, Bozzolo EP, Praderio L, et al. Meningeal involvement in Wegener's granulomatosis is associated with localized disease. Clin Exp Rheumatol 2006;24(2 Suppl 41):S60–4.

44. Singhi P, Bansal A, Geeta P, et al. Predictors of long term neurological outcome in bacterial meningitis. Indian J Pediatr 2007;74(4):369–74.

45. Ropper AH. The Guillain-Barré syndrome. N Engl J Med 1992;326:1130–6.

46. Nagaoka U, Kato T, Kurita K, et al. Cranial nerve enhancement on three-dimensional MRI in Miller Fisher syndrome. Neurology 1996;47(6):1601–2.

47. Connor SE, Leung R, Natas S. Imaging of the petrous apex: a pictorial review. Br J Radiol 2008;81(965):427–35.

48. Yang SS, Li ZJ, Liu X, et al. Pediatric isolated oculomotor nerve schwannoma: a new case report and literature review. Pediatr Neurol 2013;48(4):321–4.

49. Elmalem VI, Younge BR, Biousse V, et al. Clinical course and prognosis of trochlear nerve schwannomas. Ophthalmology 2009;116(10):2011–6.

50. Nakaoku Y, Murakami G, Fujimoto Y, et al. A case of leptomeningeal melanomatosis presenting with right abducens nerve palsy. Rinsho Shinkeigaku 2014;54(8):675–8.

51. Liu GT, Volpe NJ, Galetta SL. Eye movement disorders: third, fourth, and sixth nerve palsies and other causes of diplopia and ocular misalignment. In: Liu GT, Volpe NJ, Galetta SL, editors. Neuro-ophthalmology diagnosis and management. 2nd edition. New York: Saunders Elsevier; 2010. p. 491–550.

52. Hunt WE, Meagher JN, Lefever HE, et al. Painful ophthalmoplegia. Its relation to indolent inflammation of the carvernous sinus. Neurology 1961;11:56–62.

53. Zhang X, Zhou Z, Steiner TJ, et al. Validation of ICHD-3 beta diagnostic criteria for 13.7 Tolosa-Hunt syndrome: analysis of 77 cases of painful ophthalmoplegia. Cephalalgia 2014;34(8):624–32.

54. Radhakrishnan K, Mokri B, Parisi JE, et al. The trends in incidence of primary brain tumors in the population of Rochester, Minnesota. Ann Neurol 1995;37:67–73.

55. Klinger DR, Flores BC, Lewis JJ, et al. The treatment of cavernous sinus meningiomas: evolution of a modern approach. Neurosurg Focus 2013;35(6):E8.

Imaging of Orbital Trauma and Emergent Non-traumatic Conditions

Blair A. Winegar, MD[a],*, Juan E. Gutierrez, MD[b]

KEYWORDS

- Orbital emergencies • Orbital trauma • Facial fractures • Open globe injury
- Intraocular foreign body • Orbital infection • Orbital inflammation • Carotid–cavernous fistula

KEY POINTS

- Multidetector computed tomography (MDCT) has become a crucial component in the assessment of orbital trauma.
- MDCT allows for accurate characterization of the orbital fractures, orbital soft tissue injuries, and assessment of orbital foreign bodies.
- Nontraumatic orbital emergencies often present a challenge to clinical diagnosis due to overlapping symptomatology necessitating radiological evaluation.
- Contrast-enhanced MR imaging allows for detailed evaluation of the orbital soft tissues and differentiation of the multiple causes of nontraumatic orbital emergencies.
- Conventional angiography is useful for the diagnosis and treatment of vascular orbital emergencies, such as carotid–cavernous fistulae.

INTRODUCTION

Radiological imaging evaluation is crucial in the aid of clinical assessment in patients with orbital trauma or nontraumatic orbital emergencies. In the setting of orbital trauma, clinical assessment of the orbits may be hindered by extensive facial soft tissue injury, decreased level of consciousness, or life-threatening injuries to the remainder of the body. Multidetector computed tomography (MDCT) is the modality of choice in the assessment of orbital trauma[1] because of its many advantages over other imaging modalities. MDCT is superior to conventional radiography due to its faster acquisition; it may be performed concomitantly with CT imaging of additional body parts frequently obtained in the setting of multi organ injuries. Additionally, it only requires 1 head position, and it allows for the assessment of the orbital soft tissues, is more sensitive for detection of fractures, and may be reformatted in multiple projections and in 3 dimensions. Ultrasound is user dependent and contraindicated in the setting of suspected open globe injury. MR imaging cannot be performed in the setting of potential intraorbital metallic foreign body.

Patients also seek emergency care for many nontraumatic orbital conditions causing a multitude of presenting symptoms to include: vision loss, scotoma, eye pain, ophthalmoplegia, diplopia, orbital bruit, proptosis, or enophthalmos. Cross-sectional imaging with either contrast-enhanced MR imaging or MDCT is helpful in differentiating the numerous etiologies of disease states that present with these symptoms. MR imaging is particularly useful in the setting of nontraumatic emergencies due to its superior evaluation of the orbital soft tissues with respect to MDCT. In addition, conventional

Disclosure Statement: No financial interests to disclose.
a Department of Radiology, University of Utah, 30 North 1900 East, Rm 1a071, Salt Lake City, UT 84132-2140, USA; b Neuroradiology Section, Centro Avanzado de Diagnostico Medico CEDIMED, Calle 18 AA sur #29 C 340, Medellin, Colombia, South America
* Corresponding author.
E-mail address: Blair.Winegar@hsc.utah.edu

Neuroimag Clin N Am 25 (2015) 439–456
http://dx.doi.org/10.1016/j.nic.2015.05.007
1052-5149/15/$ – see front matter © 2015 Elsevier Inc. All rights reserved.

neuroimaging.theclinics.com

angiography may be indicated in select cases in which a vascular abnormality affecting the orbit is suspected, such as carotid–cavernous fistulae. Although invasive, conventional angiography has advantages over CT angiography (CTA) and magnetic resonance angiography (MRA), as it consists of real-time imaging and allows for endovascular treatment when appropriate.

ORBITAL SKELETAL TRAUMA
Orbital Blowout Fracture

Orbital blowout fracture is a displaced fracture of an orbital wall directed away from the orbit, which may be characterized as pure, if the orbital rim is spared, or impure, if the orbital rim is involved in the fracture (Fig. 1). The 2 mechanisms of the orbital blowout fracture are termed the hydraulic and the bone conduction mechanisms, which both have shown to result in orbital blowout fractures in experimental models with key differences (Box 1).[2] The inferior orbital wall is most frequently affected by the blowout fracture, followed by the medial orbital wall. Although the medial orbital wall (lamina papyracea) is thinner than the inferior orbital wall, it is supported by osseous struts of the ethmoid sinuses, likely increasing its durability against fracture. Complications that advocate for early surgical repair include extraocular muscle entrapment and enophthalmos, which are typically seen in fracture fragments of greater than 1 cm in

---

> **Box 1**
> **Mechanisms of orbital blowout fractures**
>
> - Hydraulic mechanism—posteriorly oriented force to the orbit causes an acute increase in intraorbital pressure with subsequent fracture of the weakest orbital wall to relieve this pressure.
>   - ○ Larger fracture defect
>   - ○ May affect the medial orbital wall
>   - ○ Commonly results in herniation of orbital contents
> - Bone conduction mechanism—a force applied to the orbital rim is transmitted posteriorly until eventual buckling of the affected wall occurs.
>   - ○ Smaller, anterior fracture defect
>   - ○ Never involves medial wall
>   - ○ Rarely results in herniation

size.[3–5] Internal fixation of orbital blowout fracture typically results in the placement of mesh material to restore orbital volume and provide a barrier against the herniation of intraorbital contents.

A special type of the orbital blowout fracture is the trapdoor fracture. The trapdoor fracture is an inferior orbital blowout fracture in which the inferior rectus muscle or infraorbital fat herniates through the fracture defect into the underlying maxillary sinus with return of the fracture fragment back to its original position; thus, the fracture fragment acts like a trapdoor. These patients will present with signs of entrapment caused by extraocular muscle restriction, resulting in diplopia. On coronal CT imaging, the inferior rectus muscle or extraconal fat herniates inferior to the orbital floor through a nondisplaced inferior orbital wall fracture.

Superior Orbital Wall Fracture

The superior orbital wall or orbital roof is the only wall that forms a partition between the anterior cranial fossa and intraorbital contents. Fractures through the orbital roof are typically a result of a direct blow to the forehead and usually displace into the orbit, termed orbital blow-in fracture (Fig. 2). Associated frontal sinus fracture is a common finding. Potential complications include proptosis, diplopia, orbital emphysema, dural tear with resultant cerebrospinal fluid (CSF) leak or brain herniation, cerebral contusion, and extension of fracture to the orbital apex. Repair of these potential complications may require both intracranial and extracranial approaches.[6] The fractures are best visualized on coronal reformatted CT images.

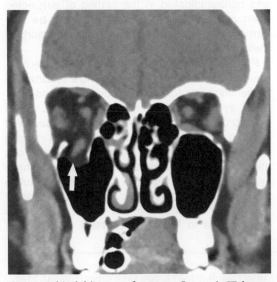

Fig. 1. Orbital blowout fracture. Coronal CT image demonstrates the inferiorly displaced fracture of the right orbital floor with herniation of intraorbital fat and inferior rectus muscle into the defect (*arrow*). Clinical correlation for entrapment should be performed.

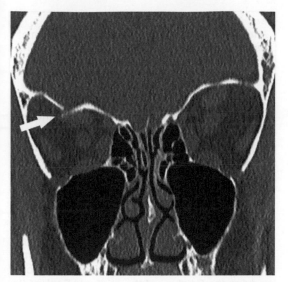

Fig. 2. Orbital blow-in fracture. Coronal CT image demonstrates comminuted and inferiorly angulated fracture of the right superior orbital wall with impingement upon the right superior rectus muscle (*arrow*).

Zygomaticomaxillary Complex Fracture

Zygomaticomaxillary complex (ZMC) fracture is caused by a direct traumatic blow to the malar eminence, resulting in diastasis through the 4 sutures that attach the zygoma to the remaining face and calvarium (Fig. 3). Historically, this fracture pattern was described by the misnomer tripod fracture, as a fracture through the zygomaticofrontal, zygomaticomaxillary, and zygomaticotemporal sutures could be discerned by conventional radiography. However, fracture additionally extends through the zygomaticosphenoid suture. The zygoma forms portions of the inferior and lateral orbital walls, anterior and posterolateral maxillary sinus walls, and zygomatic arch. Displaced ZMC fractures that rotate along the axis of the zygomaticosphenoid suture[7] or concomitant orbital floor blowout fractures can result in enophthalmos, which may necessitate intraorbital reconstruction in addition to ZMC fracture fixation.[8]

Naso-Orbitoethmoid Complex Fracture

Naso-orbitoethmoidal (NOE) complex fracture is caused by posteriorly oriented high-impact force

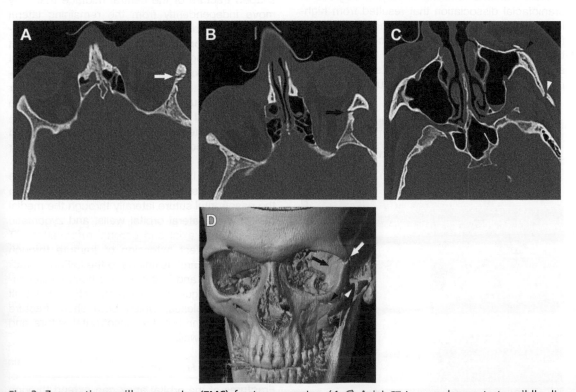

Fig. 3. Zygomaticomaxillary complex (ZMC) fracture complex. (*A–C*) Axial CT images demonstrate mildly displaced fractures through the zygomaticofrontal (*white arrow*), zygomaticosphenoid (*black arrow*), zygomaticomaxillary (*black arrowhead*), and zygomaticotemporal (*white arrowhead*) sutures, consistent with ZMC fracture pattern. (*D*) Oblique 3-dimensional volume rendered CT image demonstrates the fracture complex.

applied to the nasal region with transmission through the nasal cavity, medial orbital walls, and ethmoid sinuses (**Fig. 4**). This fracture complex typically results in severe comminution and telescoping of the bilateral nasal bones and septum, ethmoid sinuses including the cribriform plate, and medial orbital walls. Frequent complications caused by NOE fractures include proptosis due to a decrease in intraorbital volume, telecanthus from a medial canthal tendon injury, and CSF rhinorrhea caused by fracture through the cribriform plate and tear of the apposed dura. The Markowitz and Manson classification system separates NOE fracture complexes by comminution of the lacrimal fossa and involvement of the medial canthal tendon into 3 types (**Box 2**).[9] Since the medial canthal tendon is not seen by CT, description of the degree of comminution of the medial orbital wall at the expected attachment of the medial canthal tendon in the lacrimal fossa is helpful in surgical planning of potential medial canthal tendon repair.

LeFort Complex Fractures

At the turn of the twentieth century, the French surgeon Rene LeFort described 3 types of midface fracture patterns resulting in varying degrees of craniofacial dissociation that resulted from high-impact forces applied to the midface of cadavers (**Fig. 5**).[10] Disruption of the pterygomaxillary junction is the commonality shared by the 3 patterns, and it must be present to characterize a fracture pattern as a LeFort fracture. Although the 3 types

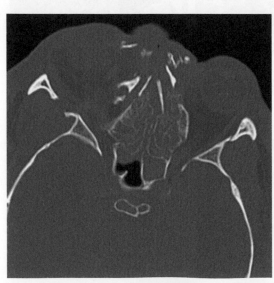

Fig. 4. NOE complex fracture. Axial CT image demonstrates comminuted and posteriorly displaced fractures of the nasal bones, medial orbital walls, and ethmoid sinus walls with resultant telecanthus.

> **Box 2**
> **Markowitz and Manson classification system of naso-orbitoethmoidal fractures**
>
> - Type I—medial canthal tendon intact and connected to single large fracture fragment
> - Type II—medial canthal tendon intact and connected to single fragment of comminuted fracture
> - Type III—medial canthal tendon disrupted with comminuted fracture of the lacrimal fossa

of complex fracture patterns described by LeFort were characterized separately and symmetrically across the midface, these fracture patterns may be seen concomitantly and/or asymmetrically involving the 2 halves of the midface. Each of the LeFort fracture types affects unique portions of the midface, which can simplify characterization (**Box 3**).[11] The LeFort type I fracture complex does not involve the orbit and will therefore not be discussed.

LeFort type II fracture complex, also known as the pyramidal fracture, results in a pyramid-shaped fracture of the central midface that may move independently from the remaining lateral face and skull base. Fracture extends obliquely inferolaterally from the nasofrontal suture (apex of pyramid) through the medial orbital walls, orbital floors, and maxillary sinus walls along the zygomaticomaxillary sutures. Involvement of the inferior orbital walls is unique to the LeFort type II fracture complex. Axial and coronal reformatted CT images enable detection of the obliquely oriented fractures extending through the medial and inferior orbital walls.

LeFort type III fracture complex produces true craniofacial dissociation. Fracture extends from the nasofrontal suture laterally through the medial orbital walls, lateral orbital walls, and zygomatic arches. Using axial and coronal reformatted CT images to detect extension of fracture through the zygomatic arch is unique to the LeFort III fracture complex, and is therefore a helpful discriminator in distinguishing between LeFort II and III fracture complexes, which both share fracture components through the nasofrontal suture and medial orbital walls.

Orbital Apex Fracture

Fractures of the orbital apex can extend through the optic canal or superior orbital fissure, resulting in damage to the cranial nerves that traverse these structures (**Fig. 6**). Fracture through the optic canal

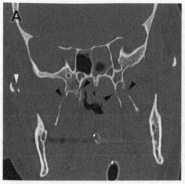
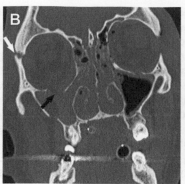
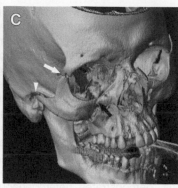

Fig. 5. LeFort complex fractures. (A) Coronal CT image demonstrates fractures through the pterygoid plates (*black arrowheads*), a requirement for LeFort complex fractures. In addition, right zygomatic arch fracture is present (*white arrowhead*). (B) Coronal CT image demonstrates obliquely oriented LeFort II fracture through the right medial orbital wall, inferior orbital wall (*black arrow*), and inferolateral maxillary sinus wall and transversely oriented LeFort III fracture through the right lateral orbital wall (*white arrow*). (C) Obliquely oriented 3-dimensional volume rendered CT of the same patient demonstrates fractures of the nasal bridge/right medial orbital wall, right inferior orbital wall (*black arrow*), right lateral orbital wall (*white arrow*), and right zygomatic arch (*white arrowhead*), consistent with a combination of right LeFort II and III complex fractures.

may result in monocular blindness from optic nerve injury caused by direct impaction from fracture fragments or subsequent compression from resultant edema or hemorrhage. In complex trauma patients in whom vision cannot be clinically assessed as a result of extensive soft tissue swelling or obtundation, detection of orbital apex fracture by MDCT may be the only method to diagnose potential vision-compromising injury.[12]

Two clinical syndromes may develop as a result of orbital apex fractures, the superior orbital fissure syndrome, and the orbital apex syndrome.[13] The superior orbital fissure syndrome is caused by fracture-related injury to cranial nerves III, IV, V_1, and VI as they traverse the superior orbital fissure, thus causing ophthalmoplegia, diplopia, and ptosis. The addition of injury to the optic nerve at the orbital apex is termed the orbital apex syndrome, and would add monocular vision loss to the patient's symptoms. On CT, special attention is needed to assess the fat about the intracanalicular optic nerve in the setting of fracture. Any soft tissue attenuation along the optic nerve should be deemed suspicious for potential edema or hemorrhage within the confined space of the optic canal. On MR imaging, replacement of the

normal T1 hyperintense fat within the optic canal or abnormal T2 hyperintensity within the optic canal or adjacent optic nerve also correlates to the injury. Injury to the optic nerve at the orbital apex is an emergency that may prompt high-dose steroid therapy or potential surgical decompression to prevent permanent blindness.

TRAUMATIC GLOBE INJURY
Ocular Hemorrhage and Detachments

Blunt and penetrating injury to the globe can result in several ocular hemorrhage patterns that are

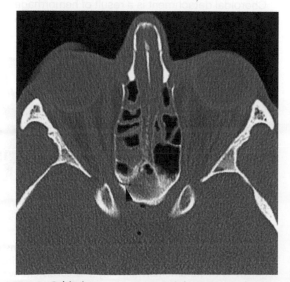

Fig. 6. Orbital apex fracture. Axial CT image demonstrates nondisplaced fracture through the medial aspect of the right optic canal (*arrowhead*), which may result in traumatic optic neuropathy.

Box 3
LeFort complex fractures unique features

- Type I—lateral margin of nasal fossa and inferior nasal septum
- Type II—inferior orbital rim
- Type III—lateral orbital rim and zygomatic arch

distinguishable on cross-sectional imaging (**Fig. 7**A). Hyphema, hemorrhage within the anterior chamber of the globe, is recognized on CT as layering hyperdensity anterior to the lens. Although hyphema is easily recognized by clinical examination and often does not require radiological diagnosis, it should prompt the radiologist to pay close attention to the posterior segment, as ophthalmoscopic examination is compromised from the intervening anterior chamber blood products.

Vitreal hemorrhage, hemorrhage within the vitreous, demonstrates heterogeneous hyperdensity as blood products mix with the vitreous humor on CT (**Fig. 7**B). Subhyaloid hemorrhage, hemorrhage external to the hyaloid membrane that covers the vitreous and separates it from the retina, is defined on CT by a layer of hyperdensity that usually pools anterior to and covers the optic disc with a sharp margin between the subhyaloid hemorrhage and vitreous (see **Fig. 7**A).

Retinal detachment, hemorrhage or fluid between the retina and choroid or between layers of the retina resulting in separation of these layers, is characterized on imaging by lentiform-shaped collections (**Fig. 8**A).[14] The retina extends to, but not across, the optic disc; thus diffuse retinal detachment gives a V-shaped appearance on axial cross-sectional images with apex at the optic disc. Choroidal melanoma is a potential malignant cause of spontaneous retinal detachment and will appear as a mushroom-shaped enhancing mass extending from the ocular wall into the vitreous (**Fig. 8**B).[15]

Choroidal detachment is a result of hemorrhage or fluid between the choroid and sclera with separation of these layers (**Fig. 9**). On CT and MR imaging, lentiform-shaped fluid/hemorrhage extends along the inner surface of the posterior aspect of the globe. In contrast to retinal detachment, choroidal detachment spares the posterior third of the globe without extension to the optic nerve insertion and may extend anteriorly to the ciliary body beyond the location of the ora serrata.[16]

Subtenon hemorrhage is a hematoma situated between the sclera and Tenon capsule (see **Fig. 7**C). On CT, subtenon hemorrhage appears as a lentiform-shaped hyperdensity along the posterior outer surface of the globe and may be difficult to distinguish from retrobulbar hematoma.

Intraocular hemorrhage may result from an acute increase of intracranial pressure that induces retinal venous hypertension from intracranial subarachnoid hemorrhage, a condition termed Terson syndrome (**Fig. 10**).[17] This finding has been linked to increased morbidity and deserves consultation with ophthalmology to prevent permanent vision impairment.

Traumatic Lens Injury

Lens subluxation or dislocation is an injury associated with partial or complete tearing of the zonular attachments to the crystalline lens, respectively (**Fig. 11**A, B). On CT, lens dislocation is recognized by abnormal positioning of the lens, which more commonly is displaced posteriorly into the dependent vitreous. Anterior lens dislocation is less common and may demonstrate subtle asymmetric decrease in anterior–posterior dimension of the anterior segment, which may be indistinguishable from anterior segment open globe injury from

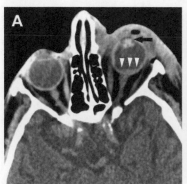 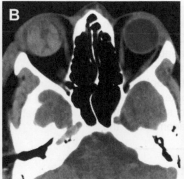 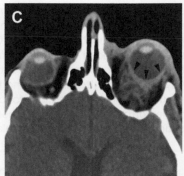

Fig. 7. Orbital hemorrhage. (*A*) Axial CT image demonstrates irregular contour of the left globe, consistent with open globe injury. Hyperattenuation within the anterior chamber and in the dependent portion of the posterior segment with fluid/hemorrhage layer is consistent with hyphema (*black arrow*) and subhyaloid hemorrhage (*white arrowheads*), respectively. (*B*) Axial CT image demonstrates heterogeneous hyperdensity within the right vitreous body, consistent with vitreous hemorrhage. (*C*) Axial CT image demonstrates hyperdensity along the outer posterior margin of the left globe, consistent with subtenon hemorrhage (*black arrowheads*). Ill-defined hyperdensity in the retrobulbar soft tissues consistent with retrobulbar hematoma resulting in proptosis.

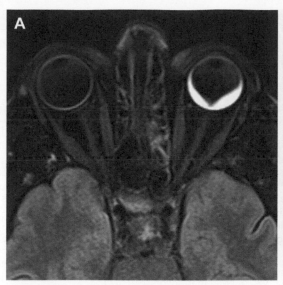

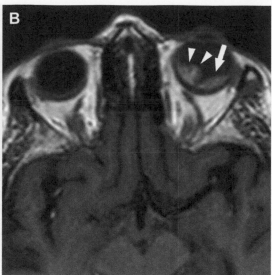

Fig. 8. Retinal detachment. (*A*) Axial T2 FLAIR MR imaging demonstrates V-shaped hyperintense collection along the posterior margin of the left globe that extends to, but not across the optic disc, consistent with retinal detachment. (*B*) Axial T1-weighted MR imaging demonstrates a hyperintense mass along the posteromedial globe with adjacent T1 hyperintense retinal detachment (*arrow*), consistent with choroidal melanoma (*arrowheads*).

corneal laceration and requires correlation with ophthalmologic examination. The most severe form of lens dislocation is lens extrusion, in which the crystalline lens is ejected from the globe through an open defect and is therefore not visualized on imaging. Lens subluxation is distinguished on CT by appropriate positioning of a portion of the crystalline lens with abnormal angulation of the portion of the lens in which the zonular attachments are disrupted.

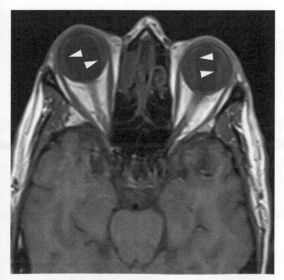

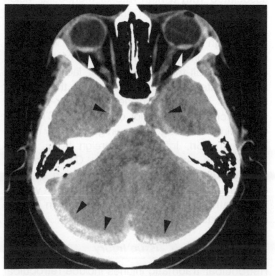

Fig. 9. Choroidal detachment. Axial T1-weighted MR imaging demonstrates bilateral biconvex hyperintense collections along the inner lateral margins of the globes, which do not extend to the optic discs, consistent with choroidal detachment (*arrowheads*).

Fig. 10. Terson syndrome. Axial CT image demonstrates hyperintensity along the posterior ocular walls that spares the optic discs, consistent with subretinal hemorrhages (*white arrowheads*). Hyperdensity throughout the extra-axial space is a result of diffuse nontraumatic subarachnoid hemorrhage (*black arrowheads*) in a patient with a ruptured posterior communicating artery aneurysm (not shown).

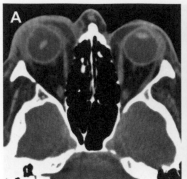
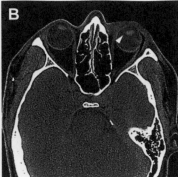
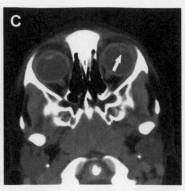

Fig. 11. Lens injury. (*A*) Lens dislocation. Axial CT image demonstrates displacement of the right crystalline lens into the vitreous body, consistent with posterior lens dislocation. (*B*) Lens subluxation. Axial CT image demonstrates posterior angulation of the medial aspect of the left crystalline lens, consistent with posterior lens subluxation (*arrowhead*). (*C*) Traumatic cataract. Axial CT image demonstrates hypoattenuation of the left crystalline lens, consistent with traumatic cataract (*arrow*).

Traumatic cataract is an opacity of the crystalline lens as a result of blunt or penetrating injury to the globe, or less commonly from electrical shock (**Fig. 11**C). On CT, decreased attenuation of the affected lens is the result of an ingress of fluid with ensuing edema.[18]

Open Globe Injury

Open globe injury or rupture is a full-thickness injury to the sclera, cornea, or both, as a result of blunt or penetrating injury to the globe, and it is associated with a high rate of monocular vision loss. On CT, when open globe injury is associated with loss of intraocular pressure, the prototypical flat tire sign is present, demonstrating a loss of volume and normal spherical shape of the globe (**Fig. 12**). Full-thickness corneal laceration can demonstrate decreased volume of the anterior segment with diminished anterior–posterior dimension of the anterior chamber on CT. Other CT findings that suggest open globe injury include lens extrusion, intraocular foreign body, vitreal hemorrhage, and intraocular air. CT is approximately 80% sensitive in the detection of open globe injury,[19] and must be used in concert with intraoperative ophthalmologic examination for the complete assessment of occult injury.

Retrobulbar Soft Tissue Injury

Retrobulbar traumatic injuries include retrobulbar hematoma, subperiosteal hematoma, orbital emphysema, extraocular muscle injury, and optic nerve injury. Retrobulbar hematoma is typically ill-defined hyperattenuation within the soft tissues posterior to the globe (see **Fig. 7**C). Subperiosteal hematoma represents a collection of blood underlying the periosteum of an orbital wall. CT shows

hyperattenuation along the affected orbital wall with convexity of hematoma projecting into the orbit, which may result in proptosis. Orbital emphysema is defined as the presence of air in the orbit, typically the result of orbital wall fracture in communication with an adjacent paranasal sinus. Orbital emphysema is typically a benign, self-limited condition; however, air tracking along the optic nerve sheath may result is optic nerve ischemia. Any space occupying material within the retrobulbar soft tissues, including retrobulbar hematoma and orbital emphysema, may result in orbital compartment syndrome, a potentially

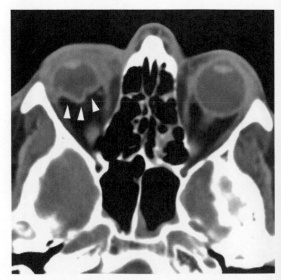

Fig. 12. Open globe injury. Axial noncontrast CT image demonstrates decreased volume and posterior contour irregularity of the right globe, consistent with the flat tire sign of open globe injury (*arrowheads*).

devastating vision-threatening complication of acutely increased intraorbital pressure. Orbital compartment syndrome is a clinical diagnosis; however, CT is helpful in defining the location of the precipitating lesion or discovering findings that are associated with poorer prognosis, such as posterior tenting of the globe.[20]

The extraocular muscles can be directly injured from orbital trauma. CT findings of increased size and/or hyperattenuation within the muscle are consistent with edema/intramural hematoma. Partial or complete disruption of the muscle may result from laceration. Avulsion from tendinous insertion on the globe may also occur. Herniation of the inferior rectus muscle into the defect is a common complication of inferior orbital blowout fracture (see **Fig. 1**).

Traumatic optic neuropathy (TON) is a condition in which direct or indirect trauma results in acute injury to the optic nerve. Most commonly, trauma results in posterior indirect optic neuropathy, thought to be caused by transmitted forces resulting in shearing injury of the intracanalicular portion of the optic nerve. TON is a clinical diagnosis in which decreased visual acuity and afferent pupillary defect are present. MDCT is helpful in cases of TON to assess for optic canal fracture, edema/hematoma within the optic canal, optic nerve sheath or intraconal hematoma, or foreign body/fracture fragments impinging upon the optic nerve that would direct potential medical (eg, high-dose steroids) or surgical intervention (eg, optic canal decompression).[21] Diffusion tensor imaging

may demonstrate reduced diffusivity within the affected optic nerve.[22] Optic nerve avulsion is an uncommon, severe injury resulting in transection of the optic nerve, which may occur at the level of the optic nerve head, intracanalicular portion, or anterior to the chiasm, thought to result from severe rotational forces to the globe.[23] MDCT or MR imaging may demonstrate subtle discontinuity of the optic nerve with an intact optic nerve sheath. Optic nerve transection, a complete disruption of the optic nerve and sheath, may occur anywhere along the course of the optic nerve, often caused by the severing action of a fracture fragment or penetrating foreign body.

Orbital Foreign Body

Radiological evaluation of the orbit for foreign bodies is crucial in the setting of orbital trauma. Although conventional radiography is able to detect the presence of an opaque intraorbital foreign body (**Fig. 13**A), it does not assess the exact location with respect to the remaining orbital soft tissues. Therefore, conventional radiography is typically reserved in the nonemergent setting to prove the presence or absence of a suspected opaque foreign body prior to MR imaging. MDCT is the modality of choice in the initial assessment of the intraorbital foreign body, as it is sensitive, allows for detection of associated injuries to the orbit and soft tissues, and allows safe detection of ferromagnetic materials unlike MR imaging (**Fig. 13**B). Second-tier imaging modalities that

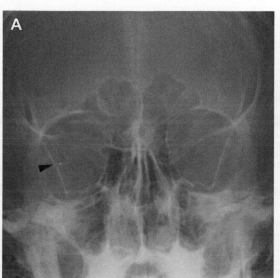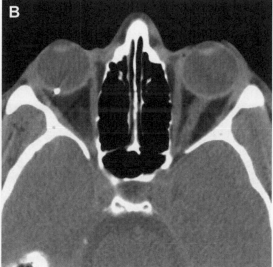

Fig. 13. Intraocular metallic foreign body. (*A*) A frontal radiograph of the orbits demonstrates a punctate metallic foreign body in the right orbit (*arrowhead*). (*B*) Axial noncontrast CT image of the same patient demonstrates a metallic intraocular foreign body.

may be used to identify foreign bodies include ultrasound and MR imaging. B-mode ultrasound is useful for detection of intraocular foreign bodies, but it is user-dependent and not typically able to characterize the foreign material. Additionally, contact ultrasonography is contraindicated in the setting of open globe injury. MR imaging is reserved as a second-line modality to detect suspected nonmetallic foreign body, if CT is negative. MR imaging is contraindicated when there is suspected metallic intraocular foreign body, since electromagnetic torque forces may cause foreign body migration and resultant ocular damage and potential vision loss.

It is useful to categorize intraocular foreign bodies as metallic (eg, iron, copper, or metal alloys), nonmetallic inorganic (eg, glass or plastic), and organic materials (eg, wood, dirt, or plant material) for the purpose of preoperative planning. Metallic foreign bodies are more hyperdense than bone on CT, with Hounsfield units in the thousands (Fig. 14). Nonmetallic foreign bodies are also typically hyperattenuating when compared with orbital soft tissues, but less than metallic materials. Organic materials can have a wide range of attenuation. In particular, wood can be air attenuation and may be confused with orbital emphysema.[24] Therefore, if the air conforms to a geometric shape or is not in a nondependent position, for the possibility of intraorbital wooden foreign body should be considered (Fig. 15).

The decision to undergo surgical extraction of intraocular foreign body depends on the size, location, foreign body material, damage to surrounding structures, and potential damage by surgical exploration.[25] Metallic foreign bodies are typically well tolerated; however, intraocular copper may result in a sterile endophthalmitis (acute chalcosis), and intraocular iron may result in siderosis bulbi. Nonmetallic inorganic foreign bodies, such as plastic, are also typically well tolerated. However, organic foreign materials typically contaminate the globe with microorganisms, thus increasing the risk of endophthalmitis and necessitating prompt surgical removal.

It is important for the radiologist to be familiar with common sites and appearances of orbital calcifications and ocular postsurgical changes that may mimic intraocular foreign bodies. Trochlear calcifications are small curvilinear calcifications in the anteromedial orbit at the site of the trochlear apparatus, the fibrous sling containing the superior oblique tendons (Fig. 16A).[26] Phthisis bulbi is the result of end-stage damage to the globe, which appears shrunken and irregular with dystrophic calcifications on CT and may mimic open globe injury with intraocular foreign body (Fig. 16B). Optic drusen are calcified mucopolysaccharides at the optic nerve heads and should not be confused with foreign bodies layering dependently in the vitreous (Fig. 16C).[27] Retinal detachment tamponade is a procedure in which the posterior segment is filled with silicone oil or gaseous compounds (eg, air or sulfur hexaflouride) in order to appose the detached ocular wall layers. On MDCT, silicone oil is hyperattenuating, and the gaseous compounds have air attenuation. These compounds may be confused with vitreous hemorrhage or

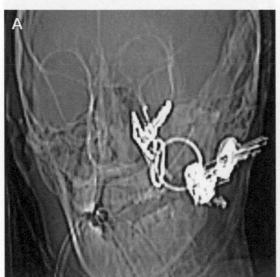
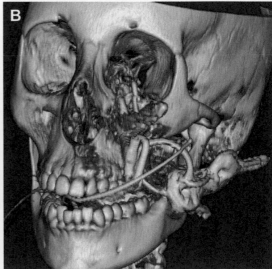

Fig. 14. Intraorbital metallic foreign body. (*A, B*) A scout image and 3-dimensional volume rendered CT images demonstrate left intraorbital extension of car keys in a patient status after motor vehicle collision.

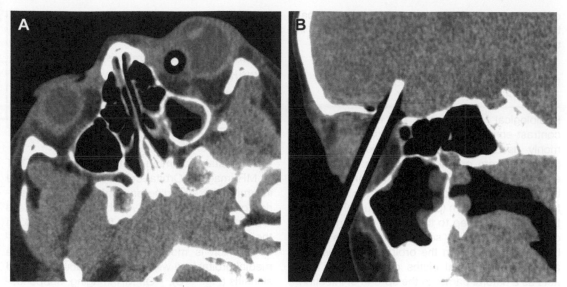

Fig. 15. Intraorbital wooden foreign body. (*A, B*) Axial and sagittal CT images demonstrate a pencil within the medial aspect of the left orbit extending into the left anterior cranial fossa. The pencil graphite is hyperdense, and the wood component is air density.

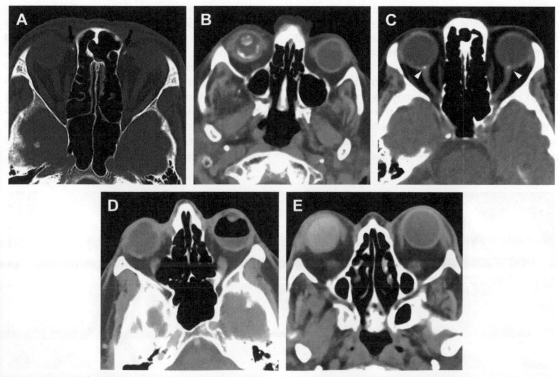

Fig. 16. Potential orbital trauma mimics. (*A*) Trochlear calcification. Axial CT image demonstrates curvilinear hyperdensities in the anteromedial orbits at the site of the trochlear apparatus, consistent with trochlear calcifications (*arrows*). (*B*) Phthisis bulbi. Axial CT image demonstrates a shrunken and partially calcified globe. (*C*) Optic disc drusen. Axial noncontrast CT image demonstrates bilateral punctate calcifications at the optic discs, consistent with optic disc drusen (*arrowheads*). (*D, E*) Retinal detachment treatment. (*D*) Axial CT image demonstrates left intravitreal air status after vitrectomy and air tamponade. (*E*) Axial CT image demonstrates hyperdensity in the right vitreous body status after vitrectomy with intravitreal silicone oil tamponade.

ocular emphysema, and thus knowing the patient's recent past surgical history is important in the setting of trauma (**Fig. 16**D, E).

NONTRAUMATIC ORBITAL EMERGENCIES
Orbital Infection

Radiological assessment of the orbit with contrast-enhanced CT or MR imaging is commonly used to differentiate preseptal cellulitis (**Fig. 17**A) from orbital cellulitis (**Fig. 17**B) in the emergency setting. These entities are stratified by infection limited to the soft tissues superficial to the orbital septum (preseptal cellulitis) or infection extending deep to the orbital septum (orbital cellulitis). The orbital septum is a fibrous membrane extending from the orbital rim periosteum and along the tarsal plates of the eyelids that acts as a natural barrier to the spread of infection. Preseptal cellulitis is a less severe infection that may be treated with oral antibiotics in an outpatient setting. On the other hand, orbital cellulitis is treated more aggressively with intravenous antibiotics, as infection may be complicated by vision loss, ophthalmoplegia, or intracranial spread of infection. The potential intracranial complications of orbital cellulitis are identifiable on MDCT or MR imaging (**Box 4**). Surgery may be required to drain concomitant subperiosteal or orbital abscesses.

The orbital septum is usually not visualized by MDCT or MR imaging, but may be imagined as a line connecting the margins of the orbital rim and anterior to the globe. Preseptal cellulitis is characterized by soft tissue swelling, stranding, and patchy enhancement of the soft tissues superficial

---

Box 4
Intracranial complications of orbital cellulitis

- Cavernous sinus thrombosis
- Intracranial abscess
- Subdural empyema
- Meningitis

---

to the orbital septum on contrast enhanced MDCT or MR imaging. Orbital cellulitis will demonstrate inflammatory stranding and enhancement posterior to the orbital septum. A subperiosteal abscess is defined as a rim-enhancing fluid collection along the orbital wall with adjacent paranasal sinus infection, which is most commonly seen along the medial orbital wall with associated acute ethmoid sinusitis (**Fig. 17**C).[28] On MR imaging, subperiosteal or intraorbital abscesses will demonstrate rim enhancement with internal T2 hyperintensity and restricted diffusion.[29]

Acute invasive fungal sinusitis is an aggressive infection with high mortality affecting immunocompromised patients, particularly those with uncontrolled diabetes or neutropenia (eg, bone marrow transplant recipients or patients on chronic immunosupression), which may result in intraorbital extension (**Fig. 18**). On contrast-enhanced MDCT, intraorbital involvement is seen as variably enhancing soft tissue within the orbit and adjacent opacification of the involved paranasal sinus with or without intervening osseous destruction. MR imaging demonstrates T2 hyperintensity and postgadolinium enhancement of the involved intraorbital soft tissues. Treatment includes radical debridement,

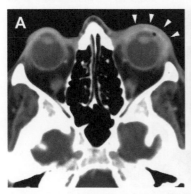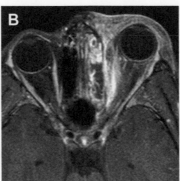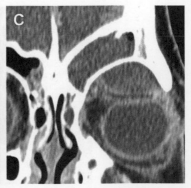

Fig. 17. Preseptal and orbital cellulitis. (*A*) Axial contrast-enhanced CT image demonstrates thickening and enhancement of the left preseptal soft tissues without extension posterior to the orbital septum, consistent with preseptal cellulitis (*arrowheads*). (*B*) Axial T1 postgadolinium fat saturation image demonstrates ethmoid sinusitis with abnormal enhancement within the preseptal and retrobulbar soft tissues, consistent with preseptal and orbital cellulitis. (*C*) Coronal contrast-enhanced CT image demonstrates frontal sinusitis with an extraconal superior orbital rim-enhancing fluid collection resulting in mass effect upon the left globe, consistent with a subperiosteal abscess.

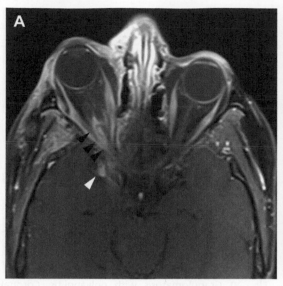

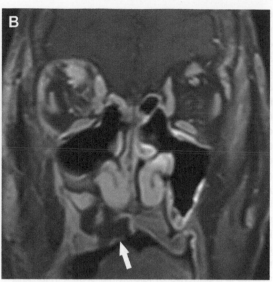

Fig. 18. Invasive fungal sinusitis. (*A*) Axial T1 postgadolinium fat saturated image demonstrates ill-defined enhancement in the right orbital apex at the optic nerve (*black arrowheads*) extending intracranially along the anterior margin of the right middle cranial fossa (*white arrowhead*). (*B*) Coronal T1 postgadolinium fat saturation image demonstrates inflammatory changes of paranasal sinuses and prior bilateral uncinectomies and ethmoidectomies. Nonenhancement of the right aspect of the hard palate is consistent with necrosis secondary to angioinvasion (*arrow*).

intravenous antifungals, and treatment of the underlying immunodeficiency.[30,31]

Orbital Inflammatory Conditions

Idiopathic orbital inflammatory syndrome (IOIS), otherwise known as orbital pseudotumor, is a nonspecific inflammation of the orbit without local or systemic causes (Fig. 19). Patients present with orbital pain and a wide variety of additional symptoms depending on the location of inflammation, including proptosis, restricted eye movement, conjunctival injection, or impaired vision.

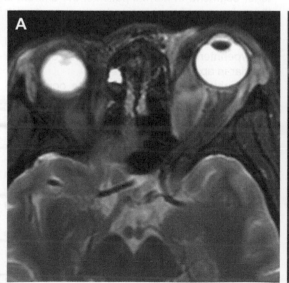

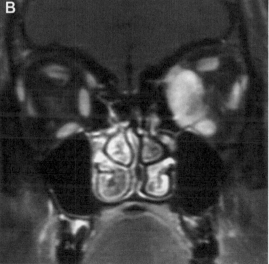

Fig. 19. IOIS. (*A*) Axial T2-weighted fat saturated image demonstrates enlargement and hyperintensity involving the left medial rectus muscle including the anterior tendinous portion, a distinction that differentiates IOIS from thyroid ophthalmopathy. (*B*) Coronal T1 postgadolinium fat saturation image demonstrates ill-defined enhancement and thickening involving the left medial rectus muscle, consistent with myositic subtype of IOIS.

Contrast-enhanced MR imaging demonstrates nonspecific, ill-defined inflammatory stranding and enhancement that may affect a number of orbital subsites, including: extraocular muscles, lacrimal glands, retrobulbar fat, ocular walls, orbital apex, optic nerve sheath (eg, optic perineuritis), or a combination of these structures. Differential diagnostic considerations of orbital inflammation include orbital cellulitis, granulomatosis with polyangiitis, sarcoidosis, and lymphoma. Apparent diffusion coefficient (ADC) values may be helpful in differentiating IOIS from lymphoma and orbital cellulitis.[32] Although idiopathic orbital inflammatory syndrome is a diagnosis of exclusion, empiric treatment with systemic steroids is attempted in suspected cases. Biopsy and second-line treatment with low-dose radiotherapy or cytotoxic chemotherapy are reserved for refractory cases. Tolosa-Hunt syndrome is a subtype of idiopathic orbital inflammatory syndrome involving the cavernous sinus, resulting in painful ophthalmoplegia.[33]

Granulomatosis with polyangiitis is a syndrome associated with granulomatous inflammation and small- or medium-sized vessel vasculitis that predominantly involves the kidneys and respiratory tracts and is associated with cytoplasmic staining antineutrophil cytoplasmic antibodies (c-ANCA). On imaging, nonspecific mass-like inflammation may involve any regions of the orbital soft tissues (Fig. 20). Attention to the adjacent paranasal sinuses and nasal cavity may demonstrate extensive mucosal inflammation with variable destruction of the nasal septum and sinus walls.[34,35]

Ocular Infection/Inflammation

Infection or inflammation may affect any of the globe layer, the anterior or posterior segment, or a combination. Scleritis, inflammation of the sclera, may be designated as anterior or posterior if the inflammation occurs anterior or posterior to the extraocular muscle attachments. Anterior scleritis results in eye pain and erythema of the visualized sclera. On the other hand, posterior scleritis presents with eye pain, but without erythema. Uveitis is defined as inflammation involving the uvea, a combination of the iris, ciliary body, and choroid. Uveitis can be subdivided into anterior, intermediate, and posterior subtypes depending on the components of the affected uvea. In general, diagnosis of inflammation of the ocular layers is determined through ophthalmologic examination with the aide of B-mode ultrasound. However, eye pain and visual disturbance in the absence of erythema, such as in cases of posterior scleritis or posterior uveitis, may prompt contrast-

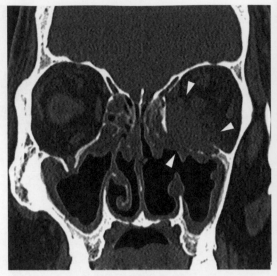

Fig. 20. Granulomatosis with polyangiitis. Coronal noncontrast CT image demonstrates paranasal sinus inflammatory mucosal thickening and destruction of the left inferior nasal turbinate, left medial maxillary sinus wall, and left orbital floor. Abnormal ill-defined inflammatory soft tissue extends into the left orbit engulfing the inferior and medial rectus muscles (arrowheads) in a patient with granulomatosis with polyangitis.

enhanced CT or MR imaging in the emergency setting. Contrast-enhanced T1 and T2 weighted sequences with fat saturation in the axial and sagittal planes are the ideal sequences to assess inflammation involving the ocular layers of the posterior segment. In normal patients, the choroid is the only normally enhancing layer, given its rich vascularity. The inflamed ocular layer will demonstrated thickening, contrast enhancement, and T2 hyperintensity, which may be focal, diffuse, or nodular in appearance (Fig. 21).

Endophthalmitis is infection of the ocular cavities and adjacent structures resulting in pain, edema, and decreased vision (Fig. 22). This condition is typically the result of direct inoculation of bacteria or fungus into the globe from ocular surgery or trauma, termed exogenous endophthalmitis, and requires surgical intervention with administration of intraocular antibiotics or potential enucleation. Rarely, hematogenous seeding of the ocular cavities may affect immunocompromised or chronically ill patients, typical in the setting of uncontrolled diabetes, termed metastatic or endogenous endophthalmitis. Panophthalmitis is the most severe form of endophthalmitis, in which the infection encompasses the entirety of the structures of the eyeball. Acute endophthalmitis may be a diagnostic dilemma, particularly in cases of endogenous endophthalmitis, given its

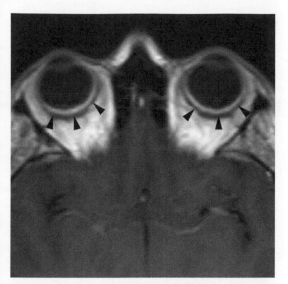

Fig. 21. Posterior uveitis. Axial T1-weighted postgadolinium MR imaging demonstrates abnormal enhancement and thickening of the bilateral choroid and retina (*arrowheads*) in a patient with Vogt-Koyanagi-Harada syndrome (granulomatous panuveitis, exudative retinal detachments with neurologic and cutaneous manifestations).

low incidence and nonspecific symptoms, prompting radiological assessment. Contrast-enhanced CT may reveal relative hyperattenuation of the affect vitreous, thickening and enhancement of the ocular wall, and/or adjacent periorbital inflammation. Contrast-enhanced MR imaging is the modality of choice in the assessment for endophthalmitis, with possible findings to include abnormal increased fluid-attenuated inversion recovery (FLAIR) signal within the vitreous, regions of restricted diffusion within the globe, ocular wall

thickening and enhancement, and/or periorbital inflammatory changes.[36]

Vascular Orbital Emergencies

Carotid–cavernous fistulae (CCF) are an abnormal communication between the carotid arterial system and the cavernous sinus, typically resulting in conjunctival chemosis, pulsatile proptosis, pain, ophthalmoplegia, and progressive vision loss (**Fig. 23**). CCF can be classified according to the cause, traumatic or spontaneous, or whether the arterial supply arises directly from the internal carotid artery or indirectly from meningeal branches of the internal carotid artery, external carotid artery, or both (**Box 5**).[37] CT angiography is more sensitive than MRA in the detection of CCF.[38] Both can demonstrate enlarged cavernous sinus with increased internal vascularity, enlarged superior ophthalmic vein, proptosis, and possible enlargement/edema within the extraocular muscles of the affected side. These findings may be unilateral or bilateral. Digital subtraction angiography (DSA) is required for definitive diagnosis and possible endovascular treatment. DSA will demonstrate retrograde flow within the superior ophthalmic vein and corresponding cavernous sinus in the arterial phase of injection and allow for identification of the site of fistula, whether directly from the internal carotid artery or internal carotid artery (ICA)/external carotid artery (ECA) feeding vessels in the case of indirect fistula. Direct CCFs may be treated endovascularly with transarterial detachable balloon occlusion, transvenous coil embolization, covered stent across the fistula, or carotid sacrifice. Indirect CCFs may be initially treated with manual carotid compression. If this is unsuccessful,

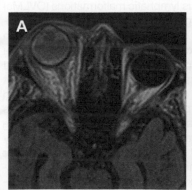 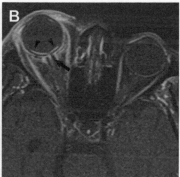 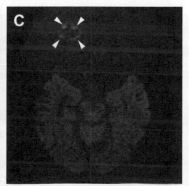

Fig. 22. Endophthalmitis. (*A*) Axial FLAIR MR imaging demonstrates hyperintense signal within the right globe with inflammatory changes in the orbital soft tissues. (*B*) Axial T1 postgadolinium fat saturation MR imaging demonstrates abnormal enhancement involving the right preseptal and retrobulbar soft tissues, optic nerve (*black arrow*), and posterior uvea (*black arrowheads*). (*C*) Axial diffusion weighted imaging demonstrates foci of hyperintensity along the ocular wall, consistent with subchoroidal abscesses (*white arrowheads*).

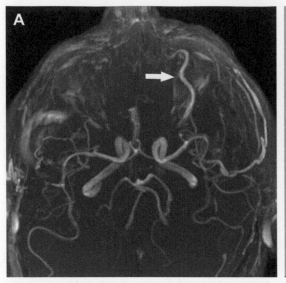
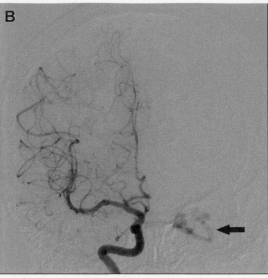

Fig. 23. Carotid–cavernous fistula. (A) 3-dimensional time-of-flight magnetic resonance angiography axial maximal intensity projection image demonstrates dilatation of the left superior ophthalmic vein (white arrow) consistent with arterialized flow. (B) Digital subtraction angiography, right internal carotid artery injection, frontal projection, demonstrates contrast opacification of the cavernous sinuses and left superior ophthalmic vein (black arrow) in the arterial phase, consistent with carotid–cavernous fistula.

endovascular treatment with transvenous coil embolization is typically curative.[39]

Orbital venous varices are congenital low-flow venous malformations with connection to the systemic venous system that dilate in the setting of increased venous pressure (eg, Valsalva maneuver, coughing, etc.) and are the most common cause of spontaneous retrobulbar hemorrhage. Patients typically exhibit reversible proptosis, elicited by increased venous pressure. Patients may present to the emergency department with sudden painful proptosis caused by non-traumatic retrobulbar hemorrhage or variceal thrombosis. Contrast-enhanced CT performed with and without

provocative maneuvers (eg, Valsalva maneuver or internal jugular vein compression) will demonstrate increased size of the enhancing intraorbital mass during the increase in venous pressure.[40] The orbital venous varix may not be visualized on the CT performed without provocative maneuver. CT may also demonstrate internal phleboliths within the varix, retrobulbar hemorrhage if present, or hyperattenuating clot without enhancement in the setting of thrombosis. Contrast-enhanced MR imaging will demonstrate variable T1 and T2 signal intensity within the varix, diffuse contrast enhancement, and enlargement of the varix with provocative maneuver.

Orbital venous lymphatic malformations (OVLMs) are benign congenital low-flow vascular malformations that may grow slowly with time, resulting in progressive proptosis (Fig. 24). OVLMs are characterized histopathologically by numerous dilated interconnecting vascular channels, which are not connected to the systemic venous system, in contrast to the previously described orbital venous varix. These masses typically demonstrate an infiltrative transspatial growth pattern in which they violate natural tissue planes that restrict other pathologies; therefore, they may involve both intraconal and extraconal compartments or preseptal and postseptal compartments. These lesions may acutely enlarge due to spontaneous internal hemorrhage or upper respiratory tract infection, resulting in sudden increase in proptosis or optic nerve injury, prompting emergent assessment.

Box 5
Barrow classification of spontaneous carotid–cavernous fistulae

- Type A—direct high-flow shunt between internal carotid artery (ICA) and cavernous sinus
- Type B—indirect low flow shunt between meningeal branches of the ICA and cavernous sinus
- Type C—indirect low flow shunt between meningeal branches of the external carotid artery (ECA) and cavernous sinus
- Type D—indirect low flow shunt between the cavernous sinus and meningeal branches of both ECA and ICA

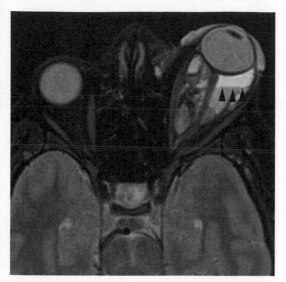

Fig. 24. Orbital venous lymphatic malformation (OVLM). Axial T2-weighted fat saturation image demonstrates a loculated left retrobulbar mass with internal fluid/fluid levels (*arrowheads*) of varying signal intensity resulting in proptosis, consistent with OVLM.

MR imaging is the modality of choice in characterization of these lesions, which typically demonstrate multiloculated, trans-spatial T2 hyperintensity with thin, barely perceptible walls. In the setting of internal hemorrhage, multiple fluid–fluid levels with variable T1/T2 signal corresponding to hemorrhage products of varying ages are present.[41] The venous components of these lesions will demonstrate enhancement, while the typically, nearly imperceptible walls and septations of the lymphatic components show thickening and enhancement in the setting of upper respiratory tract infection. Surgical removal is controversial and typically reserved for cases complicated by optic nerve compression, corneal exposure, or intractable pain, as complete resection is limited by the infiltrative, trans-spatial growth pattern; recurrence is common.[42]

SUMMARY

In conclusion, radiological imaging is essential in the assessment of orbital emergencies. Multidetector CT allows for rapid assessment of osseous and soft tissue injuries in the setting of orbital trauma and can identify orbital or ocular foreign bodies in a majority of cases. The radiologist should be familiar with the midface complex fracture types that affect the orbits and commonly associated complications (eg, medial canthal tendon injury with NOE complex fracture). Contrast-enhanced MR imaging allows for the differentiation of many etiologies of nontraumatic orbital emergencies

that present with similar clinical symptoms. Although CT angiography or MRA can typically diagnose carotid–cavernous fistula, conventional angiography is regarded as the gold standard in classification and is necessary for endovascular treatment.

REFERENCES

1. Kubal W. Imaging of orbital trauma. Radiographics 2008;28:1729–39.
2. Waterhouse N, Lyne J, Urdang M, et al. An investigation into the mechanism of orbital blowout fractures. Br J Plast Surg 1999;52:607–12.
3. Harris G. Orbital blow-out fractures: surgical timing and technique. Eye 2006;20:1207–12.
4. Cole P, Kaufman Y, Hollier L. Principles of facial trauma: orbital fracture management. J Craniofac Surg 2009;20:101–4.
5. Kummoona R. Management of injuries of the orbital skeleton. J Craniofac Surg 2009;20:762–7.
6. Antonyshyn O, Gruss M, Kassel E. Blow-in fractures of the orbit. Plast Reconstr Surg 1989;84:10–20.
7. Hopper R, Salemy S, Sze R. Diagnosis of midface fractures with CT: what the surgeon needs to know. Radiographics 2006;26:783–93.
8. Ellis E, Reddy L. Status of the internal orbit after reduction of zygomaticomaxillary complex fractures. J Oral Maxillofac Surg 2004;62:275–83.
9. Markowitz B, Manson P, Sargent L, et al. Management of the medial canthal tendon in nasoethmoid orbital fractures: the importance of the central fragment in classification and treatment. Plast Reconstr Surg 1991;87:843–53.
10. Le Fort R. Etude experimentale sur les fractures de la machoire superieure. Rev Chir 1901;23:208–27, 360–79, 479–507.
11. Rhea J, Novelline R. How to simplify the CT diagnosis of Le Fort fractures. AJR Am J Roentgenol 2005;184:1700–5.
12. Unger J. Orbital apex fractures: the contribution of computed tomography. Radiology 1984;150:713–7.
13. Yeh S, Foroozan R. Orbital apex syndrome. Curr Opin Ophthalmol 2004;15:490–8.
14. Lane J, Watson R, Witte R, et al. Retinal detachment: imaging of surgical treatments and complications. Radiographics 2003;23:983–94.
15. LeBedis C, Sakai O. Nontraumatic orbital conditions: diagnosis with CT and MR imaging in the emergent setting. Radiographics 2008;28:1741–53.
16. Mafee M, Peyman G. Choroidal detachment and ocular hypotonia: CT evaluation. Radiology 1984; 153:697–703.
17. Swallow C, Tsuruda J, Digre K, et al. Terson syndrome: CT evaluation in 12 patients. AJNR Am J Neuroradiol 1998;19:743–7.

18. Segev Y, Goldstein M, Lazar M, et al. CT appearance of a traumatic cataract. AJNR Am J Neuroradiol 1995;16:1174–5.

19. Yuan W, Hsu H, Cheng H, et al. CT of globe rupture: analysis and frequency of findings. AJR Am J Roentgenol 2014;202:1100–7.

20. Oester A, Sahu P, Fowler B, et al. Radiographic predictors of visual outcome in orbital compartment syndrome. Ophthal Plast Reconstr Surg 2012;28:7–10.

21. Bodanapally U, Van der Byl G, Shanmuganathan K, et al. Traumatic optic neuropathy prediction after blunt facial trauma: derivation of a risk score based on facial CT findings at admission. Radiology 2014; 272:824–31.

22. Bodanapally U, Kathirkamanathan S, Geraymovych E, et al. Diagnosis of traumatic optic neuropathy: application of diffusion tensor magnetic resonance imaging. J Neuroophthalmol 2013;33:128–33.

23. Arkin M, Rubin P, Bilyk J, et al. Anterior chiasmal optic nerve avulsion. AJNR Am J Neuroradiol 1996;17: 1777–81.

24. Ho V, McGuckin J, Smergel E. Intraorbital wooden foreign body: CT and MR appearance. AJNR Am J Neuroradiol 1996;17:134–6.

25. Lin T, Liao T, Yuan W, et al. Management and clinical outcomes of intraocular foreign bodies with the aid of orbital computed tomography. J Chin Med Assoc 2014;77:433–6.

26. Shriver E, McKeown C, Johnson T. Trochlear calcification mimicking an orbital foreign body. Ophthal Plast Reconstr Surg 2011;27:e143–4.

27. Ramirez H, Blatt E, Hibri N. Computed tomographic identification of calcified optic nerve drusen. Radiology 1983;148:137–9.

28. Handler L, Davey I, Hill J, et al. The acute orbit: differentiation of orbital cellulitis from subperiosteal abscess by computerized tomography. Neuroradiology 1991;33:15–8.

29. Sepahdari A, Aakalu V, Kapur R, et al. MRI of orbital cellulitis and orbital abscess: the role of diffusion-weighted imaging. AJR Am J Roentgenol 2009; 193:W244–50.

30. Aribandi M, McCoy V, Bazan C. Imaging features of invasive and noninvasive fungal sinusitis: a review. Radiographics 2007;27:1283–96.

31. Groppo E, El-Sayed I, Aiken A, et al. Computed tomography and magnetic resonance imaging characteristics of acute invasive fungal sinusitis. Arch Otolaryngol Head Neck Surg 2011;173:1005–10.

32. Kapur R, Sepahdari A, Mafee M, et al. MR imaging of orbital inflammatory syndrome, orbital cellulitis, and orbital lymphoid lesions: the role of diffusion-weighted imaging. AJNR Am J Neuroradiol 2009; 30:64–70.

33. Yousem D, Atlas S, Grossman R, et al. MR imaging of Tolosa-Hunt syndrome. AJNR Am J Neuroradiol 1989;10:1181–4.

34. Santiago Y, Fay A. Wegener's granulomatosis of the orbit: a review of clinical features and updates in diagnosis and treatment. Semin Ophthalmol 2011; 26:349–55.

35. Provenzale J, Mukherji S, Allen N, et al. Orbital involvement by Wegener's granulomatosis: imaging findings. AJR Am J Roentgenol 1996;166:929–34.

36. Rumboldt Z, Moses C, Wieczerzynski U, et al. Diffusion-weighted imaging, apparent diffusion coefficients, and fluid-attenuation inversion recovery MR imaging in endophthalmitis. AJNR Am J Neuroradiol 2005;26:1869–72.

37. Barrow D, Spector R, Braun I, et al. Classification and treatment of spontaneous carotid-cavernous sinus fistulas. J Neurosurg 1985;62:248–56.

38. Chen C, Chang P, Shy C, et al. CT angiography and MR angiography in the evaluation of carotid cavernous sinus fistula prior to embolization: a comparison of techniques. AJNR Am J Neuroradiol 2005;26:2349–56.

39. Gemmete J, Ansari S, Gandhi D. Endovascular techniques for treatment of carotid–cavernous fistula. J Neuroophthalmol 2009;29:62–71.

40. Poon C, Sze G, Johnson M. Orbital Lesions: differentiating vascular and nonvascular etiologic factors. AJR Am J Roentgenol 2008;190:956–65.

41. Smoker W, Gentry L, Yee N, et al. Vascular lesions of the orbit: more than meets the eye. Radiographics 2008;28:185–204.

42. Greene A, Burrows P, Smith L, et al. Periorbital lymphatic malformation: clinical course and management in 42 patients. Plast Reconstr Surg 2005; 115:22–30.

Imaging of the Postoperative Orbit

Kim O. Learned, MD*, Farbod Nasseri, MD, Suyash Mohan, MD

KEYWORDS

- Imaging • Orbit • Postoperative • Prosthesis • Reconstruction • Retinopexy

KEY POINTS

- Inappropriate neuroimaging preceding ophthalmology referral can lead to inappropriate use of costly resources, with a potential for overdiagnosis and false positives.
- Imaging plays a critical role in recognizing the normal postoperative appearance of the commonly encountered orbital procedures, and enables early diagnosis of complications.
- The common eye surgeries that are evident on imaging include: (1) cataract surgery and intraocular lens implant; (2) retinal detachment surgeries (retinopexy, scleral buckling, and vitrectomy); (3) glaucoma aqueous shunting; (4) evisceration and enucleation; (5) ocular prosthesis; (6) eyelid weights; (7) dacryocystorhinostomy; (8) orbital decompression; (9) maxillofacial orbital reconstruction; and (10) orbital exenteration and reconstruction.
- Silicone oil, silicone sponge and rubber band, prosthesis, and implant should not be mistaken for unintended foreign bodies. Postoperative infection should be promptly identified to avoid the devastating consequence of permanent loss of vision.
- Oncologic orbital reconstruction uses vascularized free flaps composed of skin, subcutaneous fat, or fascia, with or without muscle, and at computed tomography and MR imaging their appearance reflects the flap compositions. The expected swelling and enhancement of a normal flap as a result of denervation or adjuvant chemoradiation should not be mistaken for neoplasm. Neoplasm tends to recur at the interface of the free flap and recipient surgical bed, and demonstrates mass-like growth with an appearance similar to that of the original tumor.

INTRODUCTION

The Centers for Disease Control and Prevention report the leading causes of blindness and low vision in the United States as age-related eye diseases such as macular degeneration, cataract, diabetic retinopathy, and glaucoma.[1] Cataract is the leading cause of blindness and can occur at any age. An estimated 20.5 million (17.2%) Americans aged 40 years and older have cataract, and 6.1 million require intraocular lens (IOL) replacement. Diabetic retinopathy is the leading cause of blindness in American working-aged adults (20–74 years of age) with an estimated 4.1 million Americans affected by the disease. Vitrectomy plays a vital role in the management of severe complications of diabetic retinopathy. Glaucoma is the second leading cause of blindness worldwide in Caucasians, and the leading cause of blindness in Africans and Latinos.[2] In all ethnic groups, the prevalence of glaucoma increases dramatically with age, and the aging

Disclosures: None.
Neuroradiology Division, Department of Radiology, Hospital of the University of Pennsylvania, Perelman School of Medicine at University of Pennsylvania, 219 Dulles Building, 3400 Spruce Street, Philadelphia, PA 19104, USA
* Corresponding author.
E-mail address: Kim.Learned@uphs.upenn.edu

Neuroimag Clin N Am 25 (2015) 457–476
http://dx.doi.org/10.1016/j.nic.2015.05.008

population in the United States is expected to increase by an additional 67% by 2050. As a result, the number of persons with glaucoma is expected to increase an additional 50% from 2000 to 2020, leading to increasing utilization of aqueous shunting procedures.[2–4] The number of patients with postoperative orbital procedures encountered on head and neck imaging will also be increased because of the increasing epidemic of diabetes and our rapidly aging population.

Table 1
Common types of ophthalmologic surgeries for common diseases

Pathology	Surgery	Therapeutic Goals	Highlights of Surgical Technique
Cataract	Intraocular lens implant (IOL)	To replace the damaged lens to restore vision	IOL replaces the surgically removed cataractous lens
Glaucoma	Glaucoma shunt implant	To reduce intraocular pressure by decompression of aqueous humor	Glaucoma shunt is implanted most commonly in the superior temporal quadrant of the globe
Retinal detachment	Retinopexy Scleral buckling Vitrectomy	To reappose rhegmatogenous and or tractional retinal detachment	Scleral buckle is placed radially, segmentally, or circumferentially around the globes Intraocular injected air or silicone oil fills the vitrectomy cavity
Unsalvageable globe from trauma or infection or ocular tumor	Evisceration, enucleation and ocular implant	To eradicate the disease and provide cosmesis	Removal of the globe without (evisceration) or with (enucleation) removal of the sclera. Ocular implant is placed into the empty socket
Eyelid paralysis	Eyelid weight implant	To close the upper eyelid	Subcutaneous gold implant is secured to the tarsus in upper eyelid
Lacrimal obstruction	Dacryocystorhinostomy	To relieve lacrimal obstruction	Stent drains the lacrimal fossa to the inferior meatus
Thyroid-associated orbitopathy	Orbital decompression	To decompress the orbit for cosmesis and compressive optic neuropathy	Surgery removes the medial, inferior, or lateral orbital walls
Fracture	Orbital wall reconstruction	To restore orbital volume, cosmesis, and function	Autologous bone or cartilage, silicone, titanium plate and mesh, porous polyethylene material are used to reconstruct the orbital walls
Orbit malignancy	Orbital exenteration and reconstruction	To resect tumor and close orbital exenteration defect and restore cosmesis	Free flap is contoured to fill the exenteration defect and its vascular pedicle is reanastomosed to the available regional vessels

A variety of primary and secondary tumors affecting the orbits (retinoblastoma, rhabdomyosarcoma, uveal melanoma, orbital invasion from sinonasal and skin malignancies, or metastatic disease) require various treatment algorithms.[5,6] The data extracted from the Surveillance, Epidemiology, and End Results database show that the best relative survival of the common orbital neoplasms, including uveal melanoma, lacrimal gland tumor, and sinonasal malignancies with orbital involvement, was noted in patients treated with surgery or a combination of surgery and chemoradiotherapy.[7–11] Given the multidisciplinary medical advancements in treating orbital neoplasms, there is an increasing number of survivors who require surveillance imaging to monitor local disease control and treatment response, and to detect early recurrence and guide subsequent management.[10–13]

Other common orbital procedures include orbital decompression for thyroid orbitopathy and maxillofacial orbital reconstruction in the setting of trauma. This article is not meant to be encyclopedic, and is intended only to provide pertinent information relevant to the imaging evaluation of the commonly encountered orbital procedures, outlined in **Table 1**.

Given a gamut of orbital procedures and surgeries performed for a variety of clinical indications with a range of clinically acceptable therapeutic efficacy, the imaging interpretation of the postoperative orbit is more likely to be inaccurate if performed outside the clinical context.[14] In a symptomatic patient, the imaging may detect a new or progressive abnormality, more likely to alter the treatment, and hence contribute to the patient's well-being. On the other hand, in an asymptomatic patient, overdiagnosis with false-positive findings can induce additional workup leading to increased morbidity, anxiety, and downstream costs. For these reasons, the clinical importance of postoperative imaging of the orbit relies on the radiologist's confidence in diagnosing the normal postoperative appearance, to unequivocally identify procedural complications and detect early neoplastic recurrence in oncologic surveillance.

IMPORTANT ANATOMIC AND FUNCTIONAL CONSIDERATIONS

Vision is the most valuable sense, requiring an optimal and synchronized function of the eyelid, globe, lens, retina, and optic nerve, in addition to extraocular muscles and neurovascular structures. The commonly performed orbital procedures aim to protect and preserve the primary orbital function as a visual organ and the secondary function as the center of facial cosmesis.

Globe

To facilitate the understanding of the surgical principle of ocular surgeries, the anatomy of the globe is briefly discussed. There are 3 fluid-filled spaces in the globe: the anterior chamber, the posterior chamber, and the vitreous cavity.[15] The anterior chamber extends from the cornea to the iris and communicates, through the pupil, with the posterior chamber. The posterior chamber extends from the posterior surface of the iris to the anterior surface of the vitreous. The ciliary body, which produces the aqueous humor, and the intraocular lens are located in the posterior chamber. The anterior and posterior chambers are filled with aqueous humor. The vitreous cavity occupies the posterior globe behind the posterior chamber and contains gel-like vitreous humor.

The sclera, uvea, and retina compose the 3 layers of the globe. The sclera is a fibrous capsule around the globe contiguous with the cornea anteriorly and the dural sleeve of the optic nerve posteriorly. The uvea consists of the iris and the ciliary body anteriorly and the choroid layer posteriorly. The retina comprises the sensory retina layer supported by the retinal pigment epithelium beneath, all nourished by the choroid. Conjunctiva lines the inside of the eyelids and covers the anterior sclera.

Orbit

Orbital fractures with large floor defects may cause enophthalmos. On the other hand, increase of the intraorbital fat and enlargement of the extraocular muscles from thyroid orbitopathy result in exophthalmos, with stretching and/or compression of the optic nerve, resulting in visual compromise. At the tight orbital apex, the optic nerve is surrounded by the annulus of Zinn, rendering the optic nerve vulnerable to compression by even a small mass lesion or extraocular muscle enlargement, or by osseous narrowing. Therefore, the general role of reconstructive or decompressive surgeries of the orbit is to restore the normal orbital volume to preserve its function and cosmesis.

IMAGING PROTOCOLS

The acquisition of retinal images largely depends on fundoscopic examination and fundus photography. Ultrasonography has become an indispensable imaging adjuvant for the clinical assessment of a variety of ocular diseases by the ophthalmologist.[16,17] However, many such techniques are constrained by a relatively small field of view, and are often limited when there is disease-induced opacification of the lens or vitreous hemorrhage. Even though other imaging techniques such as computed tomography (CT) or MR imaging are more often not the first test of choice in diagnosing the common ocular disorders, these offer the ability to acquire images despite media opacification. These imaging tools are also valuable in evaluating the deep orbital structures behind the globe to define the full extent of the clinically evident infection, inflammation, or neoplasm, or in cases of blunt trauma.[18,19]

CT is the workhorse in imaging evaluation for calcification, infection, integrity of the implants, and orbital reconstruction.[18,20] The strength of CT is in evaluating the integrity of the osseous structure and the reconstructive hardware;

Table 2
Normal imaging findings of the orbital implants, prosthesis, ocular injections, and reconstructive materials

Procedure	Materials	Normal Imaging Findings
Intraocular lens implant (IOL)	Acrylic, silicone, or polymethyl methacrylate	Absence of normal lens Most IOLs are linear, thin, hyperattenuating optics placed between anterior and posterior chambers
Glaucoma shunt implant	Silicone, polypropylene, or polyethylene	The plate of the shunt is most commonly implanted on the superotemporal quadrant of the globe Silicone is homogeneously hyperdense; polypropylene is homogeneously hypodense All show low signal intensity on MR imaging A small bleb (fluid pocket) may be seen at the implant
Scleral buckling	Silicone solid rubber band, silicone sponge	The buckle may normally indent the globe Silicone rubber band shows hyperattenuating band encircling the globe. Silicone sponge shows air-density wedge on the globe
Ocular injection	Air, gas, silicone oil	Air and gas have air attenuation. Silicone oil appears homogeneously hyperattenuating
Ocular implant and eye prosthesis	Medpor[a] polyethylene, acrylic, silicone, hydroxyapatite	Medpor has hypodensity between fluid and fat. Both acrylic and silicone are homogeneously hyperattenuating Hydroxyapatite is very hyperdense with characteristic lattice pattern
Eyelid weights	Gold	Metallic plate is imbedded in the upper eyelid
Orbital reconstruction	Autologous bone graft, titanium fixation pin, plate, mesh, and porous polyethylene	Bone graft or metallic hardware is contoured to the orbital defect using osteotomies, plates, and pins Porous polyethylene has hypodensity or soft-tissue density
Orbital exenteration and free flap reconstruction	Fasciocutaneous flap Myocutaneous flap	The fatty component demonstrates fat signal characteristic on T1-weighted image The muscular component has characteristic muscular striation, T1 isointensity to muscle, and variable T2 signal intensity, and exhibits variable enhancement

[a] Implant made by Stryker, Kalamazoo, MI, USA.

3-dimensional (3D) volume rendering provides valuable assessment for the restoration of the orbital contour and volume. The superb soft-tissue characterization of MR is best used in oncologic surveillance.[19,21] General guidelines for the recognition of the normal imaging appearance of commonly used materials for routine ophthalmologic surgeries are suggested in **Table 2**.

Depending on the orbital subsites, the treated abnormality, and the clinical concern following surgical procedures, CT or MR imaging is tailored to provide high-resolution details of the orbit alone or to evaluate the regional orbital operative bed including the surrounding maxillofacial and skull base structures (**Box 1**).

URGENT POSTOPERATIVE COMPLICATIONS AND IMAGING PITFALLS

Most postoperative complications are diagnosed clinically by the ophthalmologist. Endophthalmitis is acute suppurative infection of the globe, which may occur acutely after an ophthalmologic procedure (within 6 weeks of surgery) or follow an indolent course with delayed onset (more than 6 weeks after surgery). Clinically it is characterized by ciliary injection, conjunctival chemosis, decreased visual acuity, and ocular pain.[22] Characteristic imaging of acute fulminant infection and progression of disease should not be mistaken for normal surgical sequelae (**Figs. 1** and **2**). Although procedure-related retinal detachment is mostly diagnosed clinically, new

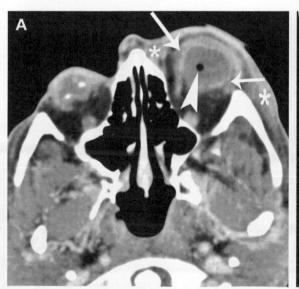
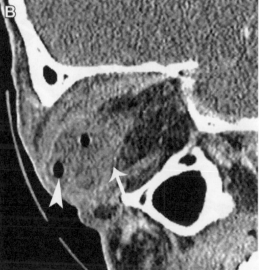

Fig. 1. Panophthalmitis. Severe eye pain, swelling, and purulent discharges 3 days after retinopexy for retinal detachment. (*A*) Axial enhanced CT image demonstrates diffuse enhancement and thickening of the uvea and sclera (*arrows*) and periorbital edema (*asterisks*). Note the residual air bubble (*arrowhead*) in the center of the vitreous chamber from pneumatic retinopexy. (*B*) Sagittal enhanced CT image shows posterior deformity of the globe (*arrow*), gas bubble migration to the anterior chamber (*arrowhead*), and nonvisualization of normal lens. The patient underwent emergent enucleation, which showed prolapsed necrotic lens, retina, and vitreous.

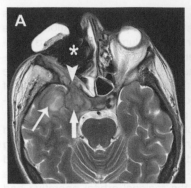
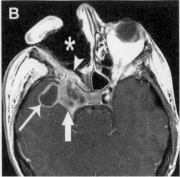
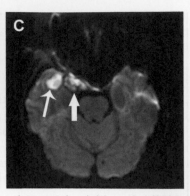

Fig. 2. *Rhizopus* fungal orbital infection. Axial T2-weighted (*A*), enhanced T1-weighted (*B*), and diffusion-weighted (*C*) images demonstrate orbital exenteration surgical bed containing surgical packing (*asterisks*). Deep to the surgical bed, the heterogeneous destructive fungal tissue directly invades the posterior orbital wall and superior orbital fissure (*arrowhead*), and spreads intracranially in the cavernous sinus (*thick arrow*) and right temporal lobe (*thin arrow*). Note the loss of the normal flow void and enhancement of the right cavernous internal carotid artery from vasoinvasive fungal occlusion.

retinal and choroidal detachments may herald an intraocular tumor (**Fig. 3**).[23]

POSTTREATMENT IMAGING FINDINGS: NORMAL AND PATHOLOGIC

To recognize the postsurgical changes and implants at imaging, one needs to understand the surgical technique and be familiar with the composition and configuration of the commonly used implants.

INTRAOCULAR LENS IMPLANTS

Cataract surgery and IOL remain the only viable alternative to preserve vision once a patient fails medical treatment. Phacoemulsification is the method of choice for removal of a cataractous lens, using ultrasonic energy to break up the cataractous lens into small fragments that are then suctioned out via a small incision.[24] Once the cataract is removed, the IOL is placed in the thin capsular bag that once housed the cataractous

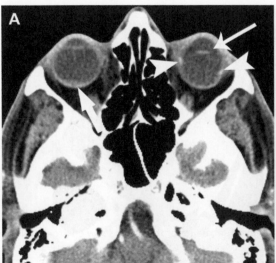
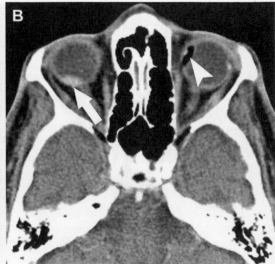

Fig. 3. Choroidal melanoma status post scleral buckling and intraocular lens replacement (IOL). (*A*) Axial enhanced CT image demonstrates silicone rubber band (*arrowheads*) encircling the left globe and left IOL (*arrow*), which is abnormally displaced posteriorly in the posterior chamber. There is subtle retinal detachment in the posterior right globe (*thick arrow*). The patient was blind on the left with decreased visual acuity on the right. (*B*) Axial enhanced CT image shows enhancing choroidal melanoma (*thick arrow*) in the upper posterior globe. Note the air-density silicone sponge (*arrowhead*) deep to the silicon rubber band at the nasal quadrant of the globe, which resulted from prior scleral buckling.

lens. The implantation of IOLs is now a highly successful operation, with well-established safety and efficacy.[25]

Many hundreds of different lens styles and designs now exist, composed of hydrophobic or hydrophilic acrylic, silicone, or polymethyl methacrylate.[24,26] The IOL comprises 2 components: the round optic, which replaces the native lens, and the loop-like haptics, which support the optic in place (Fig. 4A). Only the optic component of the lens implant is visible on CT as a hyperattenuating round disk-shaped structure with a thin profile, placed between the anterior and posterior chambers in the anatomic location of the extracted lens

(see Fig. 4B).[27] On MR imaging, this is seen as a structure of low linear signal intensity (see Fig. 4C).

An important complication related to cataract and lens implant surgery is endophthalmitis, which manifests on CT and MR as diffuse enhancement of the uvea and sclera or further involvement beyond the globe (panophthalmitis). Occasionally, dislocation or calcification of the implant can be seen on imaging (see Figs. 3A and 4D).

GLAUCOMA SHUNTING IMPLANTS

The blockage of fluid circulation in the eye leads to high intraocular pressure, which ultimately

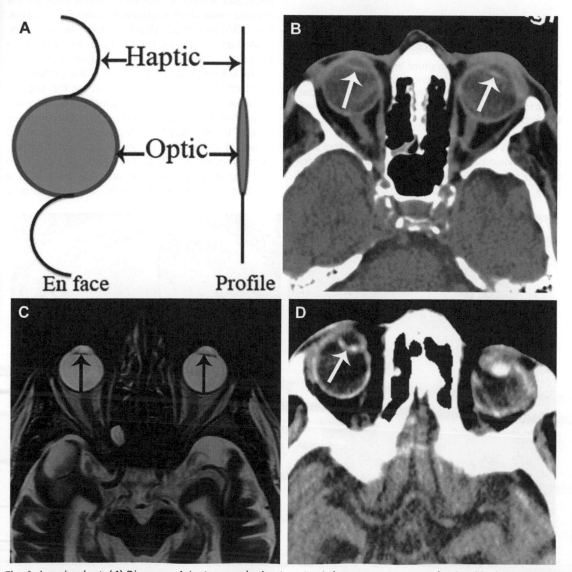

Fig. 4. Lens implant. (A) Diagram of the intraocular implant (IOL) shows round optic and string-like haptics. Axial unenhanced CT (B) and T2-weighted (C) images show normal thin profile of hyperattenuating and hypointense bilateral IOLs (arrows). (D) Axial unenhanced CT image shows abnormal calcification of the right IOL (arrow) in a patient with clinical evidence of opaque IOL and decreased visual acuity.

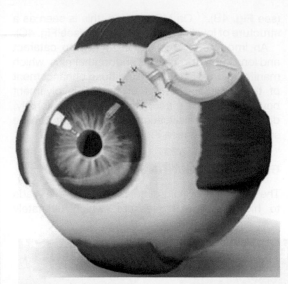

Fig. 5. Ahmed glaucoma shunt implant diagram. The plate is placed in the superior quadrant of the eye, and the tube is inserted into the anterior chamber. (*Courtesy of* New World Medical, Rancho Cucamonga, CA; with permission.)

contributes to damage of the optic nerve and subsequent vision loss. Therefore, glaucoma refractory to maximum tolerated medical therapy and laser trabeculoplasty often requires implantation

of a drainage device to lower the intraocular pressure.

There are 2 types of glaucoma shunts: valved and nonvalved. The basic requirements of any glaucoma device are the ability to remove aqueous humor from the anterior chamber without causing hypotony, and maintain long-term lower intraocular pressure. Nonvalved implants such as the Molteno (Molteno Ophthalmic Limited, Dunedin, New Zealand) and Baerveldt (Abbott Medical Optics, Santa Ana, CA, USA) offer no resistance to immediate outflow and require some forms of temporary mechanical plugging of the tube to avoid postoperative hypotony, flat anterior chambers, and choroidal effusions. Valved implants such as the Ahmed (New World Medical, Rancho Cucamonga, CA, USA) and Krupin (Eagle Vision, Memphis, TN, USA) have a one-way valve that closes below a set intraocular pressure to avoid hypotony.

The superotemporal quadrant of the globe is the most commonly chosen location for the implant because it avoids potential impingement of the oblique muscle fibers and allows for optimal exposure of the surgical field. A pocket is made in the sclera of the eye to house the plate of the glaucoma implant. A tract is then made into the anterior chamber of the eye, and the tube of the implant is then inserted (Fig. 5). The surgery

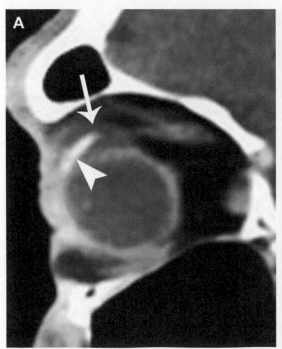
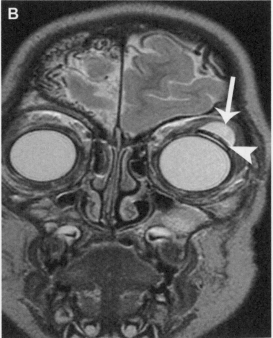

Fig. 6. Ahmed silicone glaucoma shunt implant. (*A*) Sagittal unenhanced CT image shows hyperdense silicone implant (*arrowhead*) in the superior globe surrounding by small amount of aqueous fluid density bleb (*arrow*). (*B*) Coronal T2-weighted image shows the flat hypointense plate implant (*arrowhead*) in the superotemporal quadrant of the left globe, and fluid-containing T2-hyperintense bleb (*arrow*) above the plate. The patient has glaucoma with Sturge-Weber syndrome.

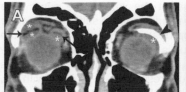
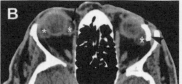
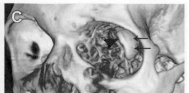

Fig. 7. Baerveldt glaucoma shunt implant. Coronal (A) and axial (B) unenhanced CT images show the large hyperdense single plate Baerveldt implant (*arrowhead*) in the superotemporal quadrant of the left globe, and smaller hypodense double-plate Ahmed implant (*arrows*) in the superotemporal and superonasal quadrants of the right globe. The implants are normally surrounded by small blebs (*asterisks*). (C) Three-dimensional (3D) volume-rendered CT image shows the characteristic larger plate surface (*arrowhead*) with fenestrations (*arrows*) of the Baerveldt implant.

creates a corneoscleral fistula that diverts the aqueous humor from the anterior chamber to a subconjunctival filtering bleb.[28] The bleb is the reservoir formed by development of fibrous capsule around the drained aqueous humor, which eventually will be absorbed by the surrounding tissue (Figs. 6 and 7).

The Baerveldt implants are composed of silicone and the Ahmed implants are either silicone, polypropylene, or polyethylene (see Figs. 6 and 7). The Baerveldt implant has fenestrations to allow ingrowth of fibrous tissue connecting the upper and lower walls of the blebs to limit their height (see Fig. 7). The implants are compatible with MR imaging and demonstrate low signal intensity surrounded by a small amount of fluid in the bleb.

The rates of reported complications range from 1% to 23%, with half of the drains failing at 5 years.[29–31] Some other common complications including shallow anterior chamber, hypotony,

postoperative elevated intraocular pressure, persistent corneal edema, choroidal effusion, hyphema, tube obstruction, and diplopia are diagnosed clinically. The rare complications of vitreous hemorrhage, retinal detachment, and endophthalmitis can be evident on CT imaging.[23] Bleb encapsulation or fibrosis, which blocks resorption of the drained aqueous humor, may be suggested on imaging in patients with clinical evidence of elevated intraocular pressure and enlarging blebs. Although late complication of bleb leak and rupture is commonly evident clinically, it may also be seen on imaging (Fig. 8).

SURGERY FOR RETINAL DETACHMENT

Retinal detachment, separation of the sensory retina from the underlying pigment epithelium, may be caused by a tear in the retina (aging-related degeneration, trauma), traction of the

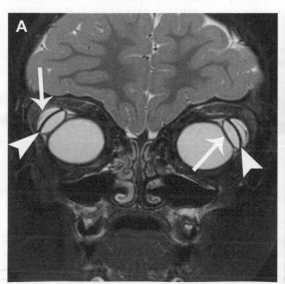
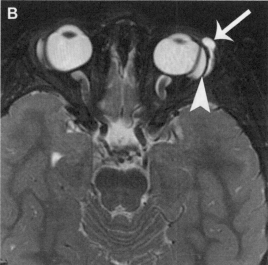

Fig. 8. Glaucoma shunt implant with bleb leak. (A) Coronal T2-weighted image shows bilateral linear low signal Ahmed valved shunts (*arrowheads*) surrounded by fluid blebs (*arrows*), which mildly indent the globes. (B) Axial T2-weighted image shows the implant (*arrowhead*) and anterior out-pouching of fluid signal in the upper outer conjunctiva of the left orbit (*arrow*), consistent with a leak.

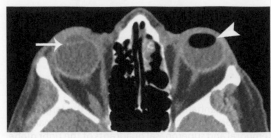

Fig. 9. Pneumatic retinopexy. Axial unenhanced CT image shows gas bubble (*arrowhead*) that tamponades the superior anterior quadrant of the left globe. Note the normal appearance of an IOL in the right globe (*arrow*).

pathologic vitreoretinal adhesion (diabetic retinopathy), or fluid exudation from ocular tumors (choroidal melanoma, metastatic disease). Exudative retinal detachment obviously needs definitive treatment of the underlying ocular neoplasm, and therefore is excluded from this discussion. Rhegmatogenous retinal detachment is treated with retinopexy, scleral buckling, and vitrectomy. Vitrectomy is also necessary for the treatment of tractional retinal detachment. Retinopexy is performed by using cryotherapy or laser photocoagulation to produce a chorioretinal scar around the retinal tear. Reapposition of the retina can be achieved with pneumatic retinopexy, scleral buckling, or both in conjunction with retinopexy.

Pneumatic Retinopexy

Intraocular injection of gas into the vitreous chamber (pneumatic retinopexy) creates the tamponade effect when the gas bubble pushes the detached retina back against the wall of the eye.[32] The most frequently used gases are sulfur hexafluoride (SF_6), perfluoropropane (C_3F_8), and sterile room air. The net result is the initial expansion of a bubble of pure SF_6 or $C_3 F_8$ within the vitreous, followed by gradual resorption (3–5 days with air, 7–10 days with SF_6, and 3–6 weeks with C_3F_8).[33,34] Cryoretinopexy is routinely performed before injection of air into the vitreous chamber, and the patient may return the next day for additional laser retinopexy as needed. Residual gas in the posterior vitreous chamber should not be mistaken for infection when there are no additional imaging or clinical findings of endophthalmitis, as discussed earlier (**Fig. 9**).

Scleral Buckling

A scleral buckle, a small synthetic band that is sutured to the sclera, exerts pressure to appose the detached layers of the retina together, resulting in normal impression on the globe. Scleral buckles are oriented either parallel or perpendicular to the rectus muscles, and focal/segmental or circumferential (**Fig. 10**). Porous silicone sponges appear as bands with air attenuation on CT, whereas the solid silicone rubber bands demonstrate hyperattenuation (see **Figs. 3** and **10**). Both are hypointense on T1-weighted and T2-weighted MR images, and are often difficult to appreciate (see **Fig. 10C**).[35] Infection, erosion, and extrusion are evident clinically, and often scleral buckles are seen incidentally on neuroimaging. Recurrent or persistent retinal detachment occurs in 9% to 25% of surgical cases.[32–35]

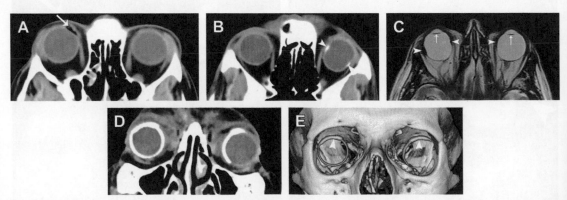

Fig. 10. Scleral buckling. (*A*) Axial unenhanced CT image shows air-density radial silicone sponge (*arrow*) in the superonasal quadrant of the right globe oriented parallel to the adjacent medial rectus muscle. The sponge was mistaken for a foreign body (wood chip). (*B*) Axial unenhanced CT image shows hyperattenuating silicone rubber band (*arrowheads*) encircling the left globe with normal mild indentation on the globe. (*C*) Axial T2-weighted image shows T2-hypointense silicone rubber band (*arrowheads*) that subtly indents the right globe and bilateral IOLs (*arrows*). Scleral buckle is difficult to identify on MR; the left scleral band is only seen along the nasal side (*arrowhead*). Coronal (*D*) and 3D volume-rendered (*E*) CT images show bilateral scleral buckling with silicone rubber bands (*arrowheads*), circumferential on the right and segmental on the left.

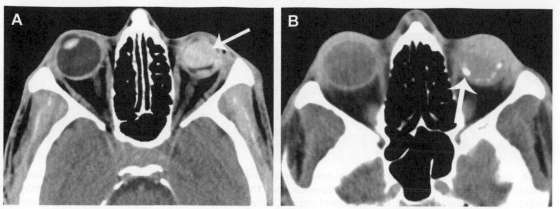

Fig. 11. Retinal detachment. (*A*) Axial unenhanced CT image shows homogeneously hyperattenuating silicone oil injection (*arrow*) in the vitreous chamber after vitrectomy and retinopexy in this patient with traction retinal detachment from diabetic retinopathy. (*B*) Axial unenhanced CT image obtained 10 years later shows removal of the hyperdense silicone oil and development of phthisis bulbi, evident by smaller globe and ocular calcifications (*arrow*). The patient had lost vision in the left eye with new eye pain related to phthisis bulbi.

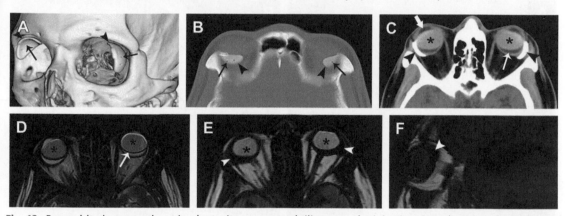

Fig. 12. Baerveldt glaucoma shunt implant, vitrectomy, and silicone ocular injection. 3D volume-rendered (*A*) and axial unenhanced (*B*) CT images show the curve profile of the Baerveldt implants (*arrowheads*) and their characteristic fenestrations (*arrows*). (*C*) Axial unenhanced CT image shows characteristic homogeneous high density of silicone injection (*asterisks*) in the posterior vitreous chamber for treatment of retinal detachment, a complication related to implant placement. Note the normal fluid density of posterior vitreous behind the silicone (*thin arrow*) and in the anterior chamber (*thick arrow*). This patient does not have visible bleb around the implants (*arrowheads*). Axial T2-weighted (*D*), axial fluid-attenuated inversion recovery (*E*), and sagittal T1-weighted (*F*) images show homogeneous signal intensity of silicone (*asterisks*), which is slightly T2-hypointense and T1-hyperintense, and demonstrates chemical shift artifact (*arrow*) at the interface between the silicone and vitreous. Note the subtle low signal intensity of the glaucoma implants (*arrowheads*).

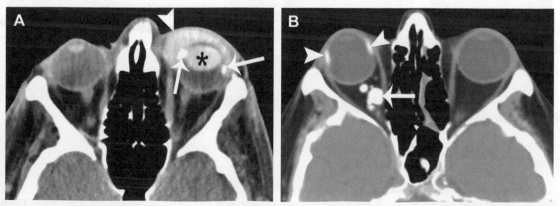

Fig. 13. Silicone migration. (*A*) Axial unenhanced CT image shows migration of silicone (*asterisk*) from the globe into the conjunctiva and periorbital soft tissue of the upper eyelid (*arrowhead*). Note the hyperdense silicone rubber band of scleral buckling (*arrows*) encircling the globe. (*B*) Axial unenhanced CT image shows abnormal location of the silicone (*arrow*) in the retrobulbar space after remote vitrectomy, intraocular silicone injection, and subsequent removal for diabetic retinopathy. Note the normal appearance of the silicone rubber band (*arrowheads*).

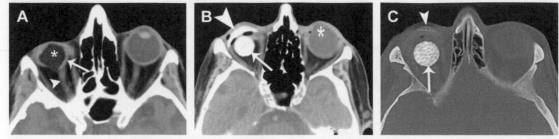

Fig. 14. Ocular implant and eye prosthesis. (*A*) Axial unenhanced CT image shows right evisceration with visible residual sclera (*arrow*) and preserved optic nerve (*arrowhead*) and the typical fluid-fat density of the porous polyethylene Medpor ocular implant (*asterisk*). (*B*) Axial unenhanced CT image demonstrates 2 components of the characteristic homogeneously hyperattenuating silicone prosthesis: the anterior scleral cover shell eye prosthesis (*arrowhead*) and the posterior sphere ocular implant (*arrow*). The left lens (*asterisk*) is absent from failed IOL. The patient lost vision from complications of diabetes. (*C*) Axial unenhanced CT image shows the very hyperdense hydroxyapatite ocular implant (*arrow*) with characteristic internal lattice and less hyperdense silicone eye prosthesis (*arrowhead*).

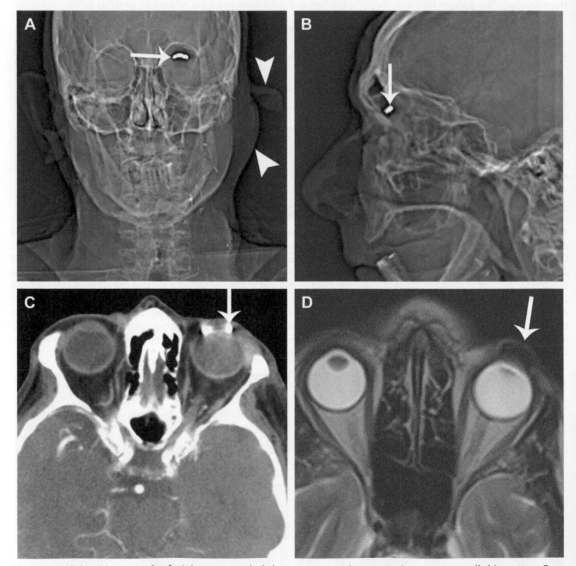

Fig. 15. Eyelid gold weight for facial nerve paralysis in a patient with metastatic squamous cell skin cancer. Frontal (*A*) and lateral (*B*) scout tomograms show the crescentic metallic weight (*arrows*), parotidectomy, and flap reconstruction (*arrowheads*). (*C*) Axial enhanced CT image accurately pinpoints the weight (*arrow*) in the upper eyelid. (*D*) T2-weighted image with fat saturation shows susceptibility artifact of the gold weight (*arrow*).

Vitrectomy

The indications for vitrectomy surgery are continuously expanding, and include the treatment of vitreous hemorrhage, infection, and retinal detachment.[34] To avoid damage to the retina, the surgical instruments are inserted into the posterior vitreous through tiny (1-mm) incisions in the posterior zone of the ciliary body (pars plana).[34,35] Initially the vitreous is completely removed from the retinal tears and any scar tissue is removed from the retina. Retinotomy is created for internal drainage of subretinal fluid. Laser retinopexy is then performed around the retinal breaks. At the conclusion of the procedure the eye is filled with gas, air, or silicone oil as a tamponade agent. Silicone oil can be removed 2 to 3 months postoperatively if the retina is completely flat. Alternatively, it can be left permanently if there is residual retraction, recurrent detachment, or hypotonia.[34,35]

Silicone oil appears homogeneously hyperattenuating to normal vitreous fluid on CT (Fig. 11), and should not be mistaken for vitreous hemorrhage.[36] Silicone oil is hyperintense to normal vitreous on T1-weighted images and variably hyperintense to hypointense on T2-weighted images (Fig. 12). The presence of chemical shift artifact and the effects of fat saturation can be used to differentiate silicone oil from vitreous hemorrhage.[35,36] Occasionally, silicone may migrate outside the globe (Fig. 13).

EVISCERATION, ENUCLEATION, OCULAR IMPLANT, AND EYE PROSTHESIS

Evisceration removes the globe content with sparing of the sclera. Enucleation removes all the content of the globe and the anterior portion of the optic nerve. Those 2 procedures are surgical treatment for unsalvageable globe rupture and intraocular malignancies.

Following evisceration and enucleation, a ball-shaped ocular implant is permanently embedded deep in the eye socket to replace the surgically removed globe.[37] Various shapes of anophthalmic sockets can be effectively reconstructed using a variety of ocular implants, resulting in various imaging appearances (Fig. 14).[27,37,38] The most commonly used ocular implant, Medpor (Stryker, Kalamazoo, MI, USA) has pore structure, which promotes native tissue ingrowth, and may be implanted without or with tissue wrap. The extraocular muscles may be sutured directly to the implant.[38] The other popular ocular implants are hydroxyapatite and nonporous alloplastic implants (acrylic and silicone). After healing is complete, a shell-shaped removable prosthetic eye is custom-made to fit over the ocular implant and under the eyelids to provide cosmesis. Alternatively, a thin scleral shell can be worn over the damaged or eviscerated eye.

In a review of 342 patients over 10 years, only 7 patients developed long-term complications

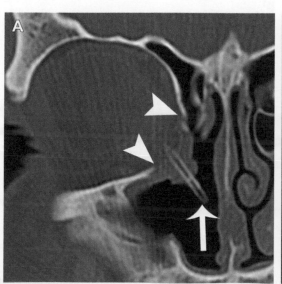
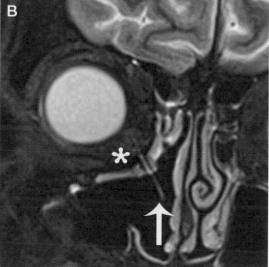

Fig. 16. Dacryocystorhinostomy and nasolacrimal duct stent. (A) Coronal unenhanced CT image shows the plastic stent (arrow) extending from the lacrimal fossa to the sinonasal cavity through the widely open dacryocystorhinostomy bone defect (arrowheads). (B) Coronal T2-weighted image with fat saturation shows the stent in place (arrow) and no evidence of dacrocystocele or collection in the lacrimal fossa (asterisk). The stent was subsequently removed.

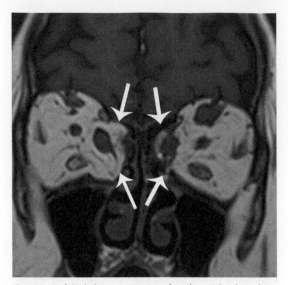

Fig. 17. Orbital decompression for thyroid-related orbitopathy. Coronal T1-weighted MR image shows endoscopic removal of the lamina papyracea along the medial and inferomedial orbital walls to decompress the orbit by allowing prolapse of the enlarged extraocular muscles and orbital fat through the defects (*arrows*).

including exposure, infection, and pyogenic granuloma.[39] Diffuse linear enhancement surrounding the implant may reflect ingrowth or granulation, and has no clinical significance.[40]

EYELID WEIGHTS

Patients affected with lagophthalmos are unable to fully close their eyelids, the causes of which include facial nerve palsy, damage to the eyelid tissues, or inhibition to proper eyelid closure as in exophthalmos or enophthalmos. Inability to fully close the eyelid exposes the cornea, leading to corneal ulceration and infectious keratitis. The commonly used gold weight, which is safe for MR imaging, is implanted subcutaneously in the upper eyelid and secured to the tarsus to enable eye closure (**Fig. 15**).[41]

LACRIMAL GLAND DACRYOCYSTORHINOSTOMY

To relieve lacrimal obstruction, the preferred surgical procedure is dacryocystorhinostomy, which entails removal of the bone from medial canthus to widely connect the nasolacrimal duct to the nasal cavity. A plastic stent can be placed in the nasolacrimal duct for temporary relief. The stents have poor long-term patency attributable to occlusion from granulation tissue or debris (**Fig. 16**).

ORBITAL DECOMPRESSION

In thyroid-associated orbitopathy, the enlargement of orbital fat and muscles within the confined bony walls causes proptosis resulting in exposure keratitis and cornea ulceration, venous congestion

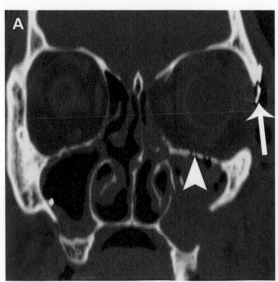

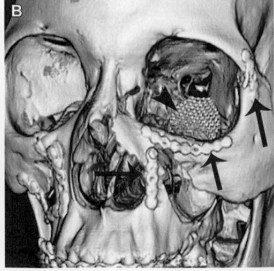

Fig. 18. Orbital reconstruction for unstable fractures. (*A*) Coronal unenhanced CT image shows reconstruction of the lateral orbital rim with pin and plate fixation (*arrow*) and the orbital floor with metallic mesh (*arrowhead*). (*B*) 3D volume-rendered CT image demonstrates reestablishment of the facial buttress and orbital contour by the pin and plate fixations (*arrows*) of left lateral and inferior orbital rims and the maxilla, and restoration of the orbital volume with normal contour of the orbital floor mesh reconstruction (*arrowhead*) to prevent enophthalmos.

resulting in edema and chemosis, and increases in orbital pressure and optic nerve compression resulting in visual impairment. The most common indications for decompression are cosmesis and compressive optic neuropathy. The postoperative outcome measures the reduction in proptosis using exophthalmometry, which measures the distance between the outer orbital rim and apex of the cornea, and the improvement in visual acuity.[42,43] Decompression is performed by fenestration of

medial, lateral, or inferior orbital wall with or without removal of the intraorbital fat.

Imaging shows reduction in proptosis, and prolapse of overgrowth orbital fat and rectus muscles into these surgically created defects of the orbital walls (**Fig. 17**). An endoscopic approach results in imaging evidence of partial ethmoidectomy and middle turbinectomy for access to the lamina papyracea. In a systematic review of 4,176 decompressions, the mean reduction of

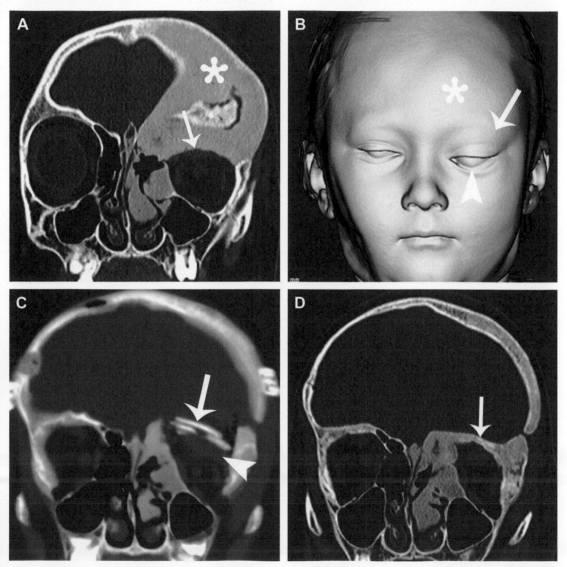

Fig. 19. Orbital reconstruction with frontal orbital advancement for fibrous dysplasia. (*A*) Coronal unenhanced CT image shows ground-glass fibrous dysplasia (*asterisk*) expanding the orbital roof compressing the superior orbit (*arrow*). (*B*) 3D volume-rendered CT image reveals the deformity with frontal bossing (*asterisk*), superior orbital roof depression (*arrow*), and resulting proptosis (*arrowhead*). (*C*) Immediate postoperative coronal unenhanced CT image shows resection of the fibrous dysplasia and orbital roof reconstruction using autologous bone grafts (*arrow*). Note that the reconstruction restores the orbital height as close as possible to the contralateral orbit. The extraconal postoperative collection (*arrowhead*) filling the fibrous dysplasia resection bed underneath the bone grafts has no clinical sequela. (*D*) Three-month follow-up unenhanced coronal CT image demonstrates osseous union of the bone grafts (*arrow*) to the orbital walls, with clinical resolution of left proptosis and optic nerve compression.

proptosis was found to be 2 to 6 mm with an overall complication rate of 9.3% (paresthesia, conjunctivitis, cerebrospinal fluid leak, vision loss, and stroke).[42]

ORBITAL WALL RECONSTRUCTION

In general, the role of surgical reconstruction of the orbit in the setting of trauma is to release entrapment and to restore orbital volume and contour, to prevent enophthalmos and cosmetic deformity.[20,44,45] The overview of orbital volume and contour and its complex bony anatomy and reconstruction is best evaluated with 3D volume-rendered CT reconstruction (**Fig. 18**). Benign neoplasms such as fibrous dysplasia and intraosseous meningioma can exert mass effect on the orbit, resulting in cosmetic deformity, proptosis,

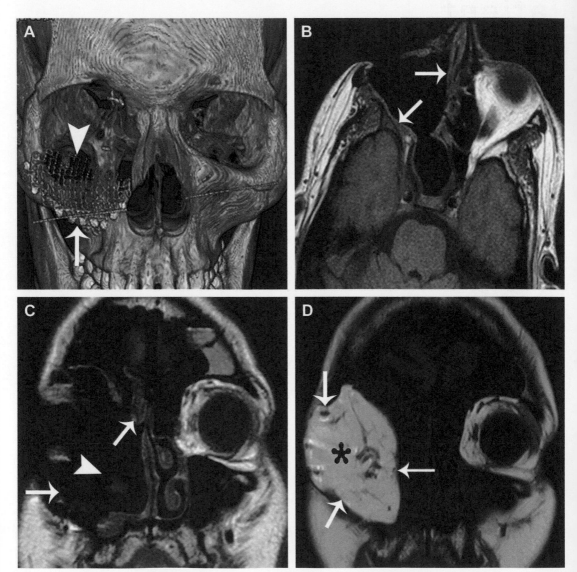

Fig. 20. Orbital exenteration and reconstruction for orbital invasion from sinonasal undifferentiated carcinoma. (*A*) 3D volume-rendered CT image shows the titanium pin and plate fixation (*arrow*) and mesh reconstruction (*arrowhead*) of the anterior maxilla and orbital rim and floor. The empty eye socket, either lined by slit-thickness skin graft or healed by granulation, serves as a cavity for orbital prosthesis. Axial (*B*) and coronal (*C*) T1-weighted MR images show empty surgical bed lined by granulation and mucosa (*arrows*) with debris and secretion (*arrowhead*) without tumor recurrence; however, imaging is not specific for detection of fistula, dehiscence, and poor wound healing, which ultimately required hardware removal and redo reconstruction in this patient. (*D*) Coronal T1-weighted MR image shows the normal fatty content (*asterisk*) of the new orbitomaxillary reconstruction using a radial forearm fasciocutaneous flap (*arrows*).

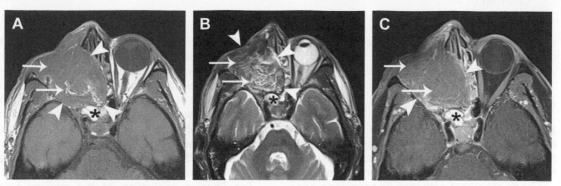

Fig. 21. Orbital exenteration and reconstruction for orbital invasion from sinonasal melanoma. Axial T1-weighted image (A), T2-weighted image (B), and enhanced T1-weighted image with fat saturation (C) show the myocutaneous flap (arrowheads) filling the orbital exenteration surgical defect. The muscle component of the flap has characteristic muscle striations (arrows) and T1-isointense to muscle with heterogeneous T2 signal intensity and enhancement similar to muscle. Secretions are trapped in the sphenoid sinus (asterisk).

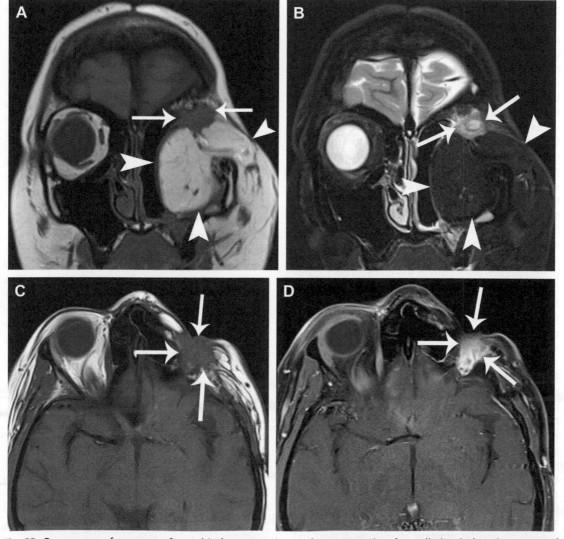

Fig. 22. Recurrence of sarcoma after orbital exenteration and reconstruction for radiation-induced sarcoma of the orbit. The patient received radiation for retinoblastoma as a child. Coronal T1-weighted (A) and short-tau inversion recovery (B) images show growing nodule (arrows) in the superior margin of fasciocutaneous flap (arrowheads) at the junction with the orbital roof resection bed. Axial unenhanced image (C) and enhanced T1-weighted image with fat saturation (D) demonstrate the solid enhancement of the recurrent sarcoma (arrows).

optic nerve compression, and extraocular muscle compression, necessitating orbital wall resection and reconstruction (**Fig. 19**).

ORBITAL EXENTERATION

Malignancies involving or invading the orbit warrant aggressive surgical management ranging from evisceration and enucleation to orbital exenteration. Orbital prosthesis has been a reasonable cosmetic solution in patients who have undergone evisceration and enucleation, as discussed earlier. The workhorse for sizable and complex orbital and facial defect reconstruction in oncologic practice is free tissue transfer flaps.[46]

Imaging is not routinely used for the assessment of common postoperative complications following flap reconstruction, such as hematomas and other collections, vascular thrombosis, infection, or flap viability.[21] The gold standard for flap monitoring remains clinical observation of the flap. The viability of the vascularized flap has a poor correlation with enhancement and the signal characteristics of the flap on imaging. Occasionally, ultrasonography or CT imaging may be indicated to identify a rapidly expanding hematoma that may need evacuation for decompression. In general, the diagnostic performance of contrast-enhanced CT for distinguishing an infected collection from a resolving hematoma/seroma without clinical input has high sensitivity but poor specificity. The edema of the flap and the surgical bed is evident up to 4 to 6 weeks following surgery, and can persist for years in patients receiving postoperative irradiation to the surgical bed. Clinicians uncommonly obtain cross-sectional imaging for fistula because its presence is usually established on clinical examination. Nevertheless, it is difficult to delineate the fistula on cross-sectional imaging (**Fig. 20**).

The primary role of follow-up CT and MR imaging is to evaluate the extent of tumor resection, monitor the response to chemoradiation, and assess for tumor recurrence or a new primary tumor. The presence of a flap is identified by the replacement of the normal anatomy by a soft-tissue mass with unique tissue composition of primarily fat or fat and muscle (see **Fig. 20**; **Fig. 21**, see **Table 2**). In general, all fasciocutaneous flaps contain nonenhancing T1 hyperintense fatty tissue (see **Fig. 20**). When the fasciomyocutaneous flap is harvested, the muscle component of the flap has characteristic striation of muscle fibers and is isointense to other muscles in the head and neck (see **Fig. 21**). However, the muscular component shows variable T2 signal intensity and degrees of enhancement relative to adjacent

normal muscle.[21] The heterogeneity of signal and enhancement of the muscle component are speculated to reflect the sequelae of vascular disruption, revascularization, or muscular denervation, and the effect of adjuvant radiation. Even though vascularized scar tissue may enhance, fibrotic scar is typically hypointense. Stability or gradual loss of volume of the enhancing flap and scar over time distinguish them from growing enhancing tumor.

The imaging evaluation of the surgical bed should begin with identification of the normal flap and delineation of its extent of coverage of the defect. Next, the border between the healthy flap and the recipient resection bed should be carefully inspected for the presence of an enlarging soft-tissue mass. New or growing mass-like tissue that is similar in appearance to the primary tumor should raise suspicion for recurrence (**Fig. 22**).[21,47]

SUMMARY

As the expected life span and cancer survival continue to improve as a result of the technological advancements in surgical techniques and the multidisciplinary treatment of orbital disease and neoplasm, imaging of the postoperative orbit will be increasingly encountered in everyday radiology practices. The altered anatomy can present a challenge to the unfamiliar radiologist, and it is of utmost importance that normal implants, prostheses, and reconstructive flaps are not mistaken for unintended foreign body or neoplasm. Fundamental knowledge of the surgical techniques and principles of common ophthalmologic surgeries and reconstructions is essential to simplify the complex imaging appearance of these postoperative cases. Postoperative imaging studies of the orbit should be interpreted with knowledge of the clinical data to avoid unnecessary incidental imaging findings and further workup or treatment of nonsymptomatic disease, which can compromise patient care.

REFERENCES

1. Centers for Disease Control and Prevention. Common eye disorders. 2015. Available at: http://wwwcdcgov/nutrition/. Accessed January 10, 2015.
2. Quigley HA, Broman AT. The number of people with glaucoma worldwide in 2010 and 2020. Br J Ophthalmol 2006;90(3):262–7.
3. Ramulu PY, Corcoran KJ, Corcoran SL, et al. Utilization of various glaucoma surgeries and procedures in Medicare beneficiaries from 1995 to 2004. Ophthalmology 2007;114(12):2265–70.

4. Minckler DS, Francis BA, Hodapp EA, et al. Aqueous shunts in glaucoma: a report by the American Academy of Ophthalmology. Ophthalmology 2008;115(6):1089–98.

5. Meltzer DE. Orbital imaging: a pattern-based approach. Radiol Clin North Am 2015;53(1):37–80.

6. Pfortner R, Mohr C, Daamen J, et al. Orbital tumors: operative and therapeutic strategies. Facial Plast Surg 2014;30(5):570–7.

7. Turner JH, Reh DD. Incidence and survival in patients with sinonasal cancer: a historical analysis of population based data. Head Neck 2012;34(6):877–85.

8. Mallen-St Clair J, Arshi A, Tajudeen B, et al. Epidemiology and treatment of lacrimal gland tumors: a population-based cohort analysis. JAMA Otolaryngol Head Neck Surg 2014;140(12):1110–6.

9. Li N, Xu L, Zhao H, et al. A comparison of the demographics, clinical features, and survival of patients with adenoid cystic carcinoma of major and minor salivary glands versus less common sites within the Surveillance, Epidemiology, and End Results registry. Cancer 2012;118(16):3945–53.

10. Tyers AG. Orbital exenteration for invasive skin tumours. Eye 2006;20(10):1165–70.

11. Hassan WM, Alfaar AS, Bakry MS, et al. Orbital tumors in USA: difference in survival patterns. Cancer Epidemiol 2014;38(5):515–22.

12. Shinohara ET, DeWees T, Perkins SM. Subsequent malignancies and their effect on survival in patients with retinoblastoma. Pediatr Blood Cancer 2014; 61(1):116–9.

13. Singh AD, Turell ME, Topham AK. Uveal melanoma: trends in incidence, treatment, and survival. Ophthalmology 2011;118(9):1881–5.

14. McClelland C, Van Stavern GP, Shepherd JB, et al. Neuroimaging in patients referred to a neuro-ophthalmology service: the rates of appropriateness and concordance in interpretation. Ophthalmology 2012;119(8):1701–4.

15. Belden CJ. MR imaging of the globe and optic nerve. Neuroimaging Clin N Am 2004;14(4):809–25.

16. Coleman DJ, Silverman RH, Rondeau MJ, et al. Explaining the current role of high frequency ultrasound in ophthalmic diagnosis (ophthalmic ultrasound). Expert Rev Ophthalmol 2006;1(1):63–76.

17. Guthoff RF, Labriola LT, Stachs O. Diagnostic ophthalmic ultrasound. In: Ryan S, editor. Retina. 5th edition. London: Saunders; 2013. p. 227–84.

18. Lee AG, Johnson MC, Policeni BA, et al. Imaging for neuro-ophthalmic and orbital disease—a review. Clin Experiment Ophthalmol 2009;37(1):30–53.

19. Wu AY, Jebodhsingh K, Le T, et al. Indications for orbital imaging by the oculoplastic surgeon. Ophthal Plast Reconstr Surg 2011;27(4):260–2.

20. Wilde F, Schramm A. Intraoperative imaging in orbital and midface reconstruction. Facial Plast Surg 2014;30(5):545–53.

21. Learned KO, Malloy KM, Loevner LA. Myocutaneous flaps and other vascularized grafts in head and neck reconstruction for cancer treatment. Magn Reson Imaging Clin N Am 2012;20(3):495–513.

22. Han DP, Wisniewski SR, Wilson LA, et al. Spectrum and susceptibilities of microbiologic isolates in the Endophthalmitis Vitrectomy Study. Am J Ophthalmol 1996;122(1):1–17.

23. LeBedis CA, Sakai O. Nontraumatic orbital conditions: diagnosis with CT and MR imaging in the emergent setting. Radiographics 2008;28(6): 1741–53.

24. de Silva SR, Riaz Y, Evans JR. Phacoemulsification with posterior chamber intraocular lens versus extracapsular cataract extraction (ECCE) with posterior chamber intraocular lens for age-related cataract. Cochrane Database Syst Rev 2014;(1):CD008812.

25. Werner L, Olson RJ, Mamalis N. New technology IOL optics. Ophthalmol Clin North Am 2006;19(4): 469–83.

26. Benjamin L. Cataract surgery. Surgical techniques in ophthalmology. Edinburgh (United Kingdom): Elsevier Saunders; 2007. Available at: http://hdl.library.upenn.edu/1017.12/1337963.

27. Adams A, Mankad K, Poitelea C, et al. Post-operative orbital imaging: a focus on implants and prosthetic devices. Neuroradiology 2014;56(11): 925–35.

28. Chen TC. Glaucoma surgery. Surgical techniques in ophthalmology. Philadelphia: Saunders Elsevier; 2008. Available at: http://hdl.library.upenn.edu/1017.12/1337969.

29. Christakis PG, Tsai JC, Kalenak JW, et al. The Ahmed versus Baerveldt study: three-year treatment outcomes. Ophthalmology 2013;120(11): 2232–40.

30. Bailey AK, Sarkisian SR Jr. Complications of tube implants and their management. Curr Opin Ophthalmol 2014;25(2):148–53.

31. Patel S, Pasquale LR. Glaucoma drainage devices: a review of the past, present, and future. Semin Ophthalmol 2010;25(5–6):265–70.

32. Chan CK, Lin SG, Nuthi AS, et al. Pneumatic retinopexy for the repair of retinal detachments: a comprehensive review (1986-2007). Surv Ophthalmol 2008; 53(5):443–78.

33. Brinton DA, Chiang A. Pneumatic retinopexy. In: Ryan SJ, editor. Retina. 5th edition. London: Saunders; 2013. p. 1721–34.

34. Bhavsar AR. Retina and vitreous surgery. Surgical techniques in ophthalmology. Philadelphia: Elsevier/Saunders; 2009. Available at: http://hdl.library.upenn.edu/1017.12/1337956.

35. Lane JI, Watson RE Jr, Witte RJ, et al. Retinal detachment: imaging of surgical treatments and complications. Radiographics 2003;23(4):983–94.

36. Mathews VP, Elster AD, Barker PB, et al. Intraocular silicone oil: in vitro and in vivo MR and CT characteristics. AJNR Am J Neuroradiol 1994;15(2):343–7.

37. Su GW, Yen MT. Current trends in managing the anophthalmic socket after primary enucleation and evisceration. Ophthal Plast Reconstr Surg 2004; 20(4):274–80.

38. Custer PL, Kennedy RH, Woog JJ, et al. Orbital implants in enucleation surgery: a report by the American Academy of Ophthalmology. Ophthalmology 2003;110(10):2054–61.

39. Christmas NJ, Gordon CD, Murray TG, et al. Intraorbital implants after enucleation and their complications: a 10-year review. Arch Ophthalmol 1998; 116(9):1199–203.

40. Barnwell JD, Castillo M. MR imaging of progressive enhancement of a bioceramic orbital prosthesis: an indicator of fibrovascular invasion. AJNR Am J Neuroradiol 2011;32(1):E8–9.

41. Kartush JM, Linstrom CJ, McCann PM, et al. Early gold weight eyelid implantation for facial paralysis. Otolaryngol Head Neck Surg 1990;103(6):1016–23.

42. Leong SC, Karkos PD, Macewen CJ, et al. A systematic review of outcomes following surgical decompression for dysthyroid orbitopathy. Laryngoscope 2009;119(6):1106–15.

43. Leong SC, White PS. Outcomes following surgical decompression for dysthyroid orbitopathy (Graves' disease). Curr Opin Otolaryngol Head Neck Surg 2010;18(1):37–43.

44. Caranci F, Cicala D, Cappabianca S, et al. Orbital fractures: role of imaging. Semin Ultrasound CT MR 2012;33(5):385–91.

45. Kolk A, Pautke C, Schott V, et al. Secondary posttraumatic enophthalmos: high-resolution magnetic resonance imaging compared with multislice computed tomography in postoperative orbital volume measurement. J Oral Maxillofac Surg 2007; 65(10):1926–34.

46. O'Connell DA, Futran ND. Reconstruction of the midface and maxilla. Curr Opin Otolaryngol Head Neck Surg 2010;18(4):304–10.

47. Lee PS, Sedrak P, Guha-Thakurta N, et al. Imaging findings of recurrent tumors after orbital exenteration and free flap reconstruction. Ophthal Plast Reconstr Surg 2014;30(4):315–21.

Imaging of Pediatric Orbital Diseases

Behroze A. Vachha, MD, PhD[a], Caroline D. Robson, MB,ChB[b],*

KEYWORDS

- Pediatric • Orbit • Ocular • CT • MR imaging • Congenital • Tumor • Vascular

KEY POINTS

- Orbital diseases in children differ from those found in adults in terms of histopathologic and imaging characteristics.
- Clinical signs are often nonspecific, and imaging is a critical step in evaluating the pediatric orbit, optic pathway, and cranial nerves that supply the orbital contents.
- High-resolution 3-T MR imaging helps characterize orbital and ocular soft-tissue lesions, permitting superior delineation of orbital soft tissues, cranial nerves, blood vessels, and blood flow and detection of intracranial extension of orbital disease.
- Computed tomography (CT) is reserved primarily for evaluation of orbital bony architecture.

INTRODUCTION

The wide spectrum of orbital disease seen in children differs substantially from that found in adults in terms of histopathologic and imaging features. Clinical symptoms and signs such as proptosis, strabismus, diplopia, and optic disc edema are nonspecific, and diagnostic imaging studies play an essential role in depicting the nature and extent of orbital abnormalities, often providing a definitive diagnosis or a relevant differential diagnosis. The information provided by imaging is also important in determining optimal medical or surgical treatment and assessing response to treatment. In this article, the salient clinical and imaging features of various pediatric orbital lesions are described, and the differential diagnoses are reviewed.

NORMAL ANATOMY

The orbital contents are contained within a bony pyramid. The orbital roof is formed by the orbital plate of the frontal bone. The lateral wall is formed by the orbital surface of the zygomatic bone and greater wing of the sphenoid. The frontal process of the maxillary bone, the lacrimal bone, lamina papyracea of the ethmoid bone, and the lesser wing of the sphenoid make up the medial wall from anterior to posterior. The orbital floor is formed by the orbital surfaces of the zygomatic, maxillary, and palatine bones. The optic foramen forms the apex of the bony pyramid and is formed by the lesser wing of the sphenoid. The superior orbital fissure is limited by the lesser wing of the sphenoid superomedially and the greater wing of the sphenoid inferolaterally. The inferior orbital fissure lies between the orbital floor and the greater wing of the sphenoid. The optic canal and superior and inferior orbital fissures transmit nerves and vessels (Table 1); spread of tumor along these conduits can occur from the orbit to extraorbital compartments including intracranial extension.

The orbital contents are divided into the intraocular compartment or globe, the muscle cone, and

Disclosures: None.
[a] Department of Radiology, Massachusetts General Hospital, 55 Fruit Street, Boston, MA 02114, USA;
[b] Department of Radiology, Boston Children's Hospital, Harvard Medical School, 300 Longwood Avenue, Boston, MA 02115, USA
* Corresponding author.
E-mail address: caroline.robson@childrens.harvard.edu

Neuroimag Clin N Am 25 (2015) 477–501
http://dx.doi.org/10.1016/j.nic.2015.05.009
1052-5149/15/$ – see front matter © 2015 Elsevier Inc. All rights reserved.

neuroimaging.theclinics.com

Table 1
Contents of orbital foramina

Foramen	Contents
Superior orbital fissure	Cranial nerves III, IV, V$_1$, VI Superior ophthalmic vein Orbital branch of middle meningeal artery
Inferior orbital fissure	Cranial nerve V$_2$ Infraorbital vein Infraorbital artery
Optic canal	Cranial nerve II Ophthalmic artery

the intraconal and extraconal spaces (**Fig. 1**A). The extraocular muscles include the superior, inferior, medial, and lateral rectus muscles and the superior and inferior obliques; all but the inferior oblique

muscles constitute the muscle cone (see **Fig. 1**B). The levator palpebrae superioris lies superior to the superior oblique muscle. The extraocular muscles converge at the orbital apex to form a fibrous connective tissue ring known as the annulus of Zinn. The nonocular compartment of the eye is divided by the muscle cone into conal (muscle cone and annulus of Zinn), intraconal, and extraconal spaces. The intraconal space contains fat, the ciliary ganglion, the ophthalmic artery and vein, and branches of the ophthalmic nerve. The ophthalmic artery and vein and cranial nerves enter the intraconal space through the annulus of Zinn. The extraconal space contains fat, the lacrimal gland, and cranial nerves (branches of the ophthalmic and trochlear nerves). The superior oblique muscles receive motor supply from the trochlear nerves (cranial nerve IV). The lateral rectus muscles are innervated by the abducens

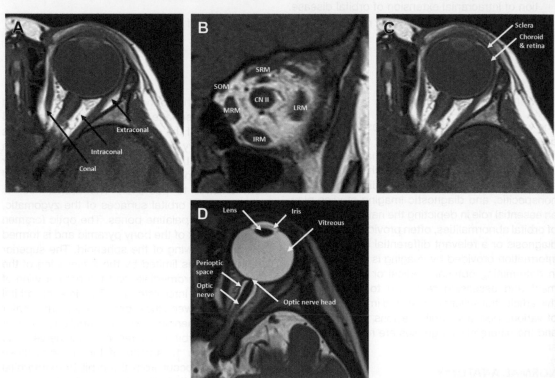

Fig. 1. Normal orbital anatomy. (*A*) High-resolution T1-weighted MR image shows the orbit divided into intraconal and extraconal spaces by the muscle cone and their relationships to the globe. (*B*) Coronal high-resolution T1-weighted MR image of the orbit shows the configuration of the extraocular muscles and the optic nerve. (*C*) High-resolution axial T1-weighted MR image and (*D*) axial T2 sampling perfection with application optimized contrasts using different flip angle evolution (SPACE) MR image showing ocular anatomy. The sclera is hypointense and continuous anteriorly with the cornea and posteriorly with dura. Normal choroid and retina are not distinguishable from each other and appear as an intermediate-intensity structure deep to the sclera on the T1-weighted image. The choroid is continuous anteriorly with the iris and ciliary body, and together, these structures make up the uvea. The lens appears hypointense on the T2-weighted image. Anterior to the lens is a faintly visible linear hypointensity, which is the iris. The iris separates the anterior segment into anterior and posterior chambers containing aqueous humor. The posterior segment lies posterior to the lens and contains the gelatinous vitreous. CN II, cranial nerve II (optic nerve); IRM, inferior rectus muscle; LRM, lateral rectus muscle; MRM, medial rectus muscle; SOM, superior oblique muscle; SRM, superior rectus muscle.

nerves (cranial nerve VI), and the oculomotor nerves (cranial nerve III) supply motor function to the remaining extraocular muscles.

The globe consists of 3 distinct layers from the outside to inside: sclera, uvea, and retina (see **Fig. 1**C, D). The choroid and retina are inseparable on routine cross-sectional imaging but can be differentiated in the presence of choroidal or retinal detachments. The uvea consists of the iris, ciliary body, and choroid (the most vascular structure of the globe). The retina continues posteriorly as the optic nerve. The collagenous sclera is continuous anteriorly with the cornea and posteriorly with the dura and appears hypointense on T1-weighted MR images at 3T (see **Fig. 1**C).

IMAGING TECHNIQUE

Imaging of the orbit is primarily accomplished by ultrasonography (US) (evaluation of the globe), CT (bony anatomy), and MR imaging (soft-tissue characterization). CT is indicated for the bony assessment in craniofacial anomalies, trauma, orbital complications of acute sinusitis (with contrast), and assessment of bony remodeling or destruction from orbital masses. Helical 2.5- to 3-mm axial images are obtained with multiplanar soft-tissue and submillimeter bone reformats. CT angiography (CTA) may be obtained for diagnosis or follow-up of suspected orbital arteriovenous malformation (AVM) or arteriovenous fistula (AVF). The parameters for CT should use the lowest dose possible while still providing diagnostic quality images.

Orbital MR imaging is optimally achieved at 3T using a 32-channel phased-array head coil or equivalent coil when possible. In some instances specialized orbital surface coils may be used. Imaging protocols depend on clinical indications. For example, suspected tumors are imaged with high-resolution, thin-section (<3 mm) axial and coronal fat-suppressed T2; axial non-echo planar diffusion-weighted imaging (DWI); axial T1 and multiplanar high-resolution, fat-suppressed, gadolinium-enhanced T1-weighted images. MR venography (MRV) and/or MR angiography (MRA) are sometimes indicated for vascular assessment. Heavily T2-weighted 3-dimensional sequences with submillimeter-thick images (eg, sampling perfection with application optimized contrasts using different flip angle evolution [SPACE], constructive interference in steady state [CISS], fast imaging employing steady state acquisition [FIESTA], sensitivity encoding [SENSE]) are of use for ocular assessment, especially for intraocular tumors such as retinoblastoma and for assessment of cranial nerves. Congenital strabismus and eye movement disorders generally require a combination of thin-section high-resolution axial and coronal T1-weighted images for assessment of the size, shape, and position of the extraocular muscles and imaging of the brain and relevant cranial nerves.

Conventional catheter angiography is reserved for the delineation of orbital AVM or AVF and sometimes for endovascular treatment.

CONGENITAL AND DEVELOPMENTAL ANOMALIES
Anophthalmos and Microphthalmos

Anophthalmos or anophthalmia refers to congenital absence of the eyes.[1,2] Anophthalmos and microphthalmos are a significant cause of congenital blindness and can be isolated or syndromic.[2–4] Several genetic mutations involving *PAX6, SOX2*, and *RAX* genes are associated with these conditions.[5]

Primary anophthalmos is bilateral in approximately 75% of cases and occurs because of failure of optic vesicle development at approximately 22 to 27 days of gestation.[6] Secondary anophthalmos is lethal and occurs when the entire anterior neural tube fails to develop. Degenerative or consecutive anophthalmos occurs when the optic vesicles form but subsequently degenerate; consequently neuroectodermal elements may be present in degenerative anophthalmos but are absent in primary and secondary anophthalmos.[7]

Microphthalmos refers to a small ocular globe with an ocular total axial length (TAL) 2 standard deviations less than that of the population age-adjusted mean.[2] Microphthalmos is further classified as severe (TAL <10 mm at birth or <12 mm after 1 year of age), simple, or complex depending on the anatomic appearance of the globe and the degree of TAL reduction.[8] Simple microphthalmos refers to an intact globe with mildly decreased TAL. Complex microphthalmos refers to a globe with anterior segment dysgenesis (developmental abnormalities of the globe anterior to the lens) and/or posterior segment dysgenesis (developmental abnormalities of the globe posterior to the lens) with mild, moderate, or severe decrease in TAL.[8] Severe microphthalmos may be difficult to differentiate from anophthalmia.[1,2] Both severe microphthalmos and degenerative anophthalmos contain neuroectodermal tissues and are considered as entities along a continuum. The diagnosis is usually based on clinical and imaging criteria.

US is used to determine the ocular TAL in microphthalmos. CT and MR imaging demonstrate an absent globe in anophthalmos (**Fig. 2**). Amorphous tissue with intermediate density on CT, intermediate signal on T1-weighted images, and low signal on T2-weighted MR images may be noted

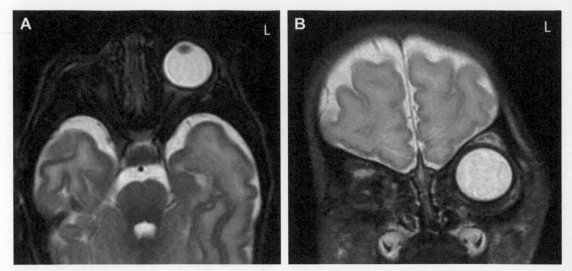

Fig. 2. Unilateral anophthalmos. A 5-day-old baby girl with unilateral right-sided anophthalmos. (A) Axial and (B) coronal T2-weighted images demonstrate complete absence of the right globe. Note the presence of amorphous tissue and structures resembling extraocular muscles within the anophthalmic right orbit. The right optic nerve is absent.

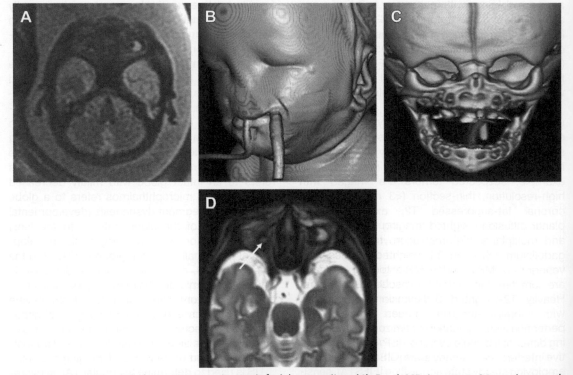

Fig. 3. Severe microphthalmos. Fetus with craniofacial anomalies. (A) Fetal MR image at 34 weeks reveals apparent right anophthalmos and left microphthalmos. The fetal nose is absent. (B) Postnatal 3-dimensional (3D) CT surface reconstruction image at 3 days of age demonstrates arrhinia and bilateral cryptophthalmos. (C) 3D CT image of the skull shows shallow malformed orbits and absence of the nares. (D) Axial T2-weighted MR image shows a rudimentary cystic structure within the right orbit (arrow), which in retrospect can be seen on the fetal MR image, and left microphthalmos. The infant was diagnosed with Bosma syndrome.

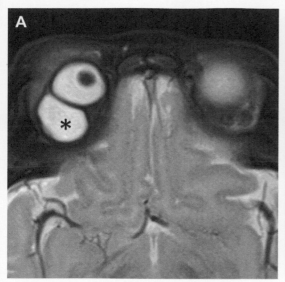
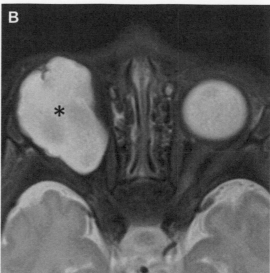

Fig. 4. Unilateral microphthalmos and cyst. A 2-month-old baby girl with persistent closure of the right eye. Clinical examination revealed right microcornea and microphthalmos with bluish discoloration of the lower eyelid thought to represent a cyst. (A, B) Axial fat-suppressed T2-weighted MR images confirm microphthalmos associated with a cyst. The globe is small, deformed, and displaced superiorly. The large cyst (asterisk) is located posterosuperior to the globe.

particularly in degenerative anophthalmos. Orbital dimensions and volumes are reduced in anophthalmos and usually in microphthalmos, unless associated with an intraorbital cyst (Figs. 3 and 4). Simple microphthalmos demonstrates a normal albeit small globe, with normal signal characteristics.

Mild to moderate microphthalmia is managed conservatively with conformers, whereas severe microphthalmia and anophthalmia are treated with endo-orbital volume replacements (implants, expanders, and dermis-fat grafts) and soft-tissue reconstruction.[2,8]

Cryptophthalmos

Embryologically, the eyelid folds appear during the seventh week and grow toward each other and fuse, with separation of lids occurring between the fifth and seventh months of development.[5,9] Cryptophthalmos is usually syndromic and results from failure of development of the eyelid folds with absence of eyebrows, eyelids, and the cornea and continuous skin extending from the forehead to the cheeks. Imaging is required to demonstrate the status of the underlying ocular globes and orbital structures before surgical intervention (see Fig. 3).

Anterior Segment Dysgenesis

Anterior segment dysgenesis results from faulty development of the anterior ocular structures, including the cornea, iris, ciliary body, lens, and anterior and posterior chambers, resulting in an increased risk of glaucoma and blindness. Anterior

segment anomalies are associated with PITX2, FOXC1 PAX6 and related mutations and produce findings such as aniridia, iris hypoplasia, primary congenital glaucoma, Axenfeld-Rieger syndrome (congenital angle anomalies with iris strands), and Peter anomaly (corneal clouding with adhesions between iris, lens, and cornea).[10] Although many of these anomalies produce ophthalmologic abnormalities that do not require further imaging, thin-section high-resolution T2-weighted 3T MR images may demonstrate abnormal size and shape of the anterior and posterior chambers and/or buphthalmos (Fig. 5).

Macrophthalmos

Elongation of the anteroposterior (AP) diameter of the posterior chamber of the globe is most frequently caused by severe myopia. Buphthalmos refers to diffuse enlargement of the AP diameter of the globe (anterior and posterior chambers) usually due to primary congenital or infantile glaucoma or due to syndromic glaucoma as seen in neurofibromatosis type I (NF-1) and Sturge-Weber syndrome.[5]

Imaging is required to differentiate macrophthalmos from other conditions resulting in enlargement of the globe such as an intraocular mass. In buphthalmos, the globe is generally uniformly enlarged but may occasionally have oval or bizarre configurations.[5] Patients with NF-1 demonstrate proptosis, sphenoid wing dysplasia, and orbital plexiform neurofibromas in addition to buphthalmos (Fig. 6).

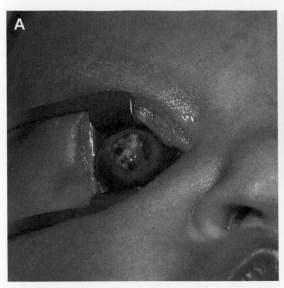

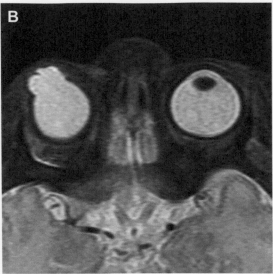

Fig. 5. Anterior segment dysgenesis. (*A*) A 1-day-old baby girl with right proptosis, elevated intraocular pressure, and scleralization with calcification on the anterior surface of the right eye. (*B*) Axial fat-suppressed T2-weighted MR image shows mild right microphthalmos with a large, irregular anterior segment consistent with the clinical finding of anterior segment dysgenesis. There is aniridia and aphakia. Progressive enlargement and exposure of the right eye occurred despite medical therapy. Subsequently, with no potential for visual rehabilitation and risk for perforation, the right eye was enucleated. ([*A*] *Courtesy of* Carolyn Wu, MD, Department of Ophthalmology, Boston Children's Hospital, Boston, MA.)

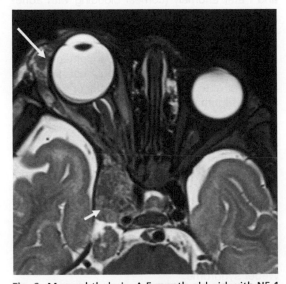

Fig. 6. Macrophthalmia. A 5-month-old girl with NF-1 and proptosis. Axial fat-suppressed T2-weighted MR image reveals enlargement of the right globe, consistent with buphthalmos. There is right sphenoid bone dysplasia with associated enlargement of the right middle cranial fossa. A plexiform neurofibroma is present within the lateral aspect of the orbit (*long arrow*). There is also a nerve sheath tumor within the right cavernous sinus (*short arrow*) and Meckel cave.

Congenital Cystic Eye

Congenital cystic eye is a rare condition resulting from failure of the optic vesicle to invaginate to form the globe. On imaging, a cystic, sometimes septated, orbital mass is seen in place of the normal globe (**Fig. 7**). The differential diagnosis includes microphthalmia with cyst, microphthalmia with cystic teratoma, ectopic brain tissue, and meningoencephalocele.[11,12]

Coloboma

Coloboma is a developmental anomaly that results from incomplete closure of the embryonic choroidal fissure, resulting in ectasia and herniation of vitreous into the retro-ocular space.[13] The developmental insult occurs during gestational days 35 to 41.[6,7] Colobomas may affect the iris, lens, ciliary body, retina, choroid, sclera, or optic nerve.[14] Colobomas may be unilateral or bilateral and can be isolated or syndromic, as seen in CHARGE syndrome (coloboma, heart defects, choanal atresia, retarded growth and development, genital malformations, and ear anomalies).[12,15] Numerous other genetic disorders are associated with coloboma, including focal dermal hypoplasia, branchio-oculofacial syndrome, trisomies 13 and 18, and Aicardi syndrome.[5]

On MR imaging, coloboma appears as a focal defect of the posterior wall of the globe, sometimes associated with microphthalmia (**Fig. 8**). A

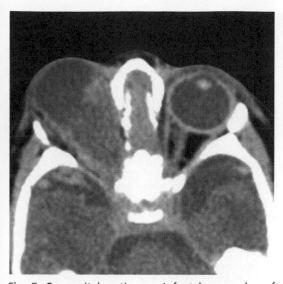

Fig. 7. Congenital cystic eye. Infant boy on day of birth noted to have a cystic orbital mass at birth. Axial contrast-enhanced CT reveals a large, heterogeneous cystic mass enlarging the orbit. In contrast to other ocular anomalies, no definite ocular structures are seen. At surgical exploration, congenital cystic eye was confirmed with only a small area of pigment consistent with uveal tissue.

minimal defect results in a small excavation along the posterior globe. A larger defect produces a retrobulbar cystic cavity outpouching from the posterior wall of the globe.[12]

Morning Glory Disc Anomaly

Morning glory disc anomaly (MGDA) is a congenital optic nerve anomaly characterized by a funnel-shaped excavation of the optic disc with a central glial tuft overlying the optic disc and an annulus of chorioretinal pigmentary changes surrounding the optic disc excavation.[16–18]

Although MGDA is usually diagnosed clinically, imaging also distinguishes MGDA from optic nerve coloboma. MGDA has 3 distinctive MR imaging findings: (1) funnel-shaped appearance of the optic disc with elevation of the adjacent retinal surface; (2) abnormal tissue associated with the ipsilateral distal intraorbital optic nerve, effacing the adjacent perioptic nerve subarachnoid space; and (3) lack of the usual enhancement at the lamina cribrosa associated with the funnel-shaped defect at the optic papilla (Fig. 9).[16] Identification of MGDA at imaging should prompt a search for associated intracranial abnormalities, including midline craniofacial and skull base defects, vascular abnormalities, and cerebral malformations.[19,20] In particular, brain MR imaging and internal carotid artery MRA should be performed because of an association with transphenoidal basal encephalocele and congenital stenoocclusive change of the internal carotid arteries (moyamoya disease) in these patients.[20] MGDA can also be seen in association with PHACES (posterior fossa anomalies, hemangioma, arterial and aortic arch anomalies, cardiac anomalies,

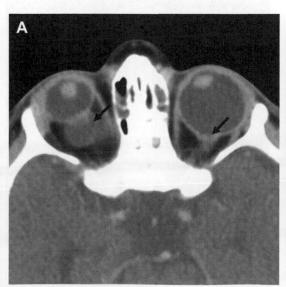
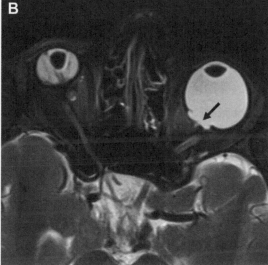

Fig. 8. Coloboma. Girl with CHARGE syndrome, right microphthalmos, and colobomata. (A) Axial contrast-enhanced CT obtained at 2 years of age reveals right micropthalmos and bilateral colobomata (arrows). (B) Axial fat-suppressed T2-weighted MR image at 16 years of age shows an interval right retinal detachment with a small residual cystic structure posterior to the right globe and a large choroidal coloboma involving the left eye (arrow).

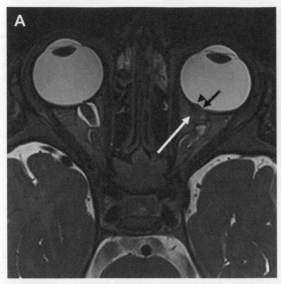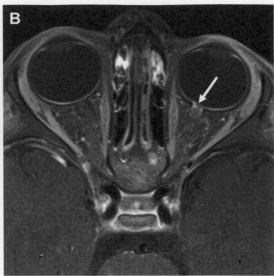

Fig. 9. Morning glory disc anomaly (MGDA). A 21-month-old boy presenting with poor vision and sensory exotropia of the left eye. Ophthalmologic examination revealed a megalopapilla with a central glial tuft and changes consistent with MGDA. (*A*) Axial 3-dimensional T2 SPACE MR image reveals a funnel-shaped appearance of the posterior optic disc (*black arrow*) with elevation of the adjacent retinal surface (*arrowhead*). There is abnormal tissue associated with the distal intraorbital segment of the ipsilateral optic nerve, with effacement of the regional subarachnoid space (*white arrow*). (*B*) Axial fat-suppressed T1-weighted MR image shows discontinuity of enhancement at the lamina cribrosa (*arrrow*), with enhancement extending along the most distal aspect of the optic nerve.

eye anomalies, and sternal anomalies and/or supraumbilical raphe).[21]

Staphyloma

Staphyloma results from thinning and stretching of the uvea and sclera and involves all layers of the globe. Risk factors include severe axial myopia, glaucoma, and severe ocular inflammation. Imaging reveals a posterior outpouching of the globe producing deformity in globe contour (**Fig. 10**).

Hypertelorism, Hypotelorism, and Cyclopia

Hypertelorism denotes increased distance between the medial orbital walls. Hypertelorism is associated with several craniofacial disorders, including cephaloceles, syndromic agenesis of the corpus callosum, and syndromic coronal craniosynostosis (**Fig. 11A**). Hypertelorism must be distinguished from dystopia canthorum in which the medial orbital walls are normally spaced but the medial intercanthal distance is increased, as seen in various types of Waardenburg syndrome.

Hypotelorism denotes decreased distance between the medial orbital walls. Hypotelorism is also associated with a variety of disorders, including the holoprosencephalies (HPE) and premature fusion of the metopic and sagittal sutures (see **Fig. 11B**). Cyclopia or cyclophthalmia

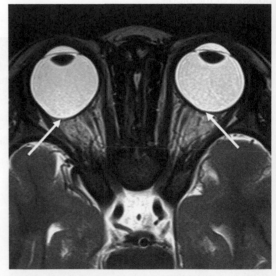

Fig. 10. Staphyloma. A 3-year-old girl with nystagmus, pale optic discs, and esotropia. Axial T2-weighted MR image shows bilateral staphylomas right greater than left. There is smooth outpouching of all layers of the globes along the temporal aspects of the optic nerves bilaterally (*arrows*). The optic nerves appear diminutive in keeping with either optic nerve hypoplasia (congenital) or atrophy (acquired).

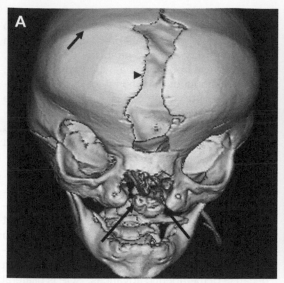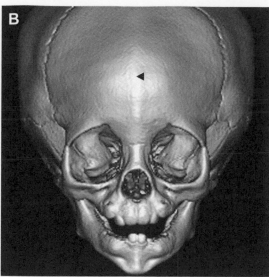

Fig. 11. Hypertelorism and hypotelorism associated with craniosynostosis. (*A*) Three-dimensional (3D) CT image in a 9-month-old girl with brachycephaly and exophthalmos reveals hypertelorism and bilateral cleft lip and palate (*long arrows*). There is bicoronal synostosis (*short arrow*) and wide patency of the metopic suture (*arrowhead*) consistent with the known diagnosis of Apert syndrome. (*B*) 3D CT image in a 7-month-old girl with trigonocephaly shows premature fusion of the metopic suture resulting in frontal ridging (*arrowhead*) associated with hypotelorism.

denotes complete fusion of the optic vesicles resulting in a single median eye. Synophthalmia represents partial fusion of the optic vesicles resulting in duplication of some anterior structures. Both cyclophthalmia and synophthalmia can be associated with HPE.[5] Other manifestations of HPE include ethmocephaly (hypotelorism with median proboscis) and cebocephaly (hypotelorism with rudimentary nose and single nostril).

Large/Small Orbit

A large orbit can be congenital or acquired and results from causes such as cephalocele, bony deformity as seen in NF-1, and bony or orbital masses (see **Figs. 6** and **7**). A small orbit accompanies anopthalmia and microphthalmia (see **Figs. 2** and **3**). Exorbitism denotes shallow orbits as seen in syndromic craniosynostosis (see **Fig. 11**). Exorbitism should not be confused with proptosis in which there is mass effect within the orbit causing ventral protrusion of the globe.

Optic Nerve Hypoplasia

Optic nerve hypoplasia (ONH) is a developmental anomaly characterized by optic nerve underdevelopment. Bilateral ONH is associated with syndromic disorders such as septo-optic dysplasia. On imaging, the affected optic nerves and part or all of the optic chiasm and tracts appear small (see **Fig. 10**). The differential diagnosis for optic hypoplasia is optic atrophy resulting from a variety

of causes such as prior infection/inflammation, trauma, irradiation, retinopathy of prematurity (ROP), and vascular insult.

Persistent Hyperplastic Primary Vitreous

Persistent hyperplastic primary vitreous (PHPV) results from failure of the embryonic hyaloid vasculature to involute, resulting in persistence of hyperplastic primary vitreous and the capillary vascular network covering parts of the lens. PHPV is typically unilateral and results in congenital microphthalmos, leukocoria, and cataract. Bilateral PHPV is associated with congenital conditions such as Norrie disease and Warburg disease.[22]

The appearance of PHPV has been likened to that of a martini glass with the glass represented by triangular retrolental fibrovascular tissue and the martini glass stem represented by the stalk of hyaloid remnant extending to the optic disc in Cloquet canal (**Fig. 12**).[23] On CT, PHPV appears as increased density of the vitreous with a V-shaped or linear structure presumed to represent a remnant of the Cloquet canal. On MR imaging, the retrolental fibrovascular tissue and stalklike hyaloid remnant are hypointense on T1- and T2-weighted images with contrast enhancement. Hemorrhage and layering vitreous debris may be seen on imaging. Absence of calcification on CT is an important distinction from retinoblastoma (**Box 1**).

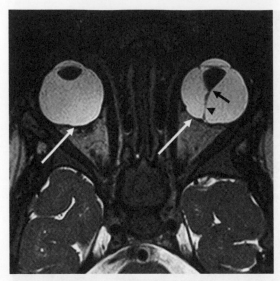

Fig. 12. PHPV. A 1-year-old girl with esotropia, nystagmus, and bilateral chorioretinal colobomas. Axial 3-dimensional T2 SPACE MR image shows a triangular deformity at the posterior aspect of the left lens (*black arrow*) that is contiguous with a linear hypointensity extending toward the optic disc representing the stalk of hyaloid remnant of the Cloquet canal (*arrowhead*). There are also bilateral chorioretinal colobomas (*white arrows*).

Coats Disease

Coats disease is a sporadic disorder characterized by a defect in retinal vascular development resulting in telangiectactic retinal vessels with vessel leakage, subretinal exudate, and retinal detachment.[22,24] Coats disease is unilateral in 80% to 90% of cases, with a male predilection. Common signs are leukocoria and strabismus.[22,24] On CT, Coats disease appears as a hyperdense exudate, typically without calcification (Fig. 13). On MR imaging, the lipoproteinaceous subretinal exudate appears hyperintense on T1- and T2-weighted images. The absence of an enhancing mass helps differentiate Coats disease from retinoblastoma (see Box 1).

Retinopathy of Prematurity

ROP or retrolental fibroplasia is a postnatal fibrovascular organization of the vitreous humor that may lead to retinal detachment. ROP is related to excessive oxygen therapy in premature, low-birth-weight infants but is now uncommon because of therapeutic advances. ROP is bilateral and asymmetric.

ROP presents with microphthalmia and a shallow anterior chamber on CT and MR imaging. On CT, there is hyperattenuation within the globe. Dystrophic calcifications are not typically a feature of ROP until late in the disease (Fig. 14A). The association of dystrophic calcifications with microphthalmia distinguishes ROP from retinoblastoma, in which there is a calcified mass or masses in a normal-sized globe (see Box 1). On MR imaging, there may be hyperintensity within the globe on T1- and T2-weighted imaging due to subretinal

---

Box 1
Differential diagnosis of leukocoria

Normal-sized eye

Calcified mass

- Retinoblastoma (single or multiple enhancing lesions, grows into vitreous or choroid)

Noncalcified mass

- Coats disease (no enhancing mass, lipoproteinaceous hyperintense subretinal exudate)

Microphthalmia

Unilateral

- PHPV (subhyaloid or subretinal blood-fluid levels, retrolental tubular mass along the hyaloid canal that enhances)

Bilateral

- ROP (no or minimal enhancement, dystrophic calcification late in disease)
- Bilateral PHPV (see earlier)

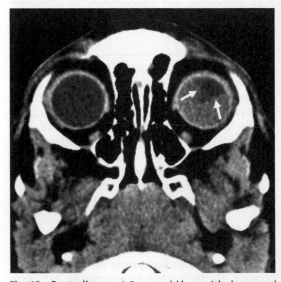

Fig. 13. Coats disease. A 3-year-old boy with decreased vision left eye. On examination, there was funnel-shaped retinal detachment and neovascular glaucoma consistent with Coats disease of the left eye. Axial CT image shows the V-shaped left retinal detachment (*arrow*). No mass lesion or calcification is seen.

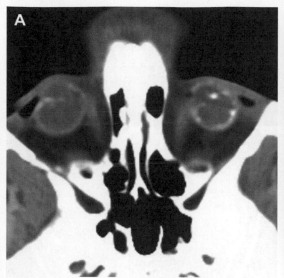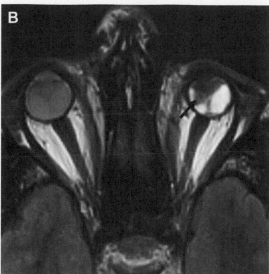

Fig. 14. Retinopathy of prematurity. A 20-year-old ex 24-week premature infant resulting in blindness. (*A*) Axial CT image reveals microphthalmia with foci of mineralization. (*B*) Axial fluid attenuated inversion recovery (FLAIR) MR image shows that there are bilateral retinal detachments with increased signal intensity compared with normal vitreous. There is a small hypointense retrolental lesion on the left (*arrow*).

hemorrhages. In addition, a hypointense retrolental mass may be noted within the globe (see **Fig. 14**B).

Orbital and Ocular Abnormalities with Central Nervous System Malformations

Orbital and ocular anomalies are a feature of several craniofacial disorders as alluded to in earlier sections. Orbital manifestations of NF-1 include spheno-orbital dysplasia, buphthalmos, optic nerve glioma, nerve sheath tumors (neurofibromas, plexiform neurofibromas, and malignant peripheral nerve sheath tumor) (see **Fig. 6**), and occasionally rhabdomyosarcoma (RMS). Orbital lesions in Sturge-Weber syndrome include buphthalmos, glaucoma, venous dysplasia, and venous hypertension (**Fig. 15**A).[25] Tuberous sclerosis is characterized by retinal neuroglial hamartoma (see **Fig. 15**B),[26] and retinal hemangioblastomas are a feature of von Hippel-Lindau disease.[27–30] Joubert syndrome is characterized by abnormal eye movements and optic nerve and/or chorioretinal coloboma, less commonly retinal abnormalities.[31] Several ocular abnormalities occur in congenital muscular dystrophies such as Walker-Warburg syndrome, including cataracts, microphthalmos, buphthalmos, retinal pigmentary changes, PHPV, retinal detachment, vitreous hemorrhage, coloboma, Peter anomaly, and ONH.[32]

Aicardi syndrome is a rare X-linked disorder characterized by agenesis of the corpus callosum, cortical malformations, and chorioretinal lacunae.[33] Additional central nervous system (CNS) and ocular findings are seen with varying frequency, including microphthalmos, anomalous retinal vessels, retinal detachment, dysplasia or coloboma of the optic nerve, persistent pupillary membrane, iris synechiae, posterior iris or choroidal staphylomas, and cataracts.[33,34] Morning glory disc–like anomalies, involving ring-shaped pigment deposits surrounding or within a colobomatous optic nerve head, have also been described in patients with Aicardi syndrome.[33,35]

Nasolacrimal Duct Cyst and Mucocele

Nasolacrimal duct (NLD) cyst and mucocele is typically congenital in nature due to failure of canalization of the distal NLD at the valve of Hasner. This common anomaly is detected incidentally or because of a cystic medial canthal swelling or neonatal nasal obstruction and respiratory distress. On imaging, there is cystic expansion of the intranasal NLD, which protrudes beneath the inferior turbinate, sometimes with enlargement of the lacrimal sac (**Fig. 16**). The differential diagnosis includes meningocele and neuroglial heterotopia, which can appear cystic but project into the nasal cavity above the inferior turbinate.

Lacrimal Gland Anomalies

Aplasia or hypoplasia of the lacrimal gland is a rare disorder that is sometimes associated with aplasia of the salivary glands in the aplasia of the lacrimal and salivary gland syndrome[36] or with abnormalities of the ears, teeth, and digits in the lacrimoauriculodentodigital syndrome.[37] Patients

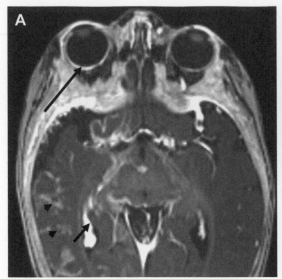
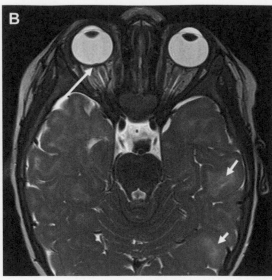

Fig. 15. Ocular abnormalities with CNS malformations. (A) Sturge-Weber syndrome (SWS) in a 3-year-old boy. Axial contrast-enhanced T1 magnetization-prepared rapid acquisition gradient-echo (MPRAGE) image shows abnormal right choroidal enhancement (*long arrow*) associated with venous dysplasia. Other typical features of SWS are demonstrated, including enlargement of the right choroid plexus (*short arrow*) and abnormal enhancement around the right temporal lobe related to abnormal venous drainage (*arrowheads*). (B) Tuberous sclerosis in a 10-month-old girl. Axial T2-weighted MR image reveals a small retinal neuroglial hamartoma (*long arrow*). Subcortical tubers are seen within the temporal lobes (*short arrows*).

present with alacrima, and imaging reveals absence or marked paucity of lacrimal tissue.

Congenital Cranial Dysinnervation Disorders

The congenital cranial dysinnervation disorders (CCDDs) result from abnormal development of cranial motor nuclei, absence or hypoplasia of affected cranial nerves, and resultant fibrosis of abnormally innervated extraocular muscles. CCDDs include congenital fibrosis of the extraocular muscles (CFEOM; *TUBB3* and other mutations), Bosley-Salih-Alorainy syndrome and Athabascan brain dysgenesis syndrome (*HOXA1*

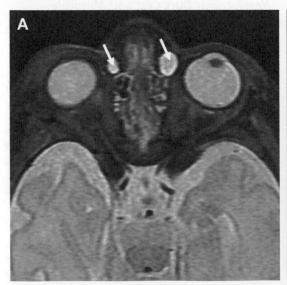
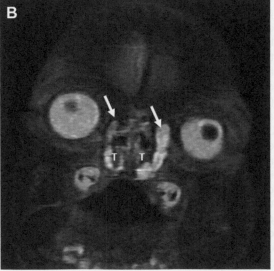

Fig. 16. Nasolacrimal duct cyst (NLDC). A 1-day-old baby girl presenting with nasal obstruction. (A) Axial and (B) coronal fast spin echo inversion recovery T2-weighted MR images reveal bilateral NLDCs, left larger than right (*arrows*). The coronal image shows that the NLDCs protrude inferior to the inferior turbinates (T). This finding is a helpful distinction from a cephalocele or neuroglial heterotopia that would reside superior to the inferior turbinate.

mutations), *HOXB1* mutations, Duane syndrome (*CHN1, SALL4* and *SALL1* mutations), Moebius syndrome, and horizontal gaze palsy with progressive scoliosis (HGPPS; *ROBO3* mutations).[38] Clinical signs depend on the underlying genetic mutation and affected cranial nerves and include strasbismus, gaze limitation or ophthalmoplegia, ptosis, and poorly reactive pupils. Imaging reveals absence or hypoplasia of the affected cranial nerves and diminutive affected extraocular muscles (**Fig. 17**). Additional malformations of the brain or inner ears occur depending on the underlying genetic mutation.

ORBITAL MASSES
Dermoid and Epidermoid

Dermoids, also known as developmental choristomas, are the most common congenital orbital masses.[13,14] These lesions likely arise from sequestered epithelial rests entrapped in orbital bony sutures and can be subcutaneous or intraorbital in location.[13,39] Both dermoids and the less common epidermoids are composed of cysts lined by keratinized, stratified squamous epithelium with dermoids also containing adnexal structures such as hair and sebaceous glands. Clinically, these lesions manifest as subcutaneous nodules adjacent to the orbital rim or as unilateral proptosis.

Imaging does not reliably distinguish between dermoids and epidermoids. On contrast-enhanced CT, these lesions present as well-defined low-density masses that remodel adjacent bone, with mild thin rim contrast enhancement. Thick, irregular rim of enhancement suggests inflammation secondary to rupture. Fatty components usually present as negative attenuation values within the mass and a fat-fluid level may occasionally be noted within a dermoid. Calcification is seldom seen in children. On MR imaging, dermoids/epidermoids typically demonstrate hypointensity on T1-weighted and variable, usually hyperintense signal on T2-weighted images with decreased diffusivity. Fat contents result in T1 shortening (**Fig. 18**). There is minimal, if any, thin peripheral contrast enhancement.

VASCULAR LESIONS

The most common vascular lesions in infants and children are infantile hemangiomas (IHs), lymphatic malformations (LMs), and venous malformations (VMs). MR imaging is the modality of choice for characterizing and distinguishing between these lesions based on degree of vascularity, the presence of a solid or cystic mass, fluid-fluid levels/hemorrhage or phleboliths, and the degree of contrast enhancement.

Lymphatic Malformation

LM is an unencapsulated mass of thin-walled lymphatic channels and represents the most common vascular malformation in childhood.[40–42] Clinically, LMs grow commensurate with growth of the

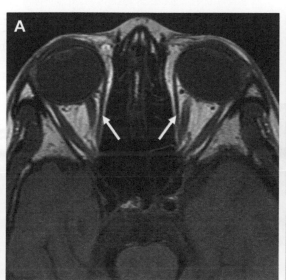
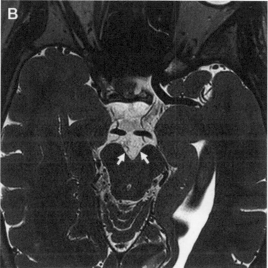

Fig. 17. Congenital cranial dysinnervation disorder. Teenaged boy with Moebius-type syndrome and TUBB 3 mutation. Clinical examination revealed facial palsy and limited adduction and elevation of the eyes. (*A*) Axial T1-weighted MR image shows diminutive medial rectus muscles bilaterally (*arrows*). The superior and inferior rectus muscles were also small (not shown). (*B*) Axial 3D T2 SPACE image at the level of the midbrain and interpeduncular cistern demonstrates absence of cranial nerve III bilaterally (*arrows*).

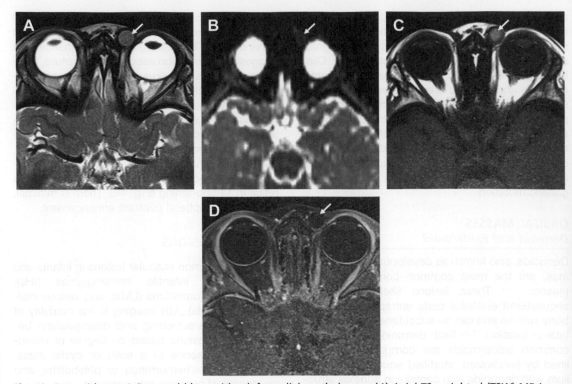

Fig. 18. Dermoid cyst. A 2-year-old boy with a left medial canthal mass. (*A*) Axial T2-weighted (T2W) MR image shows a sharply circumscribed left preseptal mass (*arrow*) that is isointense with gray matter. (*B*) Diffusion-weighted imaging apparent diffusion coefficient map reveals that the lesion has decreased diffusivity (*arrow*). (*C*) Axial T1-weighted (T1W) image demonstrates mild T1 shortening within the mass (*arrow*). (*D*) Gadolinium-enhanced fat-suppressed T1W image shows that the lesion does not enhance (*arrow*). These features are consistent with a dermoid cyst, which was confirmed following surgical excision. Dermoids have variable, typically homogeneous signal intensity on T1W and T2W images and typically show decreased diffusivity and minimal, if any, marginal enhancement.

patient but may enlarge suddenly as a result of the propensity to bleed or become infected.

On US, CT, and MR imaging, LMs appear microcystic or macrocystic, lobulated, and septated. Transpatial involvement of the intraconal and extraconal spaces may occur. Characteristic fluid-fluid levels usually associated with hemorrhage are well seen on MR imaging and are a typical feature of LM (**Fig. 19**). Hemorrhage also alters the signal intensity on MR imaging, sometimes

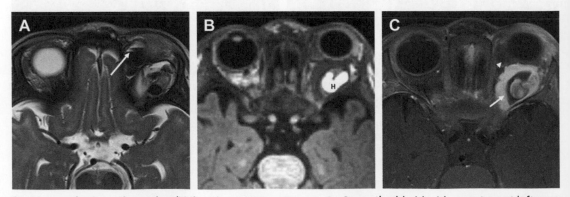

Fig. 19. Lymphatic malformation (LM) with venous component. An 8-month-old girl with recent-onset left proptosis. (*A*) Axial T2-weighted MR image reveals a macrocystic, hemorrhagic left intraconal mass that contains fluid-fluid levels (*arrow*), characteristic of LM complicated by hemorrhage. (*B*) Axial T1-weighted (T1W) MR image shows the hyperintense hemorrhage (H). (*C*) Gadolinium-enhanced fat-suppressed T1W MR image shows some enhancement of the lesion consistent with a venous component (*arrow*). Nonenhancing LM is also seen (*arrowhead*).

producing T1 and T2 shortening. Pure LMs demonstrate mild enhancement of septations only, and the contained fluid does not enhance. High flow vascularity is not a feature of LMs. Enhancement of fluid within the cystic septations is consistent with a venous component (see **Fig. 19**), as evidenced also by the presence of phleboliths. Evaluation of the brain is indicated to assess for associated intracranial venous lesions such as cavernous malformations, prominent developmental venous anomalies, and occasionally high-flow arteriovenous fistulae.[42]

Surgery to reduce compression on the optic nerve and improve cosmetic appearance may be associated with recurrence. Sclerotherapy with sodium tetradecyl sulfate or OK-432 may be helpful in the management of macrocystic LMs; however, the use of sclerotherapy in the postseptal orbit is limited because of the risk of postprocedural increased intraorbital pressure caused by swelling.[43]

Venous Malformation

Orbital VM is a distensible low-flow lesion characterized by dilated venous channels. VMs increase in size with Valsalva maneuver, crying, and straining. VMs must be distinguished from orbital varices that arise secondary to arteriovenous shunting or venous occlusive diseases such as venous sinus thrombosis.[44]

US, CT, and MR imaging show a well-defined cystic, septated lesion. The venous blood enhances gradually with contrast. VMs are sometimes complicated by thrombosis, which affects the echogenicity on US and density or signal intensity on CT and MR imaging, respectively. Phleboliths are a characteristic feature of VMs (**Fig. 20**). As with LMs, high-flow vascularity is not a feature of VMs. As mentioned, sometimes lesions demonstrate mixed characteristics of VM and LM with associated intracranial VMs.[41]

Arteriovenous Malformation and Carotid Cavernous Fistula

Orbital AVMs are uncommon high-flow vascular anomalies that may present with proptosis and orbital bruit. Imaging usually consists of MR imaging with MRA and CTA or conventional angiography to demonstrate the arterial and venous anatomy and the presence of a nidus or tangle of vessels between the enlarged arterial feeders and early draining veins. Therapeutic options vary depending on the anatomy of the lesion and can include endovascular embolization and/or surgery.

A carotid cavernous fistula (CCF) is an abnormal connection between the internal carotid arterial system and the cavernous venous sinuses. Direct CCF can be caused by craniofacial injury or trauma. Spontaneous CCF may develop from rupture of an intracavernous aneurysm or secondary to vessel weakness in conditions such as Ehlers-Danlos syndrome or fibromuscular dysplasia.[45–48] Although CCF is uncommon in children, the signs and symptoms seem to be similar to those seen in adults.[45–47]

CT and MR imaging demonstrate dilation of the superior ophthalmic vein and exophthalmos with enlarged extraocular muscles (**Fig. 21**A). On MR images, there may be distension of the cavernous sinuses with abnormal cavernous sinus flow voids. Conventional angiography identifies the exact location of the CCF so as to plan definitive treatment (see **Fig. 21**B).

NEOPLASMS

Pediatric ophthalmic tumors are classified into orbital neoplasms and intraocular tumors. Many

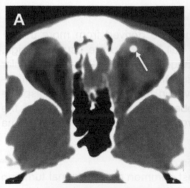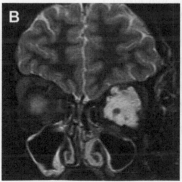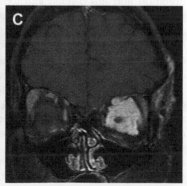

Fig. 20. Venous malformation (VM). Teenaged girl with blue rubber bleb nevus syndrome. (A) Axial CT image shows a phlebolith within the left orbit (arrow). (B) Coronal T2 short tau inversion recovery (STIR) MR image shows a large, hyperintense, multicystic intraconal lesion. (C) Coronal fat-suppressed contrast-enhanced T1-weighted MR image shows that the lesion enhances. These features are diagnostic of VM.

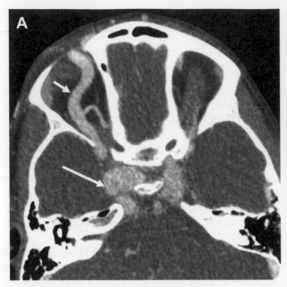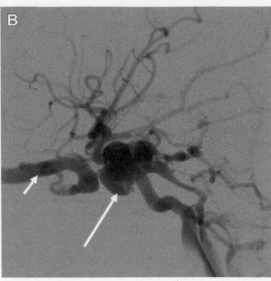

Fig. 21. Carotid cavernous fistula (CCF). A 6-year-old girl with remote eye trauma, headaches, and vertigo. (*A*) Axial contrast-enhanced CT shows marked enlargement of the right superior ophthalmic vein (SOV) (*short arrow*) and the right cavernous sinus/cavernous right internal carotid artery (ICA) (*long arrow*). (*B*) Cerebral angiography with selective right ICA injection confirms the direct CCF (*long arrow*) with principal drainage into an enlarged right SOV (*short arrow*) and both cavernous sinuses and their tributaries (*long arrow*).

of these tumors are benign; however, they have a significant impact on vision and may result in significant morbidity and mortality. This section presents common orbital and intraocular lesions.

Orbital Neoplasms

Infantile hemangioma

IH is the most common vascular tumor of infancy. Orbital hemangioma typically presents shortly after birth with proptosis and/or a strawberry red mass involving the periorbital skin. IH is characterized by proliferation with rapid growth during the first year of life followed by gradual involution by 7 to 8 years of age.[40,49] True congenital hemangiomas are uncommon and are divided into those that involute rapidly (rapidly involuting congenital hemangioma) and those that do not (noninvoluting congenital hemangioma). Imaging is indicated to detect the extent of the lesion and to distinguish IH as a cause of proptosis from other orbital masses.

The imaging features of IH are characteristic and diagnostic. US demonstrates a hyperechoic, bosselated mass with prominent high-flow vascularity noted on color Doppler US. CT demonstrates a well-defined mass with intense homogeneous enhancement. MR imaging demonstrates a solid, circumscribed, and somewhat lobulated mass that is isointense with white matter on T2-weighted images. Characteristic signal voids are a feature of proliferating IH and reflect prominent vascularity. Proliferating IH also demonstrates

intense, homogeneous contrast enhancement (**Fig. 22**). Involution is associated with decreased vascularity and enhancement and increasing fibrofatty matrix. Bony remodeling may occur. IH must be distinguished from cystic lesions such as LMs, VMs, or mixed low-flow vascular anomalies and from solid tumors such as RMS. The key feature distinguishing IH from RMS is the intense enhancement and vascularity of IH. Orbital hemangioma can be associated with other anomalies as a manifestation of PHACES association.[21]

Most hemangiomas are treated conservatively anticipating involution. However, tumors that compromise vision can be treated with systemic propranolol.

Teratoma

Orbital teratomas are derived from more than 1 primitive germ cell layer and are usually benign. CT and MR imaging demonstrate a multilocular cystic and solid mass (comprising fat, calcification, or both) within the orbit that may displace the normal globe and result in expansion of the bony orbit. Surgical resection of benign teratoma is curative.

Rhabdomyosarcoma

RMS is the most common mesenchymal tumor in children[50–52] and the most prevalent pediatric extraocular orbital malignancy.[53,54] Two histologic subtypes of RMS are prevalent in children: the embryonal subtype is the most common orbital

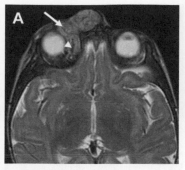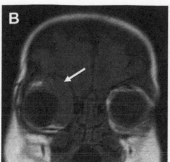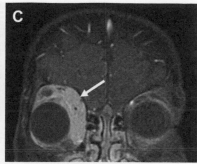

Fig. 22. Infantile hemangioma. A 4-month-old girl with ptosis. (A) Axial T2-weighted MR image shows a sharply marginated extraconal, preseptal, and frontonasal mass (*arrow*) that is isointense with white matter and contains vascular signal voids (*arrowhead*). (B) Coronal T1 precontrast and (C) postcontrast fat-suppressed T1-weighted images demonstrate the avidly enhancing soft-tissue mass (*arrow*) centered within the medial aspect of the right orbit. These findings are characteristic of proliferating infantile hemangioma.

variant and is the least aggressive subtype; the more aggressive alveolar subtype is less prevalent in the orbit.[55] Orbital RMS typically presents with rapidly progressive, unilateral proptosis and diplopia. The median age of presentation is 6 to 8 years,[56] although the alveolar subtype generally affects older children or adolescents.[43]

CT, PET-CT, and MR imaging are important in the preoperative evaluation and staging of orbital RMS and provide complementary information. CT demonstrates osseous erosion and/or remodeling, whereas MR imaging demonstrates soft-tissue characterization and intracranial extension. MR imaging and PET-CT are used for follow-up and assessment of therapeutic response.

On CT images, orbital RMS generally appears as an extraconal, ovoid, well-circumscribed mass that is isodense relative to muscle, with moderate to marked contrast enhancement. Remodeling of bone or frank aggressive bony destruction can occur. Eyelid thickening is a common associated finding whether or not the tumor extends to the eyelid.

On MR imaging, RMS is isointense to muscle on T1-weighted images and hyperintense to muscle on T2-weighted images, often appearing isointense with cerebral cortex, with decreased diffusivity and moderate to marked contrast enhancement (Fig. 23). The mass may distort or displace but does not typically invade the globe. The extraocular muscles are similarly distorted and are sometimes inseparable from tumor. Invasion of adjacent paranasal sinuses or intracranial contents may be seen, and comparison of nonenhanced and enhanced T1-weighted images helps distinguish tumor extension into the paranasal sinuses from trapped sinus secretions.

Many benign and malignant entities share clinical features of RMS. Proliferating IH presents in younger children and demonstrates characteristic

vascular flow voids and more intense and homogeneous enhancement. RMS may appear indistinguishable from orbital lymphoma, which is the chief differential diagnostic consideration.

Orbital RMS treatment usually consists of surgical resection, followed by radiation therapy and chemotherapy. Prognosis depends on histologic and molecular subtype and feasibility of complete surgical resection. Parameningeal spread of tumor suggests a worse prognosis. The 5-year survival rates for embryonal and alveolar subtypes are 94% and 74%, respectively.[51]

Langerhans cell histiocytosis

Langerhans cell histiocytosis (LCH) represents a spectrum of disease ranging from benign unifocal bone disease to more aggressive multisystem disease.[57] Eosinophilic granuloma, the most localized and benign form of LCH often presents as unifocal bone disease with orbital bone involvement; the lesion usually manifests in children (boys > girls) younger than 4 years with proptosis, ptosis, erythema, and enlarging palpebral fissures.[53]

CT and MR imaging help delineate the extent of disease and bony involvement. On CT, LCH typically appears as a well-defined, moderately to markedly enhancing osteolytic soft-tissue mass. Bony margins are characteristically sharply defined with beveled edges (Fig. 24A).

On MR images, the soft-tissue component can be heterogeneous or homogeneous on T1-weighted images and hyperintense, isointense, or hypointense relative to cerebral cortex on T2-weighted images. Moderate to marked homogeneous or heterogeneous enhancement occurs. MR imaging is the modality of choice for demonstrating intracranial extension. The MR features of LCH can simulate more aggressive sarcomatous lesions or metastasis; however, the CT features of LCH are usually characteristic (see

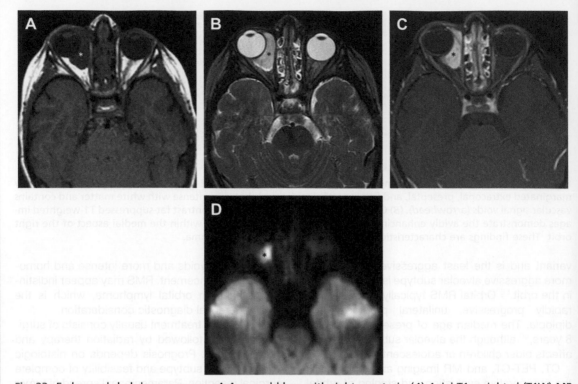

Fig. 23. Embryonal rhabdomyosarcoma. A 4-year-old boy with right proptosis. (*A*) Axial T1-weighted (T1W) MR image shows a mass (*asterisk*) along the medial aspect of the orbit, which is isointense to muscle. (*B*) Axial T2-weighted MR image shows that the mass is hyperintense to muscle. (*C*) Axial fat-suppressed contrast-enhanced T1W image demonstrates moderate tumoral enhancement. (*D*) Diffusion-weighted imaging shows that there is decreased diffusivity within portions of the mass (*asterisk*). The lack of vascular flow voids distinguishes rhabdomyosarcoma from hemangioma.

Fig. 24). In young children, the differential diagnosis includes other histiocytic tumors such as juvenile xanthogranuloma. Surgical resection of isolated lesions is usually curative.

Leukemia

Chloroma (granulocytic sarcoma) represents the most common form of acute myelogenous leukemic involvement of the orbit.[13,58] These solid tumors typically present in children with proptosis and diplopia. These lesions may be bilateral in contrast to RMS.[13]

On CT, chloroma presents as an irregular mass of homogeneous density with poor contrast enhancement and frequent lytic, permeative bony erosion. On MR imaging, the lesion is isointense to muscle on T1- and T2-weighted images with decreased diffusivity and variable, homogeneous enhancement (Fig. 25). In addition to chloromas, orbital leukemia may result in optic nerve infiltration; intraocular involvement of the choroid, retina, or anterior chamber; and infiltration of extraocular muscles. The differential diagnosis includes RMS, lymphoma, and metastatic neuroblastoma.

Treatment of chloroma is usually systemic chemotherapy and bone marrow transplantation.[13] Leukemic infiltration of the optic nerve is a medical emergency because of the potential for permanent visual loss if left untreated. The treatment in such cases is low-dose radiation therapy often combined with intrathecal chemotherapy.[13]

Lymphoma

Lymphoproliferative disease accounts for approximately 10% of pediatric orbital tumors; lymphoid hyperplasia accounts for 10% to 40% of the lesions, whereas non-Hodgkin lymphoma accounts for 60% to 90% of the lesions.[59] Patients typically present with gradual, painless progressive proptosis.

On CT and MR imaging, lymphoma typically presents as a mass resulting in associated enlargement of the lacrimal glands or extraocular muscles. Lymphoma is characteristically homogeneous on T2-weighted MR images and appears isointense with white matter, with mild homogeneous contrast enhancement (Fig. 26). The differential diagnosis for a defined mass involving the extraocular muscles is primarily RMS. However,

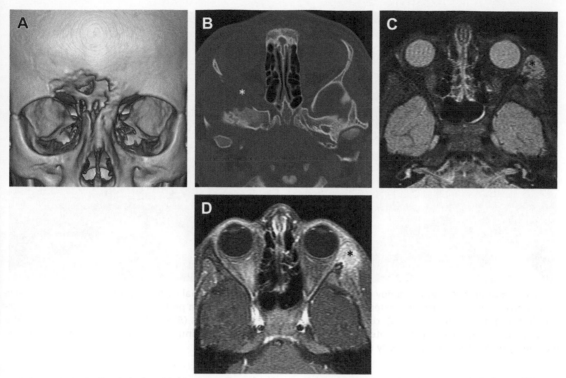

Fig. 24. Langerhans cell histiocytosis (LCH). (*A*) Three-dimensional CT in a 5-year-old boy with supraorbital LCH shows sharply marginated bony destruction with beveled edges. (*B*) Axial bone window CT in a 2-year-old boy with LCH showing sharply marginated bony destruction of the lateral wall of right sphenoid bone (*asterisk*). (*C*) Axial T2 STIR MR in a 4-year-old male with LCH shows a slightly heterogeneous mass that is isointense with cortex eroding the lateral wall of the left orbit (*asterisk*). (*D*) Contrast-enhanced axial T1-weighted MR in the same child shows that the mass enhances avidly (*asterisk*).

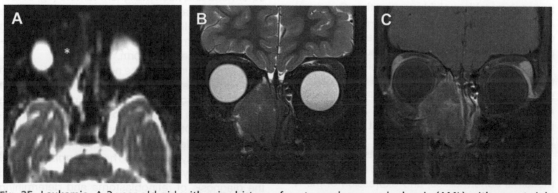

Fig. 25. Leukemia. A 3-year-old girl with prior history of acute myelogenous leukemia (AML) with recent right nasal drainage and proptosis. (*A*) Axial diffusion-weighted imaging apparent diffusion coefficient map shows a right sinonasal mass characterized by decreased diffusivity (*asterisk*). (*B*) Coronal fat-suppressed T2-weighted (T2W) MR image reveals the homogeneous, hypointense tumor that is isointense with white matter. The sinonasal tumor erodes the medial and inferior walls of the right orbit. (*C*) Coronal contrast-enhanced fat-suppressed T1-weighted image shows mild enhancement of the tumor. Chloroma was confirmed after biopsy. The homogeneous hypointensity on T2W image is indistinguishable from lymphoma.

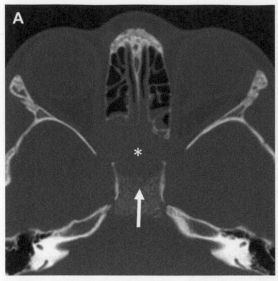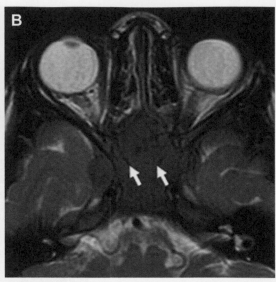

Fig. 26. Lymphoma. A 4-year-old boy with headache and vomiting. (*A*) Axial CT bone window reveals an erosive sphenoethmoidal mass (*asterisk*) extending to the orbital apices. There is a permeative pattern of bony destruction in the sphenoid bone (*arrow*), consistent with an aggressive process. (*B*) Axial T2-weighted MR shows the homogeneous and markedly hypointense tumor invading the cavernous sinuses and surrounding and compressing the optic nerves (*arrows*). Biopsy revealed Burkitt lymphoma.

the differential diagnosis for lymphoma involving the bony orbit also includes leukemia, other sarcoma, and metastasis.

Malignant lymphoproliferative lesions confined to the orbit are usually treated with radiation depending on histologic type.

Neuroblastoma metastases

Neuroblastoma is the most common primary childhood cancer to metastasize to the orbits.[60,61] The most common clinical presentation of orbital neuroblastoma metastases is unilateral or bilateral proptosis and periorbital or eyelid ecchymosis (raccoon eyes) in a child younger than 2 years.[53]

On CT, metastases appear as ill-defined, hyperdense, sometimes mineralized masses. There is permeative, lytic destruction of bone (Fig. 27A), sometimes with a characteristic spiculated periosteal reaction. On MR imaging, the lesions appear isointense with cerebral cortex on T2-weighted images, with decreased diffusivity and heterogeneous or homogeneous contrast enhancement (see Fig. 27B).

Treatment of metastatic neuroblastoma depends on clinical features, histopathologic analyses, chromosomal abnormalities, and expression of the N-Myc oncogene.[53]

Intraocular Neoplasms

Retinoblastoma

Retinoblastoma is the most common intraocular malignancy of childhood, usually manifesting before 5 years of age. Retinoblastomas are bilateral in 40% of cases.[62] Trilateral retinoblastoma (bilateral ocular tumors and a midline intracranial neuroblastic tumor, typically pineal) and quadrilateral retinoblastoma (bilateral ocular disease, pineal and suprasellar tumors) may be present.[62] There are both heritable and nonheritable forms of retinoblastoma.[62] In the heritable form, the first mutation is constitutional, whereas the second is somatic, which causes early onset of bilateral or multifocal tumors in most patients.[63] These children are at increased risk for the development of other head and neck malignant tumors (eg, osteogenic sarcoma and RMS). In the nonheritable form, both allelic mutations are somatic, resulting in unilateral tumors with an older age of presentation than the heritable form.[63]

Leukocoria, in which the normal red reflex of the retina is replaced by yellowish-white light reflecting off the tumor, occurs in 56% to 72% of patients with retinoblastoma and is the most common initial presenting sign. Other less common clinical manifestations include decreased vision, anisocoria, spontaneous hyphema, and heterochromia iridis.[62]

Imaging plays an important role in confirming the diagnosis of retinoblastoma and determining staging. CT demonstrates a hyperattenuating and typically calcified mass in the posterior globe (Fig. 28A). The mass may extend into the vitreous or subretinal space, sometimes resulting in retinal detachment. The size of the globe is normal or slightly enlarged.

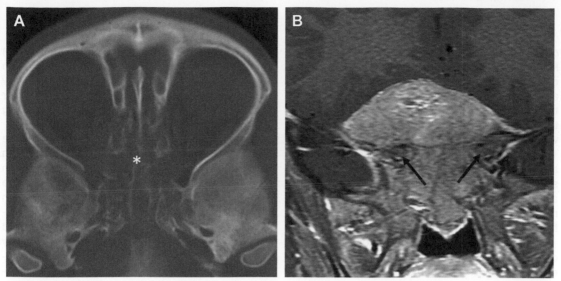

Fig. 27. Neuroblastoma. A 3-year-old boy with a headache. (*A*) Axial CT image showing lytic, permeative destruction of the sphenoid and ethmoid bones (*asterisk*). (*B*) Coronal contrast-enhanced fat-suppressed T1-weighted MR image shows a large, expansile, enhancing sphenoid bone mass encircling the optic nerves (*arrows*). Although the appearance on MR imaging could simulate a meningioma in an older child, the appearance is highly characteristic of neuroblastoma in a child of this age. The tumor demonstrated metaiodobenzylguanidine (MIBG) avidity (not shown) with a suprarenal primary neuroblastoma.

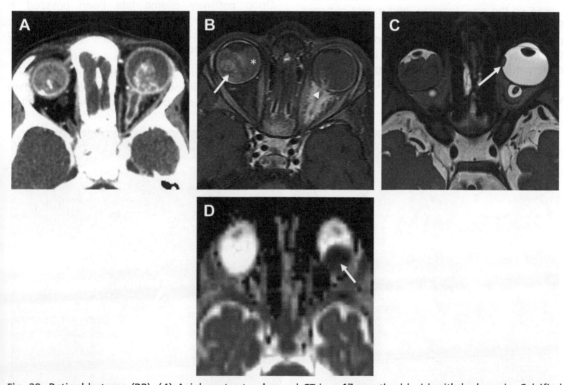

Fig. 28. Retinoblastoma (RB). (*A*) Axial contrast-enhanced CT in a 17-month-old girl with leukocoria. Calcified masses are demonstrated within the globes bilaterally consistent with RB. On the left, there is abnormal density and enhancement due to extension of tumor along the optic nerve. (*B*) Axial contrast-enhanced fat-suppressed T1-weighted MR image shows that the right ocular tumor (*arrow*) is associated with retinal detachment (*asterisk*). There is extensive enhancement around and within (*arrowhead*) the left optic nerve due to invasion by tumor. (*C*) Axial T2 SPACE MR image showing bilateral RB in a 30-month-old boy with the bilateral hypointense RB. The smaller left RB (*arrow*) is well contrasted against the hyperintense vitreous. (*D*) Axial diffusion-weighted imaging apparent diffusion coefficient map showing decreased diffusivity of a left RB (*arrow*) in a 3-month-old boy.

Three-tesla MR imaging is the modality of choice for evaluating patients with suspected or known retinoblastoma and for surveillance for synchronous and metachronous tumors of the CNS and head and neck. Retinoblastoma approximates the signal of gray matter on MR imaging, with the tumor appearing hyperintense to vitreous on T1-weighted images and hypointense to vitreous on T2-weighted images, with decreased diffusivity and contrast enhancement (see **Fig. 28**B–D). A small percentage of retinoblastomas present with a diffuse infiltrative pattern without a discrete mass or calcifications; these can be challenging to diagnose on imaging.[62]

The differential diagnosis includes other causes of leukocoria such as PHPV, Coats disease, toxocara endophthalmitis, and ROP (see **Box 1**). PHPV, Coats disease, and toxocara endophthalmitis typically lack calcifications early in the disease. ROP can be bilateral and may show calcification but is distinguished by a history of prematurity and microphthalmia (see **Fig. 14**).

Treatment of retinoblastoma is complex and is based on the size, location, and extent of tumor. Small tumors are treated with cryoablation, laser photocoagulation, chemotherapy, or plaque radiation therapy.[62] Larger tumors may be treated with chemoreduction followed by surgical resection. Tumors larger than half the globe are treated with enucleation.

Medulloepithelioma

Medulloepithelioma (diktyoma or teratoneuroma) is a rare embryonal neoplasm that arises from the primitive medullary epithelium of the ciliary body. The mean age of presentation of this tumor is 5 years, with the most common presenting symptoms being poor vision and pain.[62]

On CT, medulloepithelioma appears as a dense irregular mass arising from the ciliary body with associated dystrophic calcifications seen in approximately 30% of cases. On MR imaging, the lesion is moderately hyperintense to vitreous on T1-weighted images and hypointense on T2-weighted images with moderate to marked contrast enhancement. Tumor involving the ciliary body should suggest the diagnosis; however, if tumor arises from or spreads to the retina, histopathologic examination may be required to differentiate medulloepithelioma from retinoblastoma.

Treatment is usually enucleation to prevent local recurrence; however, distant metastasis and mortality are uncommon.

Optic pathway glioma

Optic pathway glioma has been covered in another article elsewhere in this issue by Tantiwongkosi and colleagues and is not discussed again in this section.

Papilledema and pseudopapilledema

Papilledema, defined as optic disc swelling, often occurs as a result of raised intracranial pressure

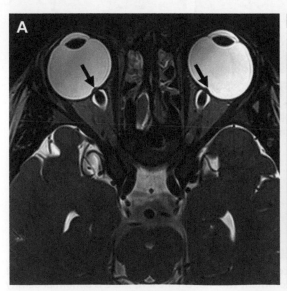
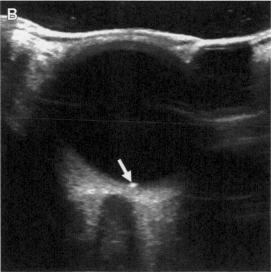

Fig. 29. Papilledema and drusen. (*A*) A 3-year-old boy with exotropia, myopia, and papilledema. (*A*) Axial 3-dimensional T2 SPACE MR image shows elevation of the optic papillae bilaterally (*arrows*). Mildly abnormal contour of the globes may be attributable to myopia with early staphyloma. No intracranial mass, hydrocephalus, or other cause for papilledema was seen. Lumbar puncture confirmed elevated opening pressure consistent with idiopathic intracranial hypertension. (*B*) Ultrasound image in an 18-year-old girl with suspected papilledema reveals an echogenic focus (*arrow*) at the optic papilla consistent with drusen.

from intracranial neoplasms, hemorrhage, idiopathic intracranial hypertension (pseudotumor cerebri), venous sinus thrombosis, or hydrocephalus.[64,65] Papilledema is usually a bilateral condition, although asymmetry may be seen on clinical examination. Imaging is indicated to evaluate the underlying cause. The modality of choice is MR imaging, as it allows visualization of the entire optic pathway, brain, and dural venous sinuses. MR imaging findings suggestive of papilledema include enlargement of the optic nerve sheaths, flattening of the posterior sclera, protrusion of the optic discs into the vitreous humor, and tortuosity of the optic nerves (Fig. 29A). Beyond evaluation of the optic pathways, MR imaging and MRV of the brain should be performed, with contrast as indicated, to evaluate for the various causes of papilledema.

Pseudopapilledema like papilledema may present with optic disc swelling but unlike papilledema is not associated with raised intracranial pressure and is typically a normal physiologic variation or secondary to causes such as Down syndrome, high hyperopia, or optic disc drusen.[64] Drusen usually presents with intraocular calcifications; when located at the optic nerve head, bulky drusen may mimic papilledema on fundoscopy and on thin-section, high-resolution T2-weighted MR images. In such patients, ocular US demonstrates the characteristic echogenic, mineralized focus at the optic papilla (see Fig. 29B), appearing as punctate increased density at the optic papilla on CT.

SUMMARY

This article discusses a wide spectrum of pediatric orbital diseases commonly encountered in clinical practice. By understanding the clinical presentation and characteristic imaging characteristics of pediatric ophthalmic disease, a narrow differential diagnosis can be formulated and appropriate timely management can be initiated.

REFERENCES

1. Albernaz VS, Castillo M, Hudgins PA, et al. Imaging findings in patients with clinical anophthalmos. AJNR Am J Neuroradiol 1997;18(3):555–61.
2. Verma AS, Fitzpatrick DR. Anophthalmia and microphthalmia. Orphanet J Rare Dis 2007;2:47.
3. Fuhrmann S. Eye morphogenesis and patterning of the optic vesicle. Curr Top Dev Biol 2010;93:61–84.
4. Voronina VA, Kozhemyakina EA, O'Kernick CM, et al. Mutations in the human RAX homeobox gene in a patient with anophthalmia and sclerocornea. Hum Mol Genet 2004;13(3):315–22.
5. Gujar SK, Gandhi D. Congenital malformations of the orbit. Neuroimaging Clin N Am 2011;21(3):585–602, viii.
6. Barkovich A. Congenital malformations of the brain and skull. In: Barkovich A, editor. Pediatric neuroimaging. 4th edition. Philadelphia: Lippincott Williams and Wilkins; 2005. p. 291–405.
7. Fitzpatrick DR, van Heyningen V. Developmental eye disorders. Curr Opin Genet Dev 2005;15(3):348–53.
8. Bardakjian T, Weiss A, Schneider AS. Anophthalmia/microphthalmia overview. In: Pagon RA, Adam MP, Ardinger HH, et al, editors. GeneReviews® [Internet]. Seattle (WA): University of Washington; 1993–2015. Available at: http://www.ncbi.nlm.nih.gov/books/NBK1378/.
9. Schoenwolf G, Bleyl S, Brauer P, et al. Development of the eyes. In: Schoenwolf G, Bleyl S, Brauer P, et al, editors. Larsen's human embryology. 5th edition. Philadelphia: Churchill Livingstone Elsevier; 2015. p. 488–500.
10. Ito YA, Walter MA. Genomics and anterior segment dysgenesis: a review. Clin Experiment Ophthalmol 2014;42(1):13–24.
11. Kandpal H, Vashisht S, Sharma R, et al. Imaging spectrum of pediatric orbital pathology: a pictorial review. Indian J Ophthalmol 2006;54(4):227–36.
12. Kaufman LM, Villablanca JP, Mafee MF. Diagnostic imaging of cystic lesions in the child's orbit. Radiol Clin North Am 1998;36(6):1149–63, xi.
13. Gorospe L, Royo A, Berrocal T, et al. Imaging of orbital disorders in pediatric patients. Eur Radiol 2003;13(8):2012–26.
14. Castillo M, Mukherji SK, Wagle NS. Imaging of the pediatric orbit. Neuroimaging Clin N Am 2000;10(1):95–116, viii.
15. Levin AV. Congenital eye anomalies. Pediatr Clin North Am 2003;50(1):55–76.
16. Ellika S, Robson CD, Heidary G, et al. Morning glory disc anomaly: characteristic MR imaging findings. AJNR Am J Neuroradiol 2013;34(10):2010–4.
17. Quah BL, Hamilton J, Blaser S, et al. Morning glory disc anomaly, midline cranial defects and abnormal carotid circulation: an association worth looking for. Pediatr Radiol 2005;35(5):525–8.
18. Kindler P. Morning glory syndrome: unusual congenital optic disk anomaly. Am J Ophthalmol 1970;69(3):376–84.
19. Traboulsi EI. Morning glory disk anomaly – more than meets the eye. J AAPOS 2009;13(4):333–4.
20. Krishnan C, Roy A, Traboulsi E. Morning glory disk anomaly, choroidal coloboma, and congenital constrictive malformations of the internal carotid arteries (moyamoya disease). Ophthalmic Genet 2000;21(1):21–4.
21. Puvanachandra N, Heran MK, Lyons CJ. Morning glory disk anomaly with ipsilateral capillary hemangioma, agenesis of the internal carotid artery, and

Horner syndrome: a variant of PHACES syndrome? J AAPOS 2008;12(5):528–30.

22. Smirniotopoulos JG, Bargallo N, Mafee MF. Differential diagnosis of leukokoria: radiologic-pathologic correlation. Radiographics 1994;14(5):1059–79 [quiz: 1081–2].

23. Kaste SC, Jenkins JJ 3rd, Meyer D, et al. Persistent hyperplastic primary vitreous of the eye: imaging findings with pathologic correlation. AJR Am J Roentgenol 1994;162(2):437–40.

24. Galluzzi P, Venturi C, Cerase A, et al. Coats disease: smaller volume of the affected globe. Radiology 2001;221(1):64–9.

25. Parsa CF. Focal venous hypertension as a pathophysiologic mechanism for tissue hypertrophy, port-wine stains, the Sturge-Weber syndrome, and related disorders: proof of concept with novel hypothesis for underlying etiological cause (an American Ophthalmological Society thesis). Trans Am Ophthalmol Soc 2013;111:180–215.

26. Robertson DM. Ophthalmic manifestations of tuberous sclerosis. Ann N Y Acad Sci 1991;615:17–25.

27. Toy BC, Agron E, Nigam D, et al. Longitudinal analysis of retinal hemangioblastomatosis and visual function in ocular von Hippel-Lindau disease. Ophthalmology 2012;119(12):2622–30.

28. Wong WT, Chew EY. Ocular von Hippel-Lindau disease: clinical update and emerging treatments. Curr Opin Ophthalmol 2008;19(3):213–7.

29. Meyerle CB, Dahr SS, Wetjen NM, et al. Clinical course of retrobulbar hemangioblastomas in von Hippel-Lindau disease. Ophthalmology 2008; 115(8):1382–9.

30. Chew EY. Ocular manifestations of von Hippel-Lindau disease: clinical and genetic investigations. Trans Am Ophthalmol Soc 2005;103:495–511.

31. Parisi MA, Doherty D, Chance PF, et al. Joubert syndrome (and related disorders) (OMIM 213300). Eur J Hum Genet 2007;15(5):511–21.

32. Kava M, Chitayat D, Blaser S, et al. Eye and brain abnormalities in congenital muscular dystrophies caused by fukutin-related protein gene (FKRP) mutations. Pediatr Neurol 2013;49(5):374–8.

33. Fruhman G, Eble TN, Gambhir N, et al. Ophthalmologic findings in Aicardi syndrome. J AAPOS 2012; 16(3):238–41.

34. Shah PK, Narendran V, Kalpana N. Aicardi syndrome: the importance of an ophthalmologist in its diagnosis. Indian J Ophthalmol 2009;57(3):234–6.

35. Aicardi J. Aicardi syndrome. Brain Dev 2005;27(3): 164–71.

36. Entesarian M, Matsson H, Klar J, et al. Mutations in the gene encoding fibroblast growth factor 10 are associated with aplasia of lacrimal and salivary glands. Nat Genet 2005;37(2):125–7.

37. Inan UU, Yilmaz MD, Demir Y, et al. Characteristics of lacrimo-auriculo-dento-digital (LADD) syndrome:

case report of a family and literature review. Int J Pediatr Otorhinolaryngol 2006;70(7):1307–14.

38. Graeber CP, Hunter DG, Engle EC. The genetic basis of incomitant strabismus: consolidation of the current knowledge of the genetic foundations of disease. Semin Ophthalmol 2013;28(5–6):427–37.

39. Bilaniuk LT, Farber M. Imaging of developmental anomalies of the eye and the orbit. AJNR Am J Neuroradiol 1992;13(2):793–803.

40. Mulliken JB, Glowacki J. Hemangiomas and vascular malformations in infants and children: a classification based on endothelial characteristics. Plast Reconstr Surg 1982;69(3):412–22.

41. Katz SE, Rootman J, Vangveeravong S, et al. Combined venous lymphatic malformations of the orbit (so-called lymphangiomas). Association with noncontiguous intracranial vascular anomalies. Ophthalmology 1998;105(1):176–84.

42. Bisdorff A, Mulliken JB, Carrico J, et al. Intracranial vascular anomalies in patients with periorbital lymphatic and lymphaticovenous malformations. AJNR Am J Neuroradiol 2007;28(2):335–41.

43. Chung EM, Smirniotopoulos JG, Specht CS, et al. From the archives of the AFIP: pediatric orbit tumors and tumorlike lesions: nonosseous lesions of the extraocular orbit. Radiographics 2007;27(6):1777–99.

44. Barnes PD, Robson CD, Robertson RL, et al. Pediatric orbital and visual pathway lesions. Neuroimaging Clin N Am 1996;6(1):179–98.

45. Kurul S, Cakmakci H, Kovanlikaya A, et al. The benign course of carotid-cavernous fistula in a child. Eur J Radiol 2001;39(2):77–9.

46. Lau FH, Yuen HK, Rao SK, et al. Spontaneous carotid cavernous fistula in a pediatric patient: case report and review of literature. J AAPOS 2005;9(3): 292–4.

47. Gossman MD, Berlin AJ, Weinstein MA, et al. Spontaneous direct carotid-cavernous fistula in childhood. Ophthal Plast Reconstr Surg 1993;9(1): 62–5.

48. Hollands JK, Santarius T, Kirkpatrick PJ, et al. Treatment of a direct carotid-cavernous fistula in a patient with type IV Ehlers-Danlos syndrome: a novel approach. Neuroradiology 2006;48(7):491–4.

49. Burrows PE, Laor T, Paltiel H, et al. Diagnostic imaging in the evaluation of vascular birthmarks. Dermatol Clin 1998;16(3):455–88.

50. Shields CL, Shields JA, Honavar SG, et al. Primary ophthalmic rhabdomyosarcoma in 33 patients. Trans Am Ophthalmol Soc 2001;99:133–42.

51. Shields CL, Shields JA, Honavar SG, et al. Clinical spectrum of primary ophthalmic rhabdomyosarcoma. Ophthalmology 2001;108(12):2284–92.

52. Crist WM, Anderson JR, Meza JL, et al. Intergroup rhabdomyosarcoma study-IV: results for patients with nonmetastatic disease. J Clin Oncol 2001; 19(12):3091–102.

53. Rao AA, Naheedy JH, Chen JY, et al. A clinical update and radiologic review of pediatric orbital and ocular tumors. J Oncol 2013;2013:975908.

54. Huh WW, Fitzgerald N, Mahajan A, et al. Pediatric sarcomas and related tumors of the head and neck. Cancer Treat Rev 2011;37(6):431–9.

55. Huh WW, Mahajan A. Ophthalmic oncology. In: Esmaeli B, editor. Ophthalmic oncology. Boston (MA): Springer; 2011. p. 61–7.

56. Shields JA, Shields CL. Rhabdomyosarcoma: review for the ophthalmologist. Surv Ophthalmol 2003; 48(1):39–57.

57. Vosoghi H, Rodriguez-Galindo C, Wilson MW. Orbital involvement in Langerhans cell histiocytosis. Ophthal Plast Reconstr Surg 2009;25(6):430–3.

58. Banna M, Aur R, Akkad S. Orbital granulocytic sarcoma. AJNR Am J Neuroradiol 1991;12(2):255–8.

59. Valvassori GE, Sabnis SS, Mafee RF, et al. Imaging of orbital lymphoproliferative disorders. Radiol Clin North Am 1999;37(1):135–50, x–xi.

60. D'Ambrosio N, Lyo J, Young R, et al. Common and unusual craniofacial manifestations of metastatic neuroblastoma. Neuroradiology 2010;52(6):549–53.

61. D'Ambrosio N, Lyo JK, Young RJ, et al. Imaging of metastatic CNS neuroblastoma. AJR Am J Roentgenol 2010;194(5):1223–9.

62. Chung EM, Specht CS, Schroeder JW. From the archives of the AFIP: pediatric orbit tumors and tumor-like lesions: neuroepithelial lesions of the ocular globe and optic nerve. Radiographics 2007;27(4): 1159–86.

63. Dimaras H, Kimani K, Dimba EA, et al. Retinoblastoma. Lancet 2012;379(9824):1436–46.

64. LaRocca V, Gorelick G, Kaufman LM. Medical imaging in pediatric neuro-ophthalmology. Neuroimaging Clin N Am 2005;15(1):85–105.

65. Passi N, Degnan AJ, Levy LM. MR imaging of papilledema and visual pathways: effects of increased intracranial pressure and pathophysiologic mechanisms. AJNR Am J Neuroradiol 2013;34(5):919–24.

Index

Note: Page numbers of article titles are in **boldface** type.

Neuroimag Clin N Am 25 (2015) 503–506
http://dx.doi.org/10.1016/S1052-5149(15)00051-9

neuroimaging.theclinics.com

Moving?

Make sure your subscription moves with you!

To notify us of your new address, find your **Clinics Account Number** (located on your mailing label above your name), and contact customer service at:

Email: journalscustomerservice-usa@elsevier.com

800-654-2452 (subscribers in the U.S. & Canada)
314-447-8871 (subscribers outside of the U.S. & Canada)

Fax number: 314-447-8029

Elsevier Health Sciences Division
Subscription Customer Service
3251 Riverport Lane
Maryland Heights, MO 63043

*To ensure uninterrupted delivery of your subscription, please notify us at least 4 weeks in advance of move.

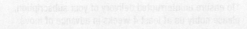

Printed and bound by CPI Group (UK) Ltd, Croydon, CR0 4YY

03/10/2016

01040714-0016

Printed and bound by CPI Group (UK) Ltd, Croydon, CR0 4YY

03/10/2024

01040374-0015